AMERICAN MADNESS

AMERICAN MADNESS

The Rise and Fall of Dementia Praecox

RICHARD NOLL

HARVARD UNIVERSITY PRESS | Cambridge, Massachusetts | London, England   2011

Library of Congress Cataloging-in-Publication Data
Noll, Richard, 1959–
American madness : the rise and fall of dementia praecox / Richard Noll.
p. ; cm.
Includes bibliographical references and index.
ISBN 978-0-674-04739-6 (alk. paper)
1. Schizophrenia—United States—Case studies.   2. Schizophrenia—Treatment—
United States—History.   I. Title.
[DNLM: 1. Schizophrenia—history—United States.   2. Schizophrenia—therapy—
United States.   3. Biological Psychiatry—history—United States.   4. History,
20th Century—United States. WM 11 AA1]
RC514.N629   2011
616.89'800973—dc22   2011012099

Much ink has been shed over dementia praecox, many contentions have ensued, and it would appear that we shall continue to regard this untimely birth as an undesirable alien.

—A. R. Urquart, *Journal of Mental Science,*
October 1908

What if dementia praecox simply does not exist?

—Oswald Bumke, at the meeting of
Central German Psychiatrists and
Neurologists in Leipzig, 28 October 1923

CONTENTS

AMERICAN MADNESS

This is a story of a madness that begins with a murder.

On the night of 25 June 1906, Harry Kendall Thaw, the thirty-five-year-old son of a Pittsburgh coal and railroad magnate, fired three shots into the face and shoulder of America's most famous architect at that time, Stanford White, age fifty-two, killing him instantly. The murder of one millionaire by another was dramatic enough. But the fact that it occurred in Manhattan in a crowded audience during a rooftop Garden Theater performance at Madison Square Garden, a luminous yellow brick and buff terra cotta Beaux Arts building that White had designed to dominate the New York skyline, electrified the nation in the days and years that followed.

In the Tower of Madison Square Garden, a structure crowned by a sensational nineteen-foot, 2,000-pound copper statue of a nude goddess Diana, White maintained a private penthouse apartment adorned with lush oriental rugs and erotic objets d'art where he would entertain friends and, especially, impressionable young women. Secreted away in other parts of the city were other rendezvous dens, including one at 22 West Twenty-fourth Street above the F. A. O. Schwartz toy store, where the charismatic White would encourage young women, after champagne or absinthe, to remove their clothes and soar, to-and-fro, almost to the ceiling, on a red velvet swing. Thaw's wife, Evelyn Nesbit, the famous twenty-one-year-old Gibson Girl model and *Florodora* showgirl, had previously been White's mistress. She had once been one of the girls on the red velvet swing.[1] But sexual jealousy was not the exclusive factor behind this very public and violent act. A smoldering madness had inflamed Thaw's brain since puberty. What was then called the "trial of the century" in 1907 ended in a hung jury after a battle of opposing expert alienists presented a confusing and professionally embarrassing array of diagnostic opinions, but in 1908 a second trial found him insane.[2] He was sent to the Matteawan Asylum for the Criminally Insane. Years later the overwhelming influence of a campaign fueled by the Thaw family's fortune finally secured his release, to the delight of the media and— amazingly—the acclaim of the public. The Thaw trials inspired numerous books, both fiction and nonfiction, and the homicide appeared in film one week after the murder, in July 1906, in an American Mutoscope and Biograph Company short, *The Thaw-White Tragedy,* which reenacted the fatal event.[3] Later more detailed versions of the story appeared in the motion pictures *The Girl in the Red Velvet Swing* (1955) and *Ragtime* (1981), which was based on the 1975 novel of the same name by E. L. Doctorow.

What does the murder of the architect Stanford White have to do with the history of psychiatry in America? And what is the connection with dementia praecox, an insanity regarded—mistakenly, as we shall see—as synonymous with the most renowned mental disease of the twentieth century, schizophrenia? The answers to these questions attest to the power of popular discourses of medicalization that operate autonomously outside the literary chatter of learned elites.[4]

Dementia praecox first came to the attention of the American public through an article about the trial published in the *New York Times* (and quoted liberally throughout the United States in other newspapers) on 5 March 1907. This was just one in a daily series of lengthy, often verbatim reports of the testimony of numerous prominent American alienists concerning the proper medical diagnosis of Thaw's "brainstorm" (as one alienist termed it) that captivated readers. It was one such expert, Charles G. Wagner, the superintendent of an asylum in Binghamton, New York, who testified that one of Thaw's possible diagnoses was "dementia praecox."[5] This novel term was repeatedly ridiculed by

Thaw's defense attorney during his closing argument as the mock diagnosis "Dementia Americana," a sarcastic attempt to deny Thaw's criminal responsibility for the murder of White by referring to "that species of insanity" which makes the protection of a man's wife and home a sacred duty above and beyond written laws (and hence justified under the "Unwritten Law").[6]

As far as can be determined, this dreadful-sounding insanity may have never been uttered before in an American courtroom, nor had it ever appeared in the pages of America's major newspapers. The introduction of this previously unknown illness during the Thaw trial induced as much mystery as fear in the fascinated public.

This terrifying new mental disease was arguably as unknown and mysterious to most of the hundreds of asylum physicians who were marooned along with a hidden nation of the insane in a loosely connected archipelago of mostly rural institutions throughout the vast forty-six United States, its territories, and Canada in March 1907. Only among a handful of the elite of the psychiatric profession who were concentrated in the northeastern states, and in a few scattered places in the Midwest such as Iowa, Michigan, and Illinois, was dementia praecox a familiar form of insanity. The widespread notoriety of the Thaw trial contributed much to change all that. With the lay public alarmed about dementia praecox thanks to increasingly more frequent reports in the popular media and, within a few years, by the publications of the mental hygiene movement (starting in 1909) and the Eugenics Record Office (founded in 1910), alienists and neurologists throughout America who may have been ignorant or critical of the newly identified mental disease faced a public who had already been educated to adopt its implicit meaning: chronic, incurable insanity.

Dementia praecox had been a diagnosis of hopelessness from its creation. It had been only a decade before the murder of Stanford White that the mental disease had first been described in full by the German psychiatrist Emil Kraepelin (1856–1926) as a deteriorating, incurable psychotic disorder in the 1896 edition of his famous textbook, *Psychiatrie*. The sixth edition in 1899, which had a profound influence on the classification of psychotic disorders throughout the twentieth century (and which continues today), expanded the disease into three subtypes.[7] In its most characteristic thumbnail manifestation most alienists and neurologists interpreted Kraepelin's concept to refer to an illness that began with an episode marked by confusion, depression, headaches, delusions (both fluid and fixed), and auditory hallucinations (usually of "voices") and soon produced gaps in attention, incoherent speech, and bizarre actions. Odd physiological manifestations, such as abnormalities in the behavior of the pupils of the eyes or abnormal reflex tension, were also posited as clinical signs of the condition. It mostly afflicted young men, and most cases began between the ages of sixteen and twenty-two. A process of cognitive deterioration followed, which Kraepelin referred to as "mental weakness" or "defect," eventually leading to permanent disability and no hope of complete recovery.

Often there was a deadness of emotional experience, a flatness of affect, an eerie remoteness that evoked an uncanny "praecox feeling" in physicians who evaluated such a patient. In patients who presented with a mélange of signs and symptoms that did not match descriptions in the textbooks—and there were many—making a diagnosis was less an explicit cognitive exercise than an experience not unlike that of recognizing a melody or a scent. Judgments based on the presumption of such tacit clinical knowledge were laden with enormous consequences for the life of the patient. In the first decades of the twentieth century dementia praecox was widely interpreted by American medical authorities and the lay public alike as the terminal cancer of mental diseases.

Not all American physicians welcomed this import from Germany, and many challenged not only the term itself but also its dire prognostic fatalism. As early as June 1906 one American alienist had sounded the alarm at a professional psychiatric conference that dementia praecox was a "new peril" of foreign origins that might too easily become a broad catch-all category that would be misapplied through careless misdiagnosis.[8] History would prove he was correct. But by World War I Kraepelin's term, if not his actual diagnostic criteria or prognostic fatalism, had gained general acceptance, and dementia praecox was identified as the primary mental health problem to be addressed in the asylum practices of alienists, in laboratory research in psychiatry, in the eugenics movement, in the mental hygiene movement, and in the courts through its infiltration into medical jurisprudence. However, after a descent that began in 1927 and was completed by 1939 dementia praecox virtually disappeared from elite literary discourses and was replaced by an alternative disease label, schizophrenia. The Swiss psychiatrist Eugen Bleuler (1857–1939)

first proposed this term in print in 1908 to refer to a new conceptualiza-
tion of the symptom picture, course, and prognosis of dementia praecox.[9] Bleuler's term—if not his essential disease concept—eventually
eclipsed Kraepelin's.

How did dementia praecox come to America? Why was it so successfully received? And why and when exactly did it fall out of favor?
Suggested answers to these questions form the core of this book.

The story of dementia praecox in America has not been told in any
other book-length treatment. This has always been surprising to me.
Dementia praecox is a term familiar to anyone who has watched old
movies (such as *The Snake Pit* [1948] and *Suddenly Last Summer* [1961]) or
even Bugs Bunny cartoons.[10] It was perhaps the most discussed mental
disease of the first half of the twentieth century. Why have scholars paid
so little attention to its history?

The reasons are varied. However, the primary obstacle to seeing
dementia praecox the way people of the past saw it is our own presentism. It is a common misconception that the currently constructed
mental disorder that we call schizophrenia is essentially the same disease
that Kraepelin named dementia praecox or what Bleuler meant by
schizophrenia. This is certainly not the case. This misreading of the past
is not entirely the fault of those of us in the present; except for a few
American alienists and neurologists engaged in an elite literary discourse
almost a century ago, most psychiatrists and lay persons of that era also
tended to use the terms interchangeably. The problem of our natural
inclination to read backward into the past from the perspective of the
present also extends to speculations concerning whether mental disorders that we now diagnose as schizophrenia are of recent origin (perhaps
as "diseases of civilization") or existed hundreds or even thousands of
years ago. Arguments can and have been made for and against this re-
cency hypothesis. Then of course there is the issue of Western ethno-
centrism and the cultural bias inherent in any attempt to see current
Western conceptions of mental disorder in non-Western cultures of the
present or the past.[11]

The argument presented here is a modified version of the "discontinuity hypothesis" of dementia praecox and schizophrenia cogently
argued by German E. Berrios, Rogelio Luque, and José M. Villagrán
in 2003. In a detailed polemic against what they term the "continuity
hypothesis" of schizophrenia, they reject the presentist assumption that

schizophrenia is a *"real, recognizable, unitary and stable* object of inquiry ('RRUS')" throughout history. According to this "myth," the view has been that "schizophrenia has always existed and in the 19th and 20th centuries alienists have polished away its blemishes and impurities, culminating in the DSM-IV definition which can therefore be considered as a real, recognizable, unitary and stable object of inquiry." Instead, based on a careful analysis of the *written* descriptions of dementia praecox, its presumed precursors or analogue psychoses, and schizophrenia by Bénédict-Augustin Morel (1809–1873), Karl Kahlbaum (1828–1899), Ewald Hecker (1843–1909), Arnold Pick (1851–1924), Emil Kraepelin, Eugen Bleuler, Carl Gustav Jung (1875–1961), Carl Wernicke (1848–1905), and Alfred Hoche (1865–1943), they conclude, "The history of schizophrenia can best be described as the history of a set of research programmes running in parallel rather than serialism and each based on a different concept of disease, of mental symptoms and of mind."[12]

The evidence for the conceptual discontinuity of dementia praecox and schizophrenia is beyond doubt. However, it should be emphasized that the discontinuities identified by these scholars existed at the level of literary discourse among members of a *European* (primarily German, Austrian, Swiss, and French) psychiatric elite. How were these divergent views received in the United States, and how were they transformed by *American* psychiatric elites? How were these ideas put into bureaucratic and clinical practice by those *not* in the elite of the psychiatric profession? How were they received in the courts and in the culture? How did they frame laboratory research? What were the continuities and discontinuities between these European and American views of dementia praecox and schizophrenia? Once dementia praecox crossed the Atlantic, how much of "Kraepelin" was actually retained in the American framing of "Kraepelin's disease"? What *was* dementia praecox in America?

What follows is an integrated intellectual and conceptual history of dementia praecox, with its rise and fall in the United States at the center of the story. The narrative was written in a style and form to reach the widest possible range of readers, from undergraduate students and nonspecialists in the history of psychiatry to the few dozen experts in the field. Because I assume no prior expertise among readers in the history of American psychiatry or medicine, the contextualizing historical information I provide regarding the backstory of certain individuals, institutions, and methodologies may be familiar to some expert historians, and I ask for their patience as the story of dementia praecox unfolds. My telling of this tale is partially informed by the years I spent as a staff psychologist on various wards of a state hospital in the 1980s, an experience I wish more historians of psychiatry would have had before writing about persons suffering from psychosis. This is a "disease history" that could have been crafted (with the selection of other sources of evidence) and told from other valid perspectives: as social history, as cultural history, as a specialized study in the evolution of American mental health policy, as a problem of the insanity concept in the history of medical jurisprudence and forensic psychiatry, as a sociological example of medicalization or the "iatrogenesis of nosology" (to use the language of the historian Charles E. Rosenberg), or strictly from the perspective of patients who were diagnosed with dementia praecox.[13] However, it is my belief that documenting the basic contours of the intellectual and chronological reception and transformation of Kraepelin's disease in America—provided here for the first time—is a necessary precondition for these other approaches and assembles a suggested organizational spine for revision in future narratives.

In the pages that follow the voices of the members of the elite members of the American psychiatric community will carry greater weight than they deserve. Historians cannot easily get around this imbalance in available evidence when trying to re-create the cognitive categories of actors acting in the past. By "elite" I mean primarily a literary elite that shaped opinion (or attempted to) through publications, although many of these individuals also held positions of localized institutional power at various times within the psychiatric community.[14] Some were superintendants of an asylum or state hospital where their power within was often regal and absolute, though constrained to a greater or lesser degree by state oversight agencies. Others were directors of research institutes and psychopathic hospitals who became politically appointed government officials with titles such as "pathologist" (New York, Michigan, Massachusetts) or "state alienist" (Illinois), and their powers extended into all institutions within a particular state. Others were neurologists in the private practice of the treatment of "nervous diseases" who were often also engaged as consultants to neurological clinics, asylums, prisons, and the courts. Many were asylum physicians, either assistant physicians in the front lines of the treatment of the insanities or pathologists who conducted autopsies and analyzed tissues and bodily fluids in asylum pathology laboratories. What distinguished them all was an intellectual impulse to publish their views, something that the overwhelming majority of neurologists and asylum alienists involved in the treatment of nervous and mental diseases did not do.

In the American psychiatry of a century ago a mark of distinction among the leaders of this elite was their ability to read German and French, and they were the conduits through which European ideas flowed into the United States. There are good reasons to believe that this literary elite was often a universe unto itself; most American physicians circa 1900, including asylum alienists and superintendents, did not read the medical literature *at all* nor participate in national professional organizations or their conferences. We tend to focus on the drama left to us through these literary remains—intellectual "crises" and other discontinuities of thought and action that, frankly, bypassed the typical asylum physician or superintendent. Still, the literary discourses of the psychiatric elite of that era have much to offer us. The cacophony of viewpoints about the classification, nomenclature, etiology, pathophysiology, course, prognosis, and rational treatment of dementia praecox reflects the place of early twentieth-century American psychiatry in the history of medicine of that era just as the arguably dissonant debate today over these same issues mirrors our twenty-first-century mystification about the current status of schizophrenia as a brain disease.

At the risk of lapsing into presentism at this point, I suggest that contemporary readers would do well to be humbled by our current state of scientific knowledge about our era's schizophrenia. Each decade the journal *Schizophrenia Research* conducts a comprehensive literature review of research findings and weighs each according to its reproducibility, whether the finding is primary to the illness, and the durability of the finding over time. More than thirty thousand published articles on schizophrenia appeared in the decade between 1998 and 2007 and now appear at the rate of more than five thousand per year. Espousing the myth of the "continuity hypothesis," in 2008 the authors of the most recent review confessed, "Despite vigorous study over the past century . . . its etiology and pathophysiology remain relatively obscure and available treatments only moderately effective." They conclude, "While many etiological and pathophysiological processes currently appear relevant to what we consider schizophrenia and it is almost certain that our construct of schizophrenia encompasses not one but several diseases, precise delineation of the constellation of distinct 'individual diseases' that are part of this entity is not possible at present."[15] As the historian Gerald Grob noted more than a quarter of a century ago, "Schizophrenia . . . may be, in fact, what 'fever' was before 1870—a general inclusive category describing a multiplicity of diseases."[16] With this in mind, the confusion of the alienists and neurologists of the past regarding dementia praecox is precisely what historians of the future will find in the literature left behind by our own psychiatric elite when they attempt to re-create the story of our era's construction of schizophrenia.

This introduction began with a murder and a trial that introduced the madness called dementia praecox to the American public. Harry Thaw's actions both during and before the murder became the focus of the much shorter second trial in January 1908 in which he was found not guilty by reason of insanity. The three experts for the defense all agreed this time: the diagnosis was manic-depressive insanity, a syndrome named and described by Emil Kraepelin in 1899. As with dementia praecox in the first trial, the second trial did much to introduce the American public to yet another of Kraepelin's concepts. These facts alone would secure Harry Thaw's footnote in the history of psychiatry. However, there is one more curious connection.

The prominent Thaw family of Pittsburgh maintained social relations with members of other wealthy families, including the family of the philanthropist Henry Phipps, a former partner of Andrew Carnegie in the steel business. On 16 June 1908, just a few months after Thaw's commitment to an asylum for the criminally insane, a short news item appeared in the *New York Times:*

PHIPPS INTERESTED IN THAW

Prisoner's Case Is Said to Have Influenced Steel Man's Donation

Pittsburg, Penn., June 15.—News that Henry Phipps, the steel magnate, had donated $500,000 to the Johns Hopkins Hospital for the purpose of making researches and effecting cures in insanity, was received with great interest in this city where Mr. Phipps ideas on insanity have long been well known. It is asserted that the case of Harry Thaw, who was a great favorite of Mr. Phipps, was mainly instrumental in Mr. Phipps making this move.[17]

The first alienist to examine Harry Thaw directly after his murder was the dean of forensic psychiatrists in New York, Allan McLane Hamilton. In his 1916 memoir Hamilton added support to this speculative story when he stated, "There is an annex to Johns Hopkins Hospital known as the Phipps Clinic which was endowed by relatives of Harry Thaw."[18] The influence of the insanity of Harry Thaw on Phipps's decision to endow a psychiatric clinic is not mentioned in any standard accounts of this signal event in the history of American medicine.[19]

The Henry Phipps Psychiatric Clinic of the Johns Hopkins Hospital held its opening exercises from 16 to 18 April 1913. Among the many distinguished speakers was Eugen Bleuler, the creator of schizophrenia. The Phipps Psychiatric Clinic was the first psychiatric training institution in an English-speaking country to be associated with a major medical school and university, an academic "university clinic" model that had long been in existence in German-speaking countries.[20] The director of the clinic was the German Swiss émigré Adolf Meyer (1866–1950), the man who, as we shall see, brought dementia praecox to America in 1896 but then later reformed Kraepelin's disease into an unrecognizable republic of "reactions."

Sometimes history has to be viewed from some very odd angles.

1

THE WORLD OF THE AMERICAN ALIENIST, 1896

In the mid-1890s most people still spoke of "alienists" and "alienism." "Psychiatrists" and "psychiatry" were unfamiliar sounds to most American ears. Over the next two decades that would change. The profession, begrudgingly, did so as well. Profound currents of modernization that had been stirring the American medical profession would eventually force their way into the cloistered world of the asylum doctors. The submission of American alienists to the overwhelming forces of history would still take decades, but arguably the process was in motion by the year 1896.

In the 1890s the teaching and practice of medicine in the United States was visibly transforming into the science-based profession that characterized the next century.[1] The opening of the Johns Hopkins Medical School in 1893 punctuated the beginning of a new era.[2] It was the first in the United States with rigorous entrance requirements and a commitment to the integration of clinical and laboratory training. It was also the first to emulate the German and Austrian model of such integration that so many thousands of American medical students had experienced in sojourns lasting from a few weeks to several years.[3] The laboratory revolution in medicine had finally reached North America after decades of exciting discoveries in physiology, anatomy, neurology, bacteriology, and chemistry had demonstrably improved clinical diagnosis—if not practice—in Europe. The *Journal of Experimental Medicine,* the first American scientific journal devoted to medical research, was founded only in 1896. Such journals had existed in Germany, France, and Austria for decades. There was no reason to assume enough laboratory research was being conducted in the United States to fill its pages, and there was certainly no reason to assume American doctors would even read it; most practicing physicians never read medical journals (many of which were in a foreign language), and fewer still had ever visited a medical library, even as students (why should they?).[4]

Though the number of American medical schools following the German model that opened in the 1890s would still be small, the direction of the future century was assured. By 1910 as many as eleven university-affiliated medical schools in the United States would be judged as excellent institutions because of their integration of clinical and laboratory training, with Johns Hopkins leading the pack.[5] Both within the American medical community and among the lay public perceptions of the core sources of the professional power and authority of physicians were being changed through the new discourses of laboratory knowledge. The laboratory functioned as a new source of elitism in the medical profession.[6]

European laboratory findings provided key evidence for a new way of thinking about disease. For thousands of years the suffering of human illness was thought to be caused by a disruption of natural balance, not only within the patient but also between the patient and his social and physical environments: something *near to* or *uniquely characteristic of* the body of an individual—perhaps a "miasma" (a foul-smelling fog or gas, often arising from the ever-present filth of times past), an imbalance (dyskrasia) of humors, or heredity ("bad blood"). Illness could also, in some instances, be interpreted as a moral, emotional and constitutional reaction to the unique circumstances or personal experiences of the life of an individual. Disease might even arise from the practice of personal habits (such as masturbation as a cause of tuberculosis or madness) or even one's occupation (such as being a cobbler, governess or scholar). Not only were notions of causality fluid, but so were the range of symptoms and outcomes. A diagnosis was usually based on the main symptom (for example, fever), modified by some salient fact about the recent life of the individual (hence "childbed fever," "jail fever," "coal lungs," "governess psychosis," and so on). Conditions of illness seemed to morph mysteriously one into the other, arising and vanishing within a visible field of activity radiating from the spatial location of the body of the individual at its center.

But by the 1860s, prior even to the germ theory of disease that took hold after 1880, a novel concept had evolved in Europe that separated the uniqueness of individual circumstances from the illnesses suffered by individuals. Diseases, it was argued, should instead be thought of as agents or entities that have distinct characteristics (a typical cluster of signs and symptoms, typical cellular pathology, typical courses, and typical outcomes) and that have an independent existence or reality *separate from* and *outside of* the body of a *particular* human being in a state of illness. Diseases became specific, and their specificity was defined by biological mechanisms (chemical and physiological abnormalities) discovered at autopsy or in the laboratory. Disease was no longer an unnatural imbalance in the life of an individual, but a deviation from fixed norms. New ways of thinking about disease led to new ways of thinking about—and relating to—diseased persons. For example, physicians who were laboratory researchers mostly interacted with specimens—bits of brain matter or other tissue samples, urine, blood, inanimate cadavers— not with patients. Furthermore, with the new concept of disease *the uniqueness of an individual human being collapsed at the moment of diagnosis.* A diseased person with a diagnosis became an example of an impersonal categorical type. The narrative of a person's life was replaced by a grander narrative of truth—a transcendent reality of categories of biological mechanisms (and all of the social interpretations associated with a specific disease diagnosis).

This new way of conceptualizing disease divided physicians. Even in Europe there was an inherent tension between laboratory researchers, whose goal of disease specificity necessarily focused them on the biological mechanisms underlying *diagnosis,* and general practitioners or alienists interested in the everyday practicalities of alleviating the suffering of individual patients and who cared little for what name an ailment might have or what may have really caused it; *treatment of symptoms* was their primary concern. The importance of the European invention of disease specificity was slowly acknowledged, to greater or lesser degree, by American doctors throughout the last third of the nineteenth century, though most general practitioners and alienists understood little and cared even less about the news from the Old World.

In truth there was considerable disarray and mediocrity in the community of American physicians. Most who were in practice in 1896 had not had the benefit of rigorous medical training unless they had spent significant time in Europe at the bench or the bedside in places like Berlin, Vienna, or Strassburg. Most of those who did have formal training had probably attended a year or two of lectures at proprietary commercial medical schools with minimal resources and little opportunity for anatomical or clinical study, later learning most of their trade in the time-honored way, in master-apprentice relationships with established doctors. Indeed many had not examined a single living patient or dissected a cadaver during their (usually quite brief) medical studies. Medical degrees were corruptly bought and sold in some of these schools, as were professorships. Although most states had licensing or certification requirements for physicians, these were loosely regulated, and infractions were rarely enforced. In 1896 American doctors were still separated into sects that referred to themselves as "regulars" (those who went to medical schools approved by the American Medical Association, which was founded in 1847) and "irregular practitioners," such as homeopaths, osteopaths, and eclectics.[7] What distinguished them was their vastly different notions of therapeutics. States that contained numerous "irregular" medical colleges either had separate licensing boards for the different sects or had members of the various sects represented on a single regulating board. The historian William G. Rothstein has estimated that in the year 1900 there were approximately 110,000 regular physicians, 10,000 homeopaths, 5,000 eclectics, and more than 5,000 other practitioners (osteopaths, herbalists, and lay healers of various sorts).[8] But of the "regulars," only 8,000 belonged to the AMA in that same year, limiting its effectiveness as a national political force.[9]

Basic laboratory science conducted mostly in Europe had revealed its potential relevance to clinical practice, but only to those American physicians open-minded enough to accept its findings. For most, knowledge gained through laboratory procedures seemed too coldly distant from the ancient doctor-patient dyad, too artificial, with its claims that life forms unseen to the naked eye caused disease; such new claims to "better" knowledge threatened the authority of the hands-on, experience-based practices that they wholeheartedly believed were "scientific." Still, to these same skeptics it was indisputably miraculous that the new science of bacteriology had discovered the causes of infectious diseases like tuberculosis and diphtheria that were formerly thought to be due to heredity, masturbation, "miasma," or a confusing variety of external, visible, and proximal causes.[10] In Berlin in late 1891 a diphtheria antitoxin had been successfully used to produce the first true cure of modern scientific medicine, but effective treatments were still lacking for other infectious diseases. The promise of the salvation of medicine through science thrilled the (mostly) young men and women who were not laden with the bad habits and mistaken notions of the older generations. The older generations of urban general practitioners and rural horse-and-buggy doctors were mostly suspicious of applied laboratory science in medical practice and viewed specialization with scorn. What was the good of knowing that tuberculosis was caused by an invisible microbe when the condition could be diagnosed by traditional signs and symptoms and the treatment remained the same? The younger generation, especially those with experience in the laboratories and university clinics of Germany, viewed their historical era differently. They hungered for the technological transcendence of human suffering. And eventually they were the ones who made it happen.

But in 1896 much of this bypassed the typical American alienist. Psychiatry was a profession unlike other medical specialties in that it arose in special institutions. Indeed it could be said it was created *by* the institutions. Asylum walls not only bonded the insane, they bounded the identity of the physicians within them. Most alienists were employed in state asylums that were deliberately built in remote areas, although some worked in their own family-run private asylums (called "sanitaria") or in county or city asylums in some of the larger urban areas such as New York, Chicago, Detroit, St. Louis, Baltimore, Pittsburgh, and Cincinnati. In fact the chasm was widening between the asylum doctors and other physicians, especially their main professional competitors for the treatment of nervous and mental diseases, the neurologists, who had conquered the lucrative domain of outpatient office practice for the treatment of less severe "nervous diseases" such as neurasthenia.[11] Indeed, claimed the Philadelphia neurologist Silas Weir Mitchell (1829–1914), American alienists had devolved into "a group of physicians who constitute almost a sect apart from our more vitalized existence."[12]

European research neurologists had defined the structural and functional hierarchy of the nervous system, providing American neurologists (a new specialty in the 1870s) with a fund of basic physiological knowledge they could apply to clinical practice. European science had also provided a halo under which American neurologists could bask, elevating their perceived status in the medical world. In addition to diagnosing and (minimally) treating well-specified neurological conditions (accident or war injuries, acute or degenerative neurological diseases such as Huntington's or Parkinson's choreas, and so on), they also claimed professional jurisdiction over the murky area of "functional" nervous diseases or "neuroses"—conditions that had signs and symptoms that seemed neurological but did not make medical sense physiologically. These were conditions that were widespread, vague, and often responsive to treatment. They were not "mental diseases" or insanity. Neurology textbooks reflected this, usually including chapters at the end of each volume on diseases such as neurasthenia, psychasthenia, hysteria, and epilepsy—but no chapters on insanity. Neurologists usually came into contact with insane patients only in their role as consultants to asylums, neurological clinics, prisons, or the courts, and their literary contributions in medical journals on the problem of insanity (including, later, dementia praecox) were based on these limited experiences.

Beginning in the 1870s neurologists pioneered private outpatient practice for the treatment of nervous and mental diseases. They could make informed diagnoses of nervous conditions and offer, in a limited way, treatments (such as hydrotherapy or electrotherapy, sedatives, or a short stay in a sanitarium). It should be remembered that, before 1940 or so, most Americans who sought out a "nerve doctor" for the outpatient treatment of their bad case of "nerves" were doing so because of distinct physical pains or other symptoms (including depression and anxiety), not to receive counseling for personal problems.

American asylum physicians were at a distinct disadvantage when compared with the neurologists. Burdened almost exclusively with the more severe and chronic mental diseases or "insanity," over which they had always claimed professional jurisdiction, they had no credible claims to therapeutic success or even laboratory-derived scientific knowledge. Did they see functional cases of neurasthenia, hysteria, and epilepsy within institutional walls? Of course they did. But the *management* of insanity remained their primary preoccupation.

By 1896 many neurological diseases had been specified in the clinics and the laboratories, thereby becoming even more organic, thus anchoring the perceived power of the neurologist in his or her ability to diagnose with scientific certainty. But not all neurologists were alike. A considerable number of physicians in outpatient private practice after 1900 who called themselves neurologists treated more nervousness than specified neurological diseases. Confusingly a neurologist could even be referred to as an alienist when in consultation or in the courts. Asylum physicians quite commonly referred to themselves as alienists—in 1896 it was not, as is commonly thought, a term to refer only to what we would call a forensic psychiatrist today—but they were more likely to apply this label to themselves when they testified in court. Outside the walls of the asylums was a world of mental health treatment in which professional fluidity reigned in the courts and in the culture.

The boundary between the actual conditions treated by neurologists and those treated by asylum physicians would become increasingly blurred between 1890 and 1920, as would their professional identities. Both treated functional and organic, nervous and mental diseases. After 1900 some asylum physicians began the slow exodus from the state hospitals to open outpatient private practices to treat the neuroses, but they did not then market themselves to the public as neurologists. For a time, beginning in World War I, "neuropsychiatrist" would serve as a blanket term to further hide the lack of distinct professional boundaries. It would only be in 1934 that the wide range of physicians who treated nervous and mental diseases formally split into the separate board-certified, licensed specialties of neurology and psychiatry. Jurisdictional disputes over what kind of doctor should treat what kind of nervous or mental disease largely ceased after that point: neurologists claimed exclusive dominion over the organic diseases of the nervous system, the psychiatrists over the functional ones that could not be satisfactorily specified by laboratory science, such as the neuroses, dementia praecox, and manic-depression.

But some early neurologists, enthused by the seemingly limitless possibilities of their new medical science, believed that jurisdiction over insanity should be entirely taken away from asylum physicians. This in part contributed to the virtual disappearance of clear professional boundaries . In the late 1870s neurologists had waged a scathing campaign against the asylum alienists, attacking them for their lassitude, therapeutic mendacity, and scientific ignorance. "The neurologists hounded the psychiatrists and the psychiatrists stayed behind their iron gates and snarled, not being able to defend themselves."[13] One of the founders of American neurology, Silas Weir Mitchell, would be invited past the iron gates to deliver the terms of surrender directly to asylum physicians.

In 1894 Weir Mitchell, an edgy, canny, literary and scientific giant in his seventh decade of life, delivered a brutally honest and thorough indictment of the alienists before a room full of their elite as an invited keynote speaker at the fiftieth annual meeting of the American Medico-Psychological Association. The AMPA was the premier national organization of alienists, comprising superintendents of institutions for the insane and the assistant physicians who did most of the actual medical work in asylums. At first Weir Mitchell had declined this invitation to address his reviled professional adversaries, but after a promise that he would be allowed to speak his mind he couldn't resist a golden opportunity to strike a blow. His remarks, although widely cited in other histories of psychiatry, are worth repeating here. Reminding the alienists of the medical advances achieved by other specialties, he then zeroed in for the kill:

> With you it has been different. You were the first of the specialists and you have never come back into line. It is easy to see how this came about. You soon began to live apart, and you still do. Your hospitals are not our hospitals; your ways are not our ways. You live out of range of critical shot; you are not preceded and followed in your ward work by clever rivals, or watched by able residents fresh with the learning of school. . . . Where, we ask, are your annual reports of scientific study, of the psychology and pathology of your patients?. . . . We commonly get as your contributions to science, odd little statements, reports of a case or two, a few useless pages of isolated post-mortem records, and these are sandwiched among incomprehensible statistics and farm balance-sheets; and this too often is your sole answer. . . . Want of competent original work is to my mind the worst symptom of torpor the asylums now present. Contrast the work you have done in the last three decades with what the little group of our own neurologists has done. . . . Even in your own line most of the text-books, many of the ablest papers, are not asylum products. What is the matter?[14]

Indeed what *was* the matter?

It is true, as other historians have noted, that in the last third of the nineteenth century public asylums in the United States underwent considerable deterioration.[15] Overcrowding was just one of the reasons, reducing these once hopeful institutions into warehouses of human degeneration. Custodial care—and at the barest minimum standard at that—replaced the midcentury hopes of administering "moral treatment" to smaller populations of inpatients who would stay for only a short time and then be "cured" by the institution as the putative therapeutic agent.[16] But by 1896 widespread apathy and a pervasive loss of confidence in the ability to effectively treat or cure insanity, termed "therapeutic nihilism," had infected most public institutions. Alcoholism, general paralysis or paresis (found later to be caused by syphilis), and a whole host of baffling conditions often casually labeled (based on the primary presenting symptom) as types of *mania* (excitement of activity) or *melancholia* (depression of activity), *primary dementia* (a dullness, mental weakness, or cognitive defect found in adolescents or adults who were not yet elderly) or *terminal dementia* (a term for burned-out, chronically insane persons)—all of these conditions seemed to produce increasingly chronic patients who defied effective treatments. By the end of the nineteenth century and into the early twentieth the average length of stay in asylums had increased compared to those treated only forty years before. And the increasingly popular notion that heredity or irreversible somatic causes were at the root of these illnesses rendered psychological or psychotherapeutic efforts futile. All of these factors were cultural and social contributors to the general malaise and inertia so forcefully illustrated by Weir Mitchell in his remarks to the psychiatric elite.

But part of the problem was the alienists themselves. The vast majority of young physicians who became alienists did so after graduating from mediocre commercial medical colleges or after an apprenticeship with a doctor, without ever having heard a single lecture on insanity or ever having examined an insane person. This is partially due to the fact that cities and towns that hosted medical schools were far away from state asylums, where most of the institutionalized insane were located, and thus there was little opportunity for in vivo instruction. This lack of training and direct experience of the insane was true even of those who had the advantage of Ivy League educations before going to medical school or—a rare experience for those who began their medical careers in institutions for the insane—the privilege of a period of training in Europe. Richard Dewey (1845–1933) knew nothing of insanity when he "finished the usual medical course, had had a year of hospital experience and practice and also a year of study and practice in Germany" before he was hired as an assistant physician at the State Hospital for the Insane at Elgin, Illinois, in 1871. "My experience was typical of the medical practitioner of that day. . . . Education in psychiatry was neglected. In most of the colleges of our land, the medical graduate could complete his entire course without ever seeing a case of mental disease."[17]

William Alanson White (1870–1937), who would become a leader in American psychiatry in the early decades of the twentieth century, had the advantage of premedical courses in anatomy, physiology, and chemistry at Cornell before completing his two years of medical instruction at the Long Island College Hospital Medical School in Brooklyn. The lecturer on nervous and mental diseases was the superintendant of the local city asylum. "He gave only one lecture that might by any chance be called a lecture in psychiatry. . . . This was my total instruction in psychiatry."[18] Like most other young alienists, he learned his craft on the job after assuming his appointment to the Binghamton State Hospital in New York in April 1892. At Harvard Medical School the young James M. Keniston had heard a few lectures on insanity delivered by the superintendant of the McLean Asylum in Massachusetts, but at the time of his appointment as assistant physician at an asylum in Providence, Rhode Island, in May 1869 he "had never seen an insane person, as no clinical demonstrations were given."[19]

Why did a young doctor decide to become an alienist? Most alienists stumbled into the profession by sheer accident: an asylum job was available and they needed a steady income that the private practice of general medicine did not provide. Although the pay was low—on average less than half of the salary of superintendents—it was reliably consistent. In comparison income from a general practice of medicine in an era of local home visits was abysmally unpredictable and often uncollectable. Furthermore in an institution free room and board for the asylum physician and his family was provided. Such security was the attraction for many, as well as the dream of one day rising to the all-powerful position of asylum superintendent, a position of paternalistic prestige and significant social status that extended outside the walls of the institution. Many asylum physicians, imbued with a Protestant religious ethic so characteristic of that era of American history, experienced a moral satisfaction from their work that offset the financial hardships, and this kept many on the wards for decades. But the duties were many, the days long (indeed, because they lived in the asylums with the patients they were always on call), and not only geographical but intellectual isolation were the norm.

Access to new medical knowledge after medical school (such as might be found in German, French, or British journals or books) and the opportunities to apply acquired knowledge were hampered by this isolation. As a rule subscriptions to foreign psychiatric journals were made only by urban specialty organizations (such as the library of the New York Academy of Medicine) and not by asylums or state hospitals nor their superintendants (who could afford them) or assistant physicians (who could not). "Even the American journals, which published abstracts of foreign work as well as American research material, must have seemed like visions of an irrelevant fairyland to assistants whose daily work was mostly composed of purely medical problems, of 'classification' of psychiatric cases, and of paperwork," observed the sociologist Andrew Delano Abbott. Prolonged isolation in largely rural asylums contributed to a lack of interest in participation in national professional organizations where new ideas from Europe were often discussed; in 1915 a full 70 percent of assistant physicians in the United States chose not to belong to the only existing national organization of psychiatrists, the American Medico-Psychological Association.[20]

New knowledge generally flowed to asylum physicians and neurologists from elite members of local or regional societies and organizations. In places like New York City, Boston, Philadelphia, Chicago, Baltimore, and Washington, D.C., where there were alienists and neurologists who could read foreign languages, European ideas were more likely to be discussed at meetings of local societies. For example, one local group, the New York Psychiatrical Society, would be the primary transatlantic conduit for the introduction of new views of dementia praecox and schizophrenia between 1907 and 1912. Presentations at the society often appeared in print within a year, in publications such as the *Journal of Nervous and Mental Disease*. But most asylums were not near these cities, nor were the journals widely read, and thus knowledge transfer from European clinics to rural American asylum wards was slow, when it existed at all.

Very few American alienists of this era left behind detailed reminiscences of their training in psychiatry. Although the experiences of

Dewey, White, and Keniston were probably typical, medical students in other colleges did indeed receive more exposure to psychiatric concepts and insane patients. In January 1893 N. Emmons Paine, a homeopathic physician who taught at the Boston University School of Medicine, sent out a "circular" to the deans of each of the 144 medical colleges in the United States and Canada as well as 170 questionnaires to superintendants of institutions for the insane "and certain other members" of the American Medico-Psychological Association. He asked three basic questions: Was psychiatry taught at the medical school? Were students examined in psychiatry as a requirement for graduation? And were the medical students exposed to clinical demonstrations involving actual insane patients?

Paine combined the information from the medical schools and the alienists in his final tabulations. Most medical colleges did not reply to the circular (only 61 of 144 responded, including 8 of the 16 homeopathic medical colleges in existence at the time), and he therefore assumed psychiatry was not taught at those schools. However, almost all of the superintendants did reply. He found that in 1893 all of the sixty-one responding colleges reported that "psychiatry is taught either by alienists or specialists." Only eight said psychiatry had been taught at their institution back in 1871 (one of Paine's auxiliary questions). Superintendants of hospitals for the insane were the teachers in 34 of the 61 colleges, and assistant physicians of these hospitals were the lecturers at two others. Twenty-four of the colleges had "filled their chairs with specialists," indicating a strong commitment to psychiatry. As to the question of whether medical students had to pass an examination on psychiatric topics as a requirement for graduation, 20 of the 61 colleges had no such exam, in 30 the examination was administered by the lecturer in his own specialty, and in 5 the students were examined on psychiatric topics but not by a specialist. Perhaps the most surprising finding was that in 42 of the 61 responding medical colleges clinics in psychiatry were held in addition to lectures: "That shows a majority, or sixty-seven percent, in favor of illustrating the lectures on insanity by cases of insanity."[21]

Paine may have been one of the most enlightened instructors in psychiatry in 1893, but he himself gave only five lectures on insanity to his medical students, each combined with a trip to the Westborough Insane Hospital, a homeopathic institution some thirty-two miles from

Boston. It is doubtful if medical students in other North American colleges received a better education in psychiatry. And why should they know anything about the insane? Certainly few young men (and fewer young women) went to medical school with the intention of becoming an alienist. Despite the security of a steady paycheck (as opposed to the insecurity of private practice), doctoring the mad in an asylum was viewed as the least desirable form of medical practice. "Positions in insane hospitals are despised now," wrote Adolf Meyer in a letter in December 1895.[22] Alienists were regarded by other physicians, especially neurologists, as occupying a position only one small grade above quacks.

Homeopaths like Paine were certainly regarded as quacks by most of the regular physicians, but such sectarian animosity did not seem to exist in the lowly community of alienists. There is no record of significant sectarian discord even though most alienists were probably trained as regular physicians. Irregulars such as homeopaths were tolerated, if not welcomed. Perhaps this was due to the fact that no one really knew what to do to make an insane person sane. It could be that experimental treatments, such as the materia medica of the homeopaths, were more likely to be tolerated by alienists than by regular physicians of other specialties. When Paine conducted his survey, six superintendents of institutions for the insane were homeopathic physicians. Furthermore, "in five States the homoeopathic medical colleges have been receiving lectures from alienists of our own school, every one a superintendant of a State hospital."[23] By 1898 New York State had two homeopathic hospitals for the insane, and other such institutions existed in Massachusetts, Minnesota, California, Michigan, and Missouri.[24] The first American homeopathic state institution for the insane was the Middletown State Homeopathic Hospital in New York, which opened in April 1874, and the last was the Allentown State Homeopathic Hospital in Pennsylvania, which opened in October 1912.

It is impossible to know how many alienists were regular or irregular physicians in 1896. We do know that, as Weir Mitchell pointed out, in 1890 there were approximately 120 public and 40 private asylums caring for more than 91,000 patients.[25] The most useful source of information about the identities of American physicians in 1896 was that year's *Medical and Surgical Register of the United States,* a directory published annually by the R. L. Polk Company since 1886. However, although Polk's *Register* identified doctors according to their sects, it did not identify their areas of specialty. The ethical code of the American Medical Association prohibited such identifications because "public identification of specialists was widely viewed as unethical advertising."[26] The same was true in Germany and Britain in 1896. Therefore there are no reliable statistics available for the exact number of physicians who identified themselves as alienists in 1896. But one estimate for the year 1895 based on the number of government-supported institutions for the insane (148), epileptics (2), and the feebleminded (42), as well as private, for-profit sanitaria (42), indicates that as many as 745 doctors did so. The actual number was probably higher.[27]

The alienists themselves did not distinguish between the regulars and the irregulars in the membership lists of their main professional organization. Founded in Philadelphia in 1844 (three years before the founding of the AMA) as the Association of Medical Superintendants of American Institutions for the Insane, the organization was an exclusive club that admitted only superintendants as members. All too often they were political appointees who did exclusively administrative, not medical, duties, and many were rarely seen by patients or staff. But the power of a superintendent was absolute within the walls of an institution, and those who were clinically engaged rendered decisions about diagnosis, treatment, and discharge with autocratic disregard of the medical opinions of the assistant physicians. After a decade of attacks by neurologists and patient advocacy groups that alienists were unresponsive to medical, scientific, and humanitarian concerns, this elite organization decided to broaden its base to include the asylum physicians who actually did have daily contact with their insane patients. Starting in 1885 assistant physicians were admitted as associate members if they had five years of experience. After the organization adopted a new constitution in 1892, the amount of time for assistant physicians to become associate members was shortened to three years of experience in an asylum. In that year the organization also changed its name to the American Medico-Psychological Association. The words "psychiatric" and "psychiatry" were regarded as terms of foreign (German) origin and use that would be too unfamiliar to the lay public and were rejected as part of the new title. Indeed it apparently wasn't until 1906 that an American alienist first used the term "psychiatrist" in print to refer to the profession, indicating its relative lack of usage among alienists at the time. This would change in 1921, with the next and final name change of the organization to the American Psychiatric Association.[28]

But the American Medico-Psychological Association was a national organization in name only. In reality it had no power to define the boundaries of the knowledge domain or practice of its members. It had virtually no budget. Although it rendered advice to state oversight boards, it was not a trade organization that lobbied politicians on behalf of its guild members. Its only function was to have an annual meeting and, after 1894, to publish the *American Journal of Insanity*. Local societies and organizations, with blended memberships composed of neurologists and asylum physicians, wielded most of the real influence over alienists until the 1930s.

Membership rolls were published in each edition of the series of *Annual Proceedings of the American Medico-Psychological Association*. In the 1896 *Proceedings* there were 219 active members listed with affiliations with American institutions, 17 in Canadian ("British America") institutions, and 15 "honorary members" from France, England, Italy, and Belgium as well as three Americans, two of whom were Silas Weir Mitchell and the psychologist and president of Clark University in Worcester, Massachusetts, G. Stanley Hall. The majority were from northeastern and midwestern states. The western and southern United States were underrepresented in the membership rolls.[29]

Adolf Meyer, the newly appointed pathologist at the Worcester Lunatic Hospital in Massachusetts, was granted full membership at the 1896 annual meeting. He had served two and a half of his three years as a pathologist at a state hospital in Kankakee, Illinois. The title of pathologist was of lower rank and status than the title of assistant physician in American asylums. But at Worcester Meyer was granted administrative powers far beyond that of any other asylum pathologist. Indeed within a few short years Meyer would emerge as the leader of psychiatry's struggle to rejoin the medical profession.

What was the occult universe that awaited the young and inexperienced physician upon first passing, no doubt with some trepidation, through the gates of the asylum? How was the passage made from newly graduated physician to experienced alienist?[30]

The first impression would have been one of both familiarity and confusion. Many of the insane looked and acted like normal people. Why were *they* here? On the other hand there were undoubtedly others engaged in extraordinary behaviors: the assumption of odd postures or stereotyped, repetitive acts that had no sensical meaning; tremors of the hands and neck that sometimes swelled into full-bodied seizures; incessant pacing, sometimes slowly, legs arced high as if stepping over bales of cotton; figures bent over in fits of vomiting, sometimes expelling a bloody froth of shards of glass mixed with the balls of cotton that were ordered as the antidote to this meal of lunacy;[31] coughing, cadaverous specters spewing phlegm into clutched cuspidors; self-directed whispering or animal-like barks; pleas of release from persecution by the Jesuits, the hounds of hell, or an absent husband; cheery words spilling forth in tortured sentences absent of logic or structure; grand introductions, a bit too loud and too pressured, from the pope or the president or God, or sincere protestations of wrongful confinement from a railroaded Vanderbilt or Carnegie; anguished, agitated, and sometimes violent gestures and cries; bodies frozen in the bedlam of despair; faces blank with alienation or contorted into skewed grimaces; sexual organs exposed and manipulated; public defecation. The strong scent of the asylum, the "odour of insanity," was an aromatic blend of rotting teeth, filthy skin, menstrual blood, ammonia, urine, feces, and the foul exhalations of paraldehyde (a sedative drug much in use by the alienists of the 1890s). Needles, sometimes hundreds of them, might be found stuck under the skin of an insane person. More than a few deliberately poisoned themselves. Many of the insane bore scars or fresh scratches or lacerations, particularly about the head, hands, and arms. Some slumped stuporously along the walls, saliva sliding over parted lips, eyelids only half-concealing the abyss of confusion.

What in god's name was wrong with these people? How could one possibly make sense out of this riot of new sensations and impressions? In time the inexperienced alienist would learn to do what generations of others had done: focus only on the familiar and immediate medical issues, keep the saner patients busy and the others drugged, and learn half a dozen diagnostic terms, each of which could be matched to a name in the records. Mania, melancholia, and dementia were the three most common diagnoses, but the new alienist was taught at the outset to disregard their importance: the patients were "insane," that is all. Many American alienists believed mania, melancholia, and dementia were merely fluid forms or expressions of the symptoms of a unitary psychosis, or "insanity." Case books from a century ago contain records of many patients who were never formally designated with a diagnosis, again indicating how irrelevant it was—but to be fair to asylum physicians, the same situation persisted in many dispensaries and hospitals and general medical practice in the United States. Despite its importance to the new scientific medicine of that time, disease specificity of the insanities was not a concern of American alienists in 1896.

Diseases that were rarely seen outside of asylums, and rarely taught in medical colleges, had to be learned quickly by the novice assistant physician. Paresis, or the "general paralysis of the insane," one of the most prevalent afflictions witnessed in asylums, was one of these. Although it had been suspected for decades that this condition was due to the ravages of syphilis, this would not be proven until the early years of the twentieth century, after which it was renamed "neurosyphilis." General paralysis cases were perhaps the most distinctive in the asylum, the most specifiable insanity—but only to the trained eye. On his very first day as assistant physician at the Binghamton State Hospital in New York, a massive facility with a census of just under one thousand insane patients, William Alanson White was met by the new superintendent, Charles G. Wagner:

> I recall my introductory walk through the wards with him. After talking with one of the patients Dr. Wagner turned to me and asked if I knew what his diagnosis was. The patient was an obvious paretic, with all the outward and evident signs of the disease, but I apparently saw none of them. So far as I can recall I had no knowledge in those days that there was such a disease as paresis. I certainly had never seen anyone with it and had had no experience with the symptoms. As we continued our way through the wards I saw any number of patients who, as far as I could determine, were perfectly all right. In other words, my attitude toward what I saw was not very different from that which I have noted constantly since then in laymen when they visit an institution of this sort.[32]

In the year 1896 only Bellevue Hospital in New York City had an insane ward or pavilion for acute cases. Acute wards for insane patients (called "psychopathic wards") in general hospitals began to appear only after 1900, with Pavilion F of the general hospital in Albany, New York, which opened in 1901, leading the trend. "Psychopathic hospitals" for acute care and, in some cases, research, would later appear in places such as Ann Arbor (1906), Boston (1912) and Baltimore (1913).

Such institutions had already existed in Europe, particularly in Germany, for many decades. But in 1896 even most state hospitals for the insane lacked a special "reception" unit for the observation of new patients, nor did many have wards for the quieter, voluntarily committed persons suffering from less severe conditions. In that era there was no system of outpatient clinics or other venues to act as mediating buffers for persons suffering from extreme emotional and cognitive duress; there were only the jail and the insane asylum.

When the new assistant physician witnessed the arrival of an admission to the asylum he would see an individual at his or her worst, often writhing in a camisole (straitjacket) or shackled and bitterly protesting his or her enslavement—unless of course the individual had been heavily drugged prior to transport, which also happened. Humiliated and angry relatives would also sometimes arrive at the asylum at the same time, creating a mournful clamor. In a searing polemic penned in 1912 by Edward Kempf (1885–1971) but never published during his lifetime, he deplored the arrest of "some sick man or woman as though they were guilty criminals." At the time he wrote these words, the twenty-seven-year-old Kempf had graduated from medical school only two years earlier and was an assistant physician at the Central Hospital for the Insane at Indianapolis. Noting that "the practice of arrest etc. is common in most of our states," he described the typical course of events: "Very often the sick patient is locked in jail for one day to several weeks. After due permission is granted by the superintendent of some institution, the patient is escorted to the Insane Asylum by the sheriff and deputy and locked behind bars as a fitting climax for his outraged emotions."[33] (The young Kempf would not have to toil in the belly of the beast much longer after putting his rage to paper: the following year, 1913, he was hired by Adolf Meyer to be an assistant resident at the newly opened Henry Phipps Psychiatric Clinic at Johns Hopkins.)

The State of California, teeming with immigrants and transients searching for a better life, had the worst reputation for such railroading. State officials vigorously arrested vagrants, drunkards, eccentrics, paupers, and other undesirables and dispatched them "with railroad speed" through the jails and courts to state asylums. In the late 1890s California had a higher proportion of insane residents than any other state, in part due to these practices.[34] Streets, jails, and almshouses were purged of such inconvenient individuals. In truth, however, across the United States the process of railroading was most often initiated by family members, and government officials were usually quite responsive to their wishes.

What was the typical workday like for an American alienist in the 1890s?

The assistant physician would be expected to assume his duties immediately upon hire. Because most state insane hospitals or asylums (the words were used interchangeably in this decade, although "asylum" was still the preferred term) were being flooded with new admissions, the overall census of the institution might be counted in the thousands. The new assistant physician would be assigned a portion of the caseload that would be roughly equal to that of his colleagues. When the twenty-nine-year-old Adolf Meyer left his pathologist position at the Illinois Eastern Hospital for the Insane in Kankakee in 1895 there were 2,100 patients who were tended by only a "few physicians." The superintendent there "used to brag with the fact that in 1875 he had 300 patients to look after and kept his notes well" and expected the assistant physicians at Kankakee to be personally responsible for the care of a comparable, if not higher number. A ratio of one alienist to 200 to 300 patients was the generally accepted standard in American asylums in the 1890s. Meyer was of the opinion that "to-day it is an impossibility to look after more than 100 patients or 150 at the outside and to do all that should be done for the patient and for the profession." In his new pathologist position at the Worcester Lunatic Hospital in Massachusetts he found "4 physicians who have never had any special training" responsible for "between 900 and 1000 patients."[35] Given the staggering number of insane patients for whom an assistant physician would bear responsibility—the actual caseload at Kankakee was between 300 and 500 per alienist[36]—it is no wonder that patient care suffered and therapeutic nihilism, a pervasive loss of confidence in the standard treatments of insanity, settled into the world of the American asylum.

In a typical institution for the insane an assistant physician might appear on the wards for only an hour in the morning and perhaps an hour in the evening, unless there was a medical emergency. During those short blocks of time he would rapidly observe the physical condition of hundreds of patients. The alienist walked quickly and did not have time to linger. Only the most obvious medical problems were noted and received attention. Sometimes attending to the multitude of medical problems of varying severity might occupy an entire day. An alienist did not usually engage in discussions with the patients—after all, they were insane, weren't they?—but would receive verbal reports from the nurses and attendants as he made his rounds. The remainder of his day would be consumed with two other activities, clerical and pharmaceutical.

Individual files containing all the medical records of a single patient did not exist in American asylums in the 1890s. Even in general medical practice this familiar procedure was coming into use only in a few innovative hospitals. Instead alienists would spend much of their day making notes (sometimes days or weeks late) in large leather-bound case books that resembled accounting ledgers. General medical hospitals were quicker to adopt the individual case file method, but such case books were still in use in many American institutions for the insane as late as 1918.[37] In a case book each patient was assigned his or her own page. Since medical information was recorded infrequently in asylums and general hospitals in that era, it might take many months, or a year or more, to fill a page. Once the page was filled another would be started, but it might be dozens of pages deeper into the volume, or in another case book entirely. These methods made it difficult, if not impossible in the instance of multiple case books, for an alienist to keep track of the case of an individual patient without considerable effort. And there was simply no time for such effort.

On the initial page started upon admission there often would be the expected personal information—name, address, family contacts, occupation, and so on—and a word or a phrase indicating the probable cause of the patient's insanity (disappointed affections, religious excitement, masturbation, fright and nervous shock, overwork, menstruation, intemperance, grief, childbirth, financial misfortune, and heredity were common) and perhaps a diagnosis (usually some form of mania, melancholia, dementia, or idiocy) accentuated by a variety of modifiers ("acute," "terminal," and so on), but it really didn't matter: the fact that a person was judged insane, not that he or she had a particular diagnosis, was the main thing. This page, and those that followed, would be filled in, line by line, with the record of any unusual medical or behavioral events, drugs prescribed and administered, indications of contact with family members or friends of the patients, and notations of transfers between wards or discharge. Even when an individual patient's entire medical record in an asylum could be pieced together page by page, case book by case book, there was really very little detailed information to indicate the range of signs and symptoms, or if the diagnosis was correct or not, or if the treatments really worked, or if indeed the patient was really insane at all. Historians today who undertake such projects in state archives are continually confronted with how unenlightening these case book records are when it comes to fathoming the true picture of an individual patient from that era. The voices of the mad were rarely recorded with much detail in asylum records.

Assistant physicians were also expected to respond to correspondence from the friends and family of the 100 to 500 or more patients who were under their direct care on any given day. When not writing notes in the case books, alienists were writing such letters by hand, without the assistance of stenographers or typewriters.

Many asylums for the insane did not employ druggists or apothecaries. When an assistant physician ordered a particular sedative, emetic or "tonic" or other substance to be given to a particular patient he often had to prepare the medications himself. This was a common practice of American physicians in private general practice, especially in rural areas, well into the twentieth century. It was viewed as an expected role of a doctor, and this expectation followed physicians through the gates of the asylums. This activity also took considerable time, and it was not uncommon for fatal mistakes in dosages of opiates and other drugs to occur when the alienist was rushed (or impaired by alcohol or opiates himself). "The public here believe in drugs and consider prescription as the aim and end of medical skill," wrote Adolf Meyer of asylum treatment in August 1894, "whereas in Germany and in many other places, the people regard the drugs as quite as great an affliction as the disease itself."[38]

In late nineteenth-century America asylum patients were heavily drugged with sedatives and hypnotics as an alternative to physical restraints. In the twenty-page entry on sedatives in the second volume of Daniel Hack Tuke's *A Dictionary of Psychological Medicine* of 1892—a fascinating, encyclopedic work that documented the world of alienism as it existed just before the dawn of the twentieth century—there are descriptions of the nature and recommended dosages of eleven different bromides (including the best known, potassium bromide, and the bromide of lithium, which would be rediscovered, in a sense, in the mid-twentieth century), camphor, chloroform, ether, paraldehyde, chloral hydrate, sulphonal, hypnal, opium, morphine, codeine, hyoscine and hyoscyamine (in extensive use in the 1890s, injected hypodermically), cannabis indica (to be sprinkled on sugared bread crumbs for the patient to eat), conium (hemlock), and at least a dozen other drugs. The pharmacologic treatment of insanity was not an innovation of the late twentieth century by any means.[39]

This was not true for all institutions for the insane. Homeopathic asylums arose to meet a demand, often from the wealthier classes, for an alternative to the excessive sedation relied upon so readily by regular alienists. Many persons in 1896 still had a lingering distrust of regular doctors due to the horrific results of their former reliance on "heroic medicine"—the bleeding and poisonous purging of the sick, often to the point of death. When it came to making decisions about the treatment of insane loved ones, irregulars such as homeopaths were viewed by some as a safer alternative. The herbal and mineral materia medica of homeopathy, combined with a restatement of the ideals of moral medicine, made these few institutions attractive to many. Homeopathic alienists also claimed higher recovery rates and lower death rates for their patients. According to George Allen, a homeopathic alienist at the Middletown State Homeopathic Hospital, for the year ending 30 September 1892 there were 1,104 patients at his institution. Comparing the recovery rate favorably in contrast to other New York State institutions, Allen argued that this meant that "the hypnotics, opiates and neurotics, and multitudinous drug-preparations of our Old-School brethren are, to say the least, unnecessary in the treatment of insanity."[40]

Very few institutions for the insane had pathologists or laboratory facilities for the analysis of blood, urine, feces, or sputum. But in 1896 there were very few diagnostic examinations or analyses to be made anyway, at least none for conditions that could be treated or cured in an asylum. Basic scientific "instruments of precision" (as equipment such as thermometers and microscopes were called) were practically nonexistent, and medical tools were in short supply. Hypodermic needles were often reused with little or no attempt at proper sterilization. Basic medical care of the insane generally declined at the same time that some institutions began changing their official names from "asylums" to "hospitals"—a grim irony. These conditions continued to exist into the next century. "One institution of more than 1,000 patients did not have a functioning microscope for several months. One psychopathic institute did not have a microscope, a manometer or an urinalysis outfit in the institution," the Chicago surgeon Bayard Taylor Holmes (1852–1924) wrote in 1911. "It was as devoid of diagnostic instruments of precision as a Christian Science temple."[41]

Given the overcrowded and unsanitary conditions, the ignorance of the causes or vectors of transmission of many diseases, the lack of responsiveness to the crusade of the public health movement, and the inability or unwillingness of assistant physicians to conduct thorough medical examinations of the patients, the insane were sometimes ravaged by epidemics of various infectious diseases. Diphtheria, typhoid fever, and dysentery commonly stormed through asylums. Tuberculosis—sometimes still referred to as consumption, graveyard cough, or the white plague (a reference to the cadaverous complexion of its victims)—was also a particularly persistent affliction. Even though the laboratory procedures for identifying the pathogenic bacterium were well known by the end of the century, few asylums had the facilities or even the desire to identify infected patients and separate them from others, despite the numerous deaths that could be attributed to this disease. Although some asylums had special tuberculosis wards (or tents placed at some distance from the main buildings), most didn't, including the Indiana state hospital where the alienist Edward Kempf worked. "This indifference to the health of the patients, attendants and physicians is intolerable and a positive criminal neglect," he wrote in 1912, adding:

> Many patients persistently spit upon the floors, bedding, rugs, couches, into the radiators and on their clothes, wholly indifferent and ignorant to the awful havoc they cause. I saw a patient whose sputum swarmed with tubercle bacilli empty her cuspidor on the floor, as she expressed it, that others might suffer with her. Is there the slightest justification for the arrest and forcible confinement of any human being to months of such exposure to the white plague?[42]

Alienists relied heavily on the nurses and attendants for observational information about the patients and for the behavioral control of the wards. Discipline was needed if a ward full of insane or physically ill persons were to be clothed, fed, and put to bed. The attendants were responsible for maintaining the cleanliness of the physical environment of their wards as well as the bodies of their patients. However, sanitary conditions varied from ward to ward and institution to institution. Ammonia was used for cleaning clothes as well as floors, but some attendants who did not believe in germs or extra effort simply had the patients sweep the wards with a broom. Unless they soiled themselves— and each asylum had its own reviled infestation of what were called the "filthy insane"—patients were usually bathed only once a week (if that) in most asylums. The inmates wore clothing from home or provided (usually) by the county or by charitable organizations. The attendants were also responsible for administering the drugs ordered and prepared by the physician. Single doses contained in cups labeled with the patient's name were carried on trays to the wards. Nurses and attendants were also be responsible for the hypodermic injections of hyoscyamine, morphine, and other drugs. All work and entertainment activities for the patients were organized by the attendants. And of course the attendants were expected to de-escalate conflicts on the wards and calm or restrain agitated or violent patients, yet at the same time maintain their composure.

Then, as now, this was a formidable challenge. An 1898 training manual for asylum nurses and attendants appealed to their better angels:

> The position of attendants is often a trying one; they are liable to misrepresentation when they have faithfully done their duty; they must learn to receive with calmness a blow or an insult, or even so great an indignity as being spit upon; they must bear with provocations that come day after day, and are seemingly as malicious as they are ingenious and designing; they must watch over the suicidal with tireless vigilance, control the violent, and keep the unclean clean.
>
> To do all this requires the exercise of self control and kindness; the putting a curb upon the temper; the education of judgment and tact; faithfulness in the performance of duty, and a knowledge of what to do and what to avoid.[43]

Formal training schools for nurses and attendants were started in 1882 at the McLean Asylum in Somerville, Massachusetts, and in 1883 at the Buffalo State Asylum for the Insane in New York. Twenty-eight other institutions had such training programs in place by 1895, but these were the exceptions, and, as with the psychiatric training of medical students, the quality of instruction varied. Most newly hired attendants had no previous experience and received no formal instruction once on the job. They lived on the asylum grounds, worked eleven- to fourteen-hour shifts six days a week (four hours off was granted one day a week in most institutions, meaing a shift of perhaps only seven hours on the seventh day of work) and were meagerly paid. Turnover rates were high. Sometimes they were not paid at all; some asylums, notably those in New York City for a time, occasionally used prisoners from the local jails and penal colonies to provide free labor as attendants.[44] The effectiveness of alienists therefore depended primarily on their working relationships with nurses and attendants who were often illiterate, uneducated, indifferent, and, at times, abusive to the patients.

It was an impossible job. Over time many alienists adopted the very same sequence of behaviors exhibited by the troubled persons reacting in a natural fashion to their loss of personal liberties: confusion, fear, and anger followed by occasional rages, then resignation and withdrawal. As the years passed an understandable disinterest in their activities, coupled in some instances with alcohol and opiate abuse, psychologically cushioned many assistant physicians. What was perceived as laziness and ignorance by dynamic young physicians fresh from medical school or training in Europe was in fact learned helplessness. When these young reformers offered new ideas for the care or study of the asylum insane their older colleagues would inevitably ask, "What is that good for?"[45]

This, then, was the world of the American alienist in 1896. Asylum doctors had long been reluctant to form close bonds with the larger medical profession, fearing a loss of autonomy, but by the early 1890s this traditional attitude began to be viewed as detrimental to their future professional status as physicians. Given such a state of affairs, how could psychiatry ever reenter a medical profession itself engaged in a momentous revolution? How could alienists ever match the trajectory of other physicians who were pulled toward the future of a rationalized, disease-specified, laboratory-science-driven medicine?

A handful of young men took up this challenge. And for many the vector of their efforts would be defined by a new conception of insanity that would arrive from Germany, a protean construct unknown to American alienists in 1896: dementia praecox.

2

ADOLF MEYER BRINGS
DEMENTIA PRAECOX TO AMERICA

"Of course Baltimore has the greatest attraction for me, as it is, or certainly will be, the center of medical instruction."[1]

When he wrote these words in a letter in April 1892, Adolf Meyer was a twenty-five-year-old graduate of the University of Zurich Medical School who had just completed his doctoral thesis on the forebrain of reptiles, had never held formal employment as a clinician or researcher, did not enjoy treating living patients during his medical training, preferred to spend his time studying the brains of the dead, and had little formal training in psychiatry. This inexperienced young man would become the most influential psychiatrist in the United States for, depending on which author one reads, either the first three or the first four decades of the twentieth century.[2] He attained such prominence and power largely because he was appointed to two of the most powerful administrative posts in American psychiatry: first, in 1902, as director of the New York Pathological (later Psychiatric) Institute, where he transformed the entire system of New York state hospitals; then, in 1910, as a professor of psychiatry and chief of the Henry C. Phipps Psychiatric Clinic at the Johns Hopkins Hospital in Baltimore. From these exalted posts he was able to systematically train all asylum physicians under his administrative command and recommend them for prominent new positions in psychiatry opening up on both sides of the Atlantic, thereby assuring his influence. It is believed that at one point or another Meyer had personally trained almost every psychiatrist who rose to senior institutional positions of power in American institutions in the first half of the twentieth century.[3]

As we shall see, the story of Adolf Meyer is intertwined with the story of dementia praecox at every major juncture in its narrative. His own story is one of ambition, luck, and a knack for bureaucratic creativity.

Without any firm prospect of employment, Meyer left his mother and brother in Switzerland and emigrated to America in September 1892. He was among the first of a small reverse migration of physicians from German-speaking countries to the United States that began in 1890. Between 1890 and 1914 "many of the great figures in German medicine began to explore the medical world on this side of the Atlantic," noted the historian Thomas Bonner, and they were responsible for sparking the interest of their students about opportunities in America.[4] The mythic allure of the New World would prove to be irresistible for ambitious young men from Switzerland, Germany, and Austria as well as those from France, England, and particularly Scotland. He convinced his widowed mother to put up her house as security against a personal loan from a family friend so that he could do this. Left alone by her beloved son with the financial and moral responsibility of paying back this loan while he struggled for the next year to find a source of income, his mother sank into what we might call a major depressive episode with psychotic features, but that at the time was termed "melancholia with fancies of persecution."[5] By Christmas 1892 she was institutionalized at the famous Burghölzli mental hospital in Zurich and was placed under the care of its chief, August Forel (1848–1931), one of Meyer's former professors.

The insanity of his mother must have confirmed what Meyer already feared about himself: that he carried within him the taint of hereditary degeneration. As a widely accepted medical and moral theory that caused widespread professional and public concern, the theory of degeneration has been called, and rightly so, "the Christian notion of original sin embodied in the nervous system."[6] Degeneracy (immorality, insanity, vulnerability to develop diseases, and so on) was literally thought to be transmitted in the protoplasm of the father (in particular) and mother to their progeny, and the physical and mental stigmata of degeneration were thought to worsen with each new generation, leading to insanity, criminality, idiocy, further vegetation, and eventually death, until the family line died out. Although the progression of degeneracy within a family could be halted through "therapeutics" (halting substance abuse, adopting a moral lifestyle, moving away from toxic urban centers, and so on), the weakness was still passed on to the next generation. August Forel was a major proponent of degeneracy theory and forbade his assistant physicians from drinking alcohol. During these years Adolf Meyer was a documented believer in degeneration as well.[7]

Meyer came from what would then be called a "neuropathic family." We know this from a revealing letter of March 1893 that he sent to the man who loaned him the money to emigrate, the pastor J. C. Sheller (a friend of Meyer's deceased father, who had also been a Zwinglian minister). Meyer suffered from "an inherited tremor" of the hands, which he said was a "defect" that "pushed me out of surgery and obstetrics to the nerve clinic where relatively few fine manipulations are necessary." He said he was told that his "physical inadequacy made a career impossible." He confessed to being a "bungler" when attempting to systematically examine patients in medical school clinics and suffered from a "chronic feeling of inadequacy." Furthermore, prior to medical school, while he was a teenager in the Gymnasium, he suffered from an "inherited and . . . considerably developed neurasthenia" and worried that his "sickness" would return later in life when he suffered from the stresses of "bad times."[8] Meyer was well aware that all of these facts led to one conclusion only: he was tainted from birth and would have to find a path that would liberate him from his feelings of inadequacy, if not his degeneracy. Fleeing to America held out this hope for him. "I can perhaps free myself from the inheritance on both sides of our family," he confessed to his younger brother in December 1892.[9]

But Meyer could not free himself from some distinctly entrenched habits of personality that would follow him to the end of his days. He was prone to a (perhaps compensatory) confidence that outstripped his competence. This was evident even in his early years and would prove to be a gift in his later years, when he took on the challenge of making clinical and administrative reforms in seemingly hopeless asylums and state hospitals. For a young man who had never held formal employ-

ment in medicine or scientific research, Meyer repeatedly showed in-
credible pluck while job hunting in America: he always wanted to start
at the top. On at least three occasions in 1892, both before and shortly
after arriving in America, rather than asking for an entry-level job he
wrote to prominent academic and medical men offering to "establish an
institution for the anatomy of the nervous system" at Clark University;
to start a neurology subdivision (headed by him of course) in the pathological laboratory of a medical school ("It would be a great honor for
Chicago if Rush College were to go ahead" with his plan); and to found
a "Brain Institute" at the University of Chicago. Needless to say all of
these proposals from the inexperienced immigrant were turned down.[10]

Other lifelong habits of personality were also present in these early
years. Meyer manifested an obsessive acquisitiveness that, in his twenties, compelled him to collect prepared anatomical and pathological
specimens of the nervous system and entire brains. In his later psychiatric
career he became a relentless "fact" collector. "Meyer fetishized 'the
facts.'"[11] It led him to preach that *all* the "facts" of a person's life must be
documented without prejudging which ones were relevant and which
ones were irrelevant. Museums fascinated him, and his wish to establish
a museum-like "Brain Institute" would be echoed in his proposal in the
late 1930s to establish a "Hall of Man" or "Science of Man" that would
visually demonstrate "man confronted with his everyday problems."[12]
Such a display would no doubt be based on the innumerable "facts" collected by him and his colleagues. Meyer thought, spoke, and wrote in a
ruminative, tangential, and elusive (some of his contemporaries would
say evasive) manner. Many of his later disciples attributed this to the fact
that English was not his first language, but these habits of thought and
expression were evident when he spoke and wrote in German as well.
He was particularly self-conscious of this fact in his youth: "I remember
that even in 1892 I definitely rejected the advice to take up psychiatry in
Switzerland because I felt it required much more ability than I had for
verbal expression, rather than opportunity for concrete demonstration
through action."[13]

Meyer was diminutive in stature, with an olive complexion, dark
eyes and hair, and well-tended goatee. Especially later in life he could
appear quietly charming, kindly, patient, and generous with his time.
To Americans in awe of German medicine, he with his German accent
and fastidious manner represented the superior Old World of learning

and culture—and he certainly used this projection by others to his advantage. But even at a young age Meyer did not suffer fools gladly, and he expressed his rage or disdain coldly rather than heatedly. His occasional lack of tact and his ever-present undertone of arrogance extended to his writings. His intellectual gifts allowed him to seize upon the weakness of any theory or method, but his manner of expressing such insights could sometimes be quite harsh. "You know, Dr. Meyer must restrain himself from belittling other writers so much," August Forel told Anna Meyer in 1892 after reading her son's dissertation on lizard brains.[14]

After a few weeks in New York Meyer found his way to Chicago. He applied for an Illinois medical license and, after paying the fee, got it within two weeks. Desperate for money, he rented a small office near Rush Medical College and attempted to establish a private practice, but was unsuccessful. Part of the reason was no doubt his discomfort with treating living patients. Because his goal was to be in a laboratory where he could study the anatomy and pathology of the nervous system—conducting autopsies, dissecting brains, preparing slides—being forced to practice medicine in order to eat and pay rent was an annoyance, if not an insult. Perhaps another reason his practice was not successful was his office decor; in addition to his books, his consulting room was lined with shelves groaning under the weight of jars of brains. He was oblivious to the impression this might make on his patients.

Finally Meyer had a lucky break. A new pathologist position was opening up at the Illinois Eastern Hospital for the Insane in Kankakee. The institution was noted for its "cottage" structure, a novel architectural feature that was regarded as more humane than the typical gothic Kirkbride-style asylum. The superintendant of Kankakee, Richard Dewey, hired Meyer but was himself fired shortly thereafter due to a change in the political winds. Meyer started his new position on 1 May 1893. For the first time since arriving in America he would have a steady income and be the boss of his own laboratory (though it would be in the basement morgue). Looking back on the two and a half years he spent at Kankakee, Meyer referred to this transformative period as his "novitiate."[15] His devoted disciple, Eunice Winters, would later write, "He came to Kankakee frankly to get brain material; he left it two and a half years later with a professional commitment to the hospitalized patient."[16] A less reverent interpretation might be that Meyer hit upon a way to persuade others that his monomania for recording "facts" was a way for asylum alienists to demonstrate to the rest of the medical profession that they were "doing something" for the patients. But there is no doubt that Meyer's personal obsession eventually changed the perception of the professional status of asylum physicians. The relentless recording of the facts of a patient's life, statements, and behavior was a way to demonstrate that mental institutions "cared" for their patients by not neglecting them. In the twentieth century this would become psychiatry's response to a model of continuous monitoring that had been adopted in general hospitals through the routine graphing of temperature charts, frequent analyses of the urine, and repeated blood counts—very little of which had any direct clinical relevance to the medical diagnosis or treatment of most patients.

To Meyer's credit this was indeed a major contribution. With better record keeping, coupled with in-house training classes on brain anatomy and psychiatric concepts, intellectually and emotionally detached asylum alienists and attendants became more interested in the patients. If the confusing mass of insane patients could now be viewed in a different, more comprehensible light, the daily toil of asylum life took on new meaning for the staff. Their jobs as asylum physicians became a bit more tolerable, and perhaps even seemed important. Certainly this awakened interest in the nature of the insane must have carried with it a secondary gain: in countless minor interactions, the patients must have indeed benefited from the attention. But neither in Kankakee nor in any other institution where Meyer would later preside would any novel form of therapy be introduced that had any decisive impact on mentally ill patients. The awakening of American psychiatry through administrative and clinical reforms instigated by Meyer was a therapeutic antidote for the learned helplessness of alienists and attendants—that is all. The asylum physicians were awakened, not the patients.

It is true that the conditions Meyer found at Kankakee were deplorable—but they were standard for American asylums. Meyer performed autopsies and conducted pathological analyses that were meaningless because the clinical record keeping was so shallow. How could he match the pathological findings with the symptoms of the living patient when there were so few details in the case books? The clinical-anatomical method, as it was called, had proven its fruitfulness in the understanding of disease in nineteenth-century medicine.[17] But this method had been failing miserably to correlate diseased brain cells with the signs and symptoms of mental disease—the main obsession of much of German and French psychiatric research for decades.[18] Meyer's lack of access to data in the case book pages of living insane patients about the signs and symptoms they exhibited while alive prevented him—perhaps serendipitously, given the trajectory of his life—from tunneling down the same blind alley.

But as with the rest of the small community of asylum pathologists in American institutions, Meyer was hired primarily to conduct autopsies and issue an opinion on the cause of death. There was absolutely no connection between the activities of the pathologist and the clinical functions of the assistant physicians or the attendants. Lab work was occasionally done on blood, urine, and sputum, but these reports were merely filed away and not taken into consideration by the alienists. Superintendants of American asylums that had such pathology labs pointed with pride to their statistical tabulations of autopsies and urinalyses: wasn't this science? Didn't these laboratory activities prove that asylum medicine was a forward-thinking branch of modern medicine? The fact that these lab results shed no light on the nature of mental disease did not seem to bother them.

At Kankakee Meyer came up with a way to break down these traditional institutional barriers. This was a remarkable achievement considering that a pathologist occupied a marginal position at the bottom of the asylum hierarchy, below the ranks of assistant physician and, of course, the all-powerful superintendent. There was no precedent for such ambition and competence to be demonstrated by someone serving at such a low rank. There was no reason why this young man's suggestions should have been taken seriously by his superiors. Yet he had won the confidence of the new superintendant, Clarke Gapen. Gapen had seen Meyer's collection of pathological specimens in the pathology laboratory and was impressed; he had never seen such a thing before. He gave Meyer permission to emerge from the basement morgue and see patients in the infirmary before they died, giving Meyer a chance to observe the signs and symptoms of dying patients before he dissected their brains. Taking note of Meyer's new interest in talking to living patients, Gapen offered him the opportunity to be in charge of two wards with a combined census of about one hundred patients. This would mark a rise in rank and institutional power equal to that of assistant physician. Still unsure of himself, Meyer refused. "You know all about my irritability and nervousness," he wrote to his brother on 21 August 1893. "It is better not to fly if the wings are too weak."[19]

Meyer also got permission to construct a document containing a structured interview for an alienist to follow when conducting the initial evaluation. Such interviews were usually conducted when the patient was placed in the bathtub directly after admission, and some alienists spent no more than three to five minutes recording a history from new patients. Meyer's structured interview required between one and two hours to complete—which did not exactly endear him to his colleagues. "He wants to work and may even try to make us work," they grumbled.[20]

What did finally win them over, however, were some informal clinics that Meyer held, demonstrating to the Americans how they should conduct an examination of the patient. Meyer soon began giving classes to the physicians on brain anatomy and basic neurological principles, and then, in early January 1894, lectures on psychiatric topics such as the acute psychoses.[21] Meyer, it should be remembered, had attended only a few lectures on psychiatry from August Forel in 1888. So he had to cobble together his material from the confusing and sometimes contradictory array of opinions he found in the psychiatric literature. Each author seemed to have his own terminology (nomenclature) and classification (nosology) of insanity. Which to choose? "Uncriticalness and dreary confusion in the nomenclature!" he complained in a letter to his old professor Forel the week before his first psychiatry lectures commenced.[22] Despite this challenge Meyer seemed to have found his niche: the classes were a success. The alienists seemed to relish learning neurological and psychiatric material from this young "German" doctor with a professorial bearing. They had a newfound respect for themselves, and a growing respect for him. And Meyer loved it.

Meyer's mother had fallen ill with melancholia six months before he began working in an insane asylum. The tragic irony of his fate was not lost on him. But it also humanized the emotionally detached young man. Aware of his family's hereditary taint and the devastating psychological effect his unpaid debt and emigration had on his mother, as he voraciously read the psychiatric literature he also began to speculate on the interplay of such factors in the insane patients he had initially avoided. "I was also personally sensitized concerning the blending and differentiation of possible hereditary and constitutional factors with definitely psychogenic, i.e., life-experienced, and somatic ones, on account of an attack of depression in my mother shortly after my emigration to the United States," he reflected much later in life, "and so I was bound to cultivate a very concrete and intimate concern for the genetic-dynamic developments in the individual patient and life-situations."[23]

In the spring of 1894 Gapen had returned from Philadelphia, where he had heard Silas Weir Mitchell's thunderous polemic against the alienists. It made an impact on him, and it made him grateful that his own institution had a "German" doctor of the caliber of Meyer. He provided Meyer with a copy of Weir Mitchell's address to the American Medico-Psychological Association. Meyer viewed this as an opening wedge that would not only bring about reforms at Kankakee, but could also elevate his own personal status. Meyer, it seemed, always had his gaze turned upward, toward the next level of power, no matter what position he was currently in. He decided to write a long report to Governor Altgeld of Illinois on current conditions at Kankakee and a description of his own views of how to integrate pathological and clinical activities in a manner resembling the model used in Germany. He also elaborated his own reform efforts: the tutorials for the staff, changes in history taking and record keeping, the clinical demonstrations. In August, with his superintendent's blessing, he sent this report to the governor along with a copy of Weir Mitchell's address. With these missives, which were shrewdly self-promoting, Meyer got the attention of the governor and his staff. From this point on Meyer would be well-known at the highest administrative levels in the state and be viewed as a welcome anomaly, a rare reformer from within who brought with him all the wisdom and learning of German medicine as well as someone who had a keen grasp—and he certainly did—of administrative and managerial issues. He demonstrated remarkable initiative for an asylum physician. This reputation would eventually be recognized by others in the medical profession outside of Illinois. And it directly led to his next job: pathologist at the Worcester Lunatic Hospital in Massachusetts.

Hosea M. Quinby, the superintendent at Worcester, was in search of a new pathologist for his institution. Meyer's neurological publications had caught his attention, as well as reports of his reform efforts at Kankakee. Quinby asked the superintendent of the McLean Hospital, Edward Cowles, to interview Meyer on his behalf at the annual meeting of the American Medico-Psychological Association, which was held in Denver in 1895. At the time Cowles was arguably the most respected man in American psychiatry. His reforms at McLean had made it the premier small asylum in the United States, and in 1895 he was president of the AMPA. Cowles interviewed Meyer and passed on a favorable recommendation to Quinby. Meyer then initiated an exchange of letters with Quinby and convinced him that his role should be more than that of a mere pathologist. Quinby agreed, a decision that changed the course of institutional psychiatry in America.

When Meyer assumed his new position at the asylum in Worcester in November 1895 he was given free rein to make changes in its administrative and procedural structure. He abolished the case books in favor of flexible files that would contain the individual records of a single patient. As at Kankakee he instituted a series of clinical demonstrations and daily clinical case conferences at which patients would be discussed. For the next three years he stressed in his annual reports that instituting the new procedures for the detailed record keeping of facts was the main focus of his efforts, even putting it above laboratory research or innovations in treatment. The resulting level of clerical intensity had never been seen before in American asylums, although similar reforms in record keeping on a smaller scale had already been instituted by J. M. Mosher, the first assistant physician at the St. Lawrence State Hospital in Ogdensburg, New York.[24]

Meyer found the same deplorable asylum conditions at Worcester that he had encountered at Kankakee. He doubled the staff of four alienists by adding four junior physicians, including one female—a rarity in the medical profession as a whole, but more common among alienists. He insisted that they be men and women of education and promise. Unlike the vast majority of American alienists, he insisted that they either already have a good reading knowledge of German and French or develop it in their (few) spare hours, when not engaged in both clinical and laboratory work at Worcester. This eventually opened the world of European psychiatry to the Americans, and many who would go on to form the elite class of American psychiatry in the early twentieth century were able to do so in part because they could read German and French psychiatric texts; some even became proficient enough to translate them into English. Many of the men who served under Meyer in Worcester went on to become superintendents of their own insane hospitals and make major contributions to American psychiatry in the decades that followed.

Despite his extensive reading in the subject, Meyer knew nothing about psychiatry, and he knew that he knew nothing. As a trained neurologist and neuropathologist he knew how to observe patients for signs of neurological impairment, take careful histories, and perform autopsies and examine specimens under a microscope. At Kankakee he had taken these skills and tried to integrate them into the asylum practice of the alienists. This gave his bosses and his minimally educated American alienist colleagues the impression that he knew more about psychiatry than he did. But the nature of mental disease? This was a problem. He needed to educate himself. After spending his first winter at Worcester, the twenty-nine-year-old bachelor was granted leave to make a tour of European psychiatric facilities and gather ideas for improvements that he could make at Worcester. This would actually be Meyer's crash course in psychiatry. It was during this fateful journey in the spring and summer of 1896 that he believed—for a time—that he had hit upon a possible solution of a problem that continued to bedevil American alienists: the classification and nomenclature of insanity.

Imagine the first impressions and sensations of a new assistant physician on the wards in an American asylum. How could one possibly see order in madness? The insanities were fluid, mercurial, occult. The observable signs and symptoms of diseases such as pneumonia, tuberculosis, and asthma were easily identified. But not insanity. There was nothing in American asylum medicine that even remotely approached the disease specificity found in the other branches of medicine. Read the text of one authority on insanity and the spectacle on the wards might crystallize into one form. Read another, and the signs and symptoms of the insanities would separate into entirely different clusters. Relying on the publications of the experts was like peering into a kaleidoscope: aim the instrument at the patients, and they would differentiate into one pattern; turn the barrel of the scope, and suddenly the groupings would change. Did the patients suffer from one general disease of "insanity," or were there specific diseases? Physicians were trained to use their five senses to diagnose and treat illness, but alienists needed a sixth sense. Where would it come from?

To accommodate this cognitive blind spot, alienists could magically squeeze an asylum of more than two thousand patients into half a dozen boxes, each defined by a single primary symptom.[25] William Alanson White vividly described the situation when he began his career as an asylum alienist in 1892:

The simplistic state of psychiatry as practiced in the state hospitals is perhaps best illustrated by our system of classification. Patients were either acute, chronic or subacute mania or melancholia—so much for the excitements and depressions. They had paresis or senile dementia, or they were deteriorated as the result of chronic mental disease, in which case they were classified as terminal dementias, or as primary dementia if the mental disease was of short duration. In addition to these there was the defective group, of which there was, as a rule, quite a contingent in the state hospitals. Finally there was an occasional para-noiac, though paranoia was a diagnosis that had only recently been elaborated. Of course we systematically labeled each patient according to the diagnosis that we thought best fitted him, but I am quite sure nobody felt that he had accomplished much in so doing. The fact that whenever a physician from another institution visited the hospital one of the first questions was, "What classification do you use?" indicates to my mind the very serious discontent with this state of affairs.[26]

What books would a typical American alienist consult in 1896, if he or she were so inclined? The most commonly available works from Europe were those by British alienists such as Thomas Clouston (1840–1915), Henry Maudsley (1835–1918), and the encyclopedic two-volume reference work edited by Daniel Hack Tuke (1827–1895). The most common American textbooks in general usage were written by two New York neurologists, Edward C. Spitzka (1852–1914) on insanity and Charles L. Dana (1852–1935) on nervous diseases. A neurology text by the British neurologist W. R. Gowers (1845–1915) was also widely used.[27] In both theory and practice, most American alienists held to an idea that originated in Europe in the 1830s, that there was only *one* form of insanity, a "unitary psychosis," and that melancholia, mania, and dementia might constitute the three symptomatic stages of its course.[28] Insanity was a continuum or dimension, not a set of dis-crete disease categories. This was another reason why American asy-lum physicians disregarded the importance of distinguishing forms of insanity: insanity itself was the only sure diagnosis. Translations from French or German alienists, though available, were still few. American asylum medicine was an intellectual wasteland when Meyer set off for Europe.

Meyer's first stop was Turin, Italy, to see the legendary proponent of degeneration theory, Cesare Lombroso (1835–1909), and to tour Italian asylums. Next he visited his mother in Zurich and found, to his relief, that after three years of suffering she had finally recovered from her serious bout of melancholia. The capstone of his fact-finding mission was a six-week sojourn in the small university psychiatric clinic in Heidelberg, where the energetic Emil Kraepelin was chief. Kraepelin's clinic was already developing a reputation for being the epicenter of new ideas in psychiatric research. During Meyer's stay there the fifth edition of Kraepelin's textbook, *Psychiatrie,* appeared in print. It was a historic departure from the previous editions and a major turning point in the history of psychiatry—and despite his lack of psychiatric training, Meyer was intellectually gifted enough to realize it. He eagerly absorbed the book while in Heidelberg. He also had the enviable opportunity to engage Kraepelin in discussions about his new methods and ideas and to watch Kraepelin's staff put them into practice.

When Meyer returned to Worcester with a freshly printed copy of Kraepelin's book he immediately began to train his medical staff to use the new classification scheme and new diagnostic terms. He also instituted administrative reforms based on what he had observed in the university psychiatric clinic in Heidelberg, mimicking them as he introduced what he would later call his "Worcester plan." The Worcester Lunatic Hospital would be the first in America to use Kraepelinian concepts of insanity. "I am strickly Kraepelinianer just now," he wrote to his friend, fellow psychiatrist, and Swiss émigré August Hoch (1868–1919) on 15 October 1896. "I make my men swear by Kraepelin although I should like sometimes to do the swearing myself. The schematism hurts me considerably. I envy you for having had K. from the start. I must wean myself from my own elaborations before I can be as certain about things as a true pupil of a man should be. . . . It is really hard for me to follow laws."[29]

Somewhere among the thousand or more insane patients in the Worcester Lunatic Hospital was the first American ever diagnosed with dementia praecox. Over the next half-century hundreds of thousands more would also succumb to this affliction. And the fates of Adolf Meyer and dementia praecox in America would be intertwined for decades thereafter.

3

EMIL KRAEPELIN

In March 1891 thirty-five-year-old Emil Kraepelin found himself be-tween two lives.[1] After five years as an expatriate professor he was leav-ing Dorpat University in Estonia, huddled with his wife, daughter, and son in a railroad car that slowly carried them from Riga, Latvia, toward their bright new future in Heidelberg. Kraepelin had been awarded a professorship at the prestigious university in the verdant Neckar Valley and would be in charge of its small psychiatric clinic. He was now re-turning to his beloved Fatherland—he was an intensely patriotic North German—and would be able to combine teaching with his most pas-sionate desires: experimental psychological research and the study of the forms of insanity. The work he would do in Heidelberg would make him world famous and brand his influence on psychiatry to this day. As the historian Edward Shorter remarked, "It is Kraepelin, not Freud, who is the central figure in the history of psychiatry."[2]

But that would be a gift of the future, and Kraepelin's personal future may not have been on his mind. During that agonizingly slow railroad journey, which should have been a triumphal celebration, Kraepelin's attention was clouded by worry.

His infant son, who had been born the previous 9 November—the same day Kraepelin received word of his appointment to Heidelberg—was gravely ill. He may have caught an infection from his four-year-old sister, who had been suffering from a "purulent inflammation of the ear." In an era when antibiotics did not exist and death in childhood was commonplace, all infectious diseases were regarded with the utmost gravity. The illnesses of both of their children at the dawn of such a promising new life in Germany filled the Kraepelins with dread; their first child, a girl born in 1885, and a later additional daughter, born in 1888, both died before the age of two. As the train approached Heidelberg their son's condition was worsening, indeed had become "almost hopeless."

Within days after arriving in Heidelberg tragedy struck. "Despite all efforts, we were not able to keep the child alive and he died from a fast developing septicaemia, which I also caught," Kraepelin recalled in his memoirs.[3] He would never have another son. Pushing through the iron fog of grief, he plunged himself into a familiar refuge: his scientific work.

In a fascinating "self-assessment" that he composed at some point after World War I, Kraepelin repeatedly stressed that his life was devoted to the free expression of his "will," and that his personal relationships, even with his family, were often of secondary importance. "One of my basic traits is strong egotism," he confessed to himself. "To deny this would be senseless."

> I am filled with a natural and powerful drive to assert myself in life and in the world, and to bring my influence to bear. The main point of this for me is not, however, good living, or the pursuit of pleasure, honor and esteem, or even monetary gain; it is the freedom to act without any hinderances. My entire being is compelled to take up creative work and it is essential for me to eliminate radically all obstacles in the path of this wish. Even thoughts of my wife and children can only temporarily prevent me from obeying this almighty urge, to which I am wholly subservient. . . . It was inevitable that my emotional relationships with others would end up somewhat curtailed by my all-surmounting urge to achieve my objectives. Even if my affection for those closest to me remains unchanging and unshakable and has rendered me a dependable person for others, the real pole of my life has always been my work.[4]

Emil Kraepelin was the progeny of an unusual and inconstant father. Karl Kraepelin was an actor, opera singer, and music teacher who abandoned his family when Emil was in his late teens or early twenties.

Money was often in short supply, and his father occasionally spent what little was left on alcohol. His father died in 1882 after having achieved a certain level of fame as a storyteller on the stages of northern and eastern Germany. By that time he had become a stranger to his family. Both Emil and his older brother, also named Karl, seemed to have developed personalities that were the antithesis of their father's. Having endured the instability caused whenever their father followed the Siren's call of his own artistic "will," both boys found solace and order in the wonders of science and nature. The younger Karl Kraepelin became an accomplished botanist as an adult and eventually became the director of the Museum of Natural History in Hamburg. Emil and his brother remained close throughout their lives and traveled the world together, delighting in botanical and zoological expeditions and long hikes through foreign terrains.[5]

Although not an imaginative person (by his own admission), Kraepelin had been a vivid dreamer since childhood. When he was a teenager he recorded his dreams and tried to determine their origins. He developed a fascination with psychology and began to read the texts of philosophers on this subject, including one by Wilhelm Wundt (1832–1920), a man who would later be regarded as the father of experimental psychology. He was encouraged in these pursuits by a friend of his father's, a Dr. Louis Krueger, who proved to be the decisive influence on Kraepelin's youthful decision to study medicine and become a psychiatrist. Indeed he had already made up his mind to become a psychiatrist before he entered the University of Leipzig at the age of eighteen in 1874. He wrote that he was following his older mentor's advice: "I decided to become a psychiatrist, as it seemed that this was the only possibility to combine psychological work with an earning profession."[6]

After his initial medical instruction Kraepelin went to the university in Würzburg and became interested in the comparative anatomy of the brain. He also began to read widely in philosophy as preparation for the day when he would become a professor, his newest career goal and one he was determined to reach by age thirty. It was during this time that he read Wundt's latest book on physiological psychology and learned that Wundt would be leaving his post in Zurich and assuming a position as a professor of philosophy in Leipzig. Kraepelin had made up his mind that one day he would be working alongside Wundt as an experimental psychologist, a goal that he achieved five years later. He met Wundt for the first time during the Easter holidays of 1877 and was able to sit in on several sessions of an advanced tutorial class. The topic of one meeting was hallucinations. Kraepelin found himself in awe of Wundt, and later, during those early years of training in his twenties, he would follow Wundt's sage personal advice in the same way that he had relied on Krueger's for guidance while a teenager. When one reads Kraepelin's *Memoirs,* which records his life up to the year 1919, one is consistently struck by the repeated regrets he expressed at various stages that his psychiatric career interfered with his passion for conducting psychology experiments. One is left with the impression that Kraepelin would have been far happier, and lived a much more fulfilled scientific life, if he had become an experimental psychologist rather than a psychiatrist.

But as would happen at several junctures in his life, fate pulled him away from the psychology laboratory. While completing the requirements for his medical degree Kraepelin was offered a job as a medical assistant in a psychiatric clinic in Würzburg. Needing the money and eager to start his medical career, he accepted the position and started in July 1877. Now, finally, after having made the decision at the age of eighteen to become a psychiatrist, Kraepelin was going to have his first experience with the insane. "Apart from my psychiatric knowledge, I was completely unprepared for the task awaiting me." His first reaction was revulsion: "At the beginning, work on the ward upset me very much. I was particularly terrified of an imbecile patient, who had fierce, hysterical fits and rolled across the whole room each time I made my rounds; similarly, another uncanny case . . . an example of the strange new illness hebephrenia, displayed extremely uncontrollable agitation. The intensity of unusual, disturbing impressions and the first feeling of personal responsibility pursued me into my sleep and caused irritating dreams."[7]

Kraepelin went to his chief, a physician named Rinecker. Even though he had been there only two weeks, Kraepelin was certain he could not stand working with the insane for very much longer. Rinecker smiled and told him that his reaction was normal and that the other assistant physicians had experienced similar problems. He urged Kraepelin to stick it out, that he'd get used to it. Eventually Kraepelin did.

At one point later that year Kraepelin suffered from a spell of extreme insomnia. He conducted his clinical duties during the day and studied hard for the approaching state medical examination late at night. Tempted, as so many physicians were in those days, to sample the drugs given to the patients, Kraepelin gave himself an injection of morphine. But instead of putting him to sleep he immediately developed nausea and began vomiting. The following day he suffered from his first migraine headache. For the next twenty years he would experience a migraine headache at least one day of every week. They finally stopped when he, like August Forel, stopped drinking alcohol and became a crusader against its degenerating effects.

The fifty to sixty patients that were, on average, in the clinic were heavily drugged with sedatives, particularly chloral hydrate. In the year that Kraepelin worked at the Würzburg clinic he would spend much of his time tending to more familiar medical problems, including many cases of typhoid. He did find time for a few scientific pursuits, such as measuring the skulls of the insane and comparing them to the size of normal skulls (they were either larger or smaller than those of normal people, he concluded), and he carefully graphed the daily fluctuations in the pulse of the insane. A prominent theory at the time was that the patterns in the pulse would reveal how incurable a person's insanity might be; in other words, it was an attempt to find a biological marker for prognosis.

Kraepelin passed his state medical examinations and was ready to advance his career. In 1878 he became an assistant physician in a Munich mental asylum that was under the direction of Bernhard von Gudden, a man fascinated with neuropathological studies of insanity who is remembered more for his death than his life: he was the personal physician of mad King Ludwig II of Bavaria, with whom he was found drowned in a lake under mysterious circumstances. Kraepelin arrived by train in Munich suffering from a major migraine headache. At Gudden's asylum he was put in charge of 150 insane patients. Because the asylum was in Bavaria, beer was freely administered to the patients at the rate of about 300 liters per day.

But once again Kraepelin was tortured by nightmares: "As they had done in Würzburg, the chaotic and repulsive pictures of the day's work also followed me into the night and left me in doubt whether I could really get used to this occupation."[8] A move to Leipzig, away from asylum work, was now his goal. He remained in Munich until February 1882. He also became engaged to his future wife. Kraepelin saw the move to Leipzig as a step closer to an academic career. He had been publishing scientific papers over the past several years but felt he needed a new direction. And of course he especially wanted to work in Wundt's famous psychology laboratory, which had opened in 1879. He had written to Wundt from Munich proposing that he do his *Habilitation* (a second doctoral thesis of a more advanced nature than the first, a necessary step to becoming a professor) on reaction-time lengths of normal subjects under the influence of chloral hydrate, bromide, amyl nitrate, and hashish. Wundt saw the value of the proposal and encouraged Kraepelin to join him.[9] This move to Leipzig was one of the riskiest ever taken by Kraepelin: "As I left the clinic, I felt as though I had been rescued, although I suddenly found myself in a particularly difficult situation. I was without money and a job, without patients and without the possibility of a further medical training."[10]

At Leipzig he finally became a university lecturer, but he wasn't earning enough money to pay the bills. He reluctantly found a position as an assistant physician when a new psychiatric clinic opened in February 1882, but was fired after only four months due to what Kraepelin believed were unjustifiable allegations of incompetence. As it turned out he was fired by one of the most respected neuroanatomists and psychiatrists of that era, Paul Flechsig (1847–1929), who also happened to be the director of the clinic.

Being fired from a job he really didn't want in the first place had its advantages. In his spare time he indulged the dream of his youth: he was allowed to work under Wundt in his lab, though in an unpaid position. "Wundt's laboratory became my refuge," he would later remark. Wundt's laboratory was still in a primitive state when Kraepelin was there. It consisted of two adjoining rooms; work benches were created by wooden planks that had been laid across old tables. But Wundt had a rich assortment of instruments that more than made up for the humble surroundings, and everyone who worked under him was imbued with the spirit of pioneers. Kraepelin wrote enthusiastically, "In spite of the Spartan simplicity of the furnishings, an industrious scientific life and a great enthusiasm for the completely new field of research reigned in these rooms."[11] In Wundt's lab Kraepelin followed through with his plans to study the effect of drugs, alcohol, and other substances on mental performance; analyzed the patterns in thousands of word associations; and was engaged in preliminary experiments on the human perception of light. From Wundt he also learned to embrace the position on the mind-body problem known as "psychophysical parallelism"— that psychological events correspond with physical events, but in a parallel (not interactive) fashion. This philosophical position protected Kraepelin from making premature material reductions of psychological events to neurophysiological events, but the language and assumptions of interactionism could not but help to seep into his later work in clinical psychiatry.

At this point in his life Kraepelin wanted more than anything to remain with Wundt in Leipzig and, quite possibly, follow in his footsteps. He desired an academic career, and he vowed never to work in an asylum again. He did not want the nightmares to return.

But he was still too poor to get married, and once again fate pulled him away from experimental psychology and back toward psychiatry. Through a friend he was told that a Leipzig publisher, Johann Ambrosias Abel, was offering to pay Kraepelin to write a psychiatry textbook, a compendium. In an era when academic careers were made by the writing of textbooks and not journal articles, Kraepelin agreed to do it. Of course he sought Wundt's advice first, and the old master assured him it would be a wise choice. A poverty-stricken twenty-seven-year-old, Kraepelin had finished most of the manuscript by Easter 1883. It would become the first edition of the famous series of *Psychiatrie* textbooks that would one day transform the entire profession.

Kraepelin resented the time that writing the textbook took away from his being in Wundt's laboratory. But it was his revered mentor who delivered the heartbreaking news to Kraepelin that he should probably return to psychiatric work:

> One day in the summer of 1883 [Wundt] noticed the ring on my finger and asked me if I was engaged. I gave him a positive reply and he felt obliged to mention the problems hindering my plan. He pointed out that his field of philosophy would probably not achieve general recognition in the near future, that I would not be able to reckon with becoming professor as fast as I had hoped, and that I would probably have to postpone my marriage indefinitely.[12]

As usual with the series of fatherly mentors Kraepelin had in his life, he followed Wundt's advice and returned to psychiatry. Only a career in medicine would provide him with enough income to get married, and professorships in psychiatry were more plentiful than those in philosophy. (Experimental psychology was viewed as a branch of philosophy in those early days.) Reluctantly, with an additional promise of a lectureship at the local university, in the fall of 1883 Kraepelin returned to Gudden's asylum in Munich. There he was able to conduct microscopic studies of nerve cells using new staining techniques that were just coming into use.

Kraepelin began to notice that he had trouble seeing out of his left eye. He had noticed the trouble in Wundt's lab in Leipzig, but now the problem was more pronounced. Soon his right eye would also give him trouble. He decided he would be unfit for psychiatric research, which in Germany in the 1880s was concerned with correlating brain cells with the signs and symptoms of insanity, and hence highly dependent upon the use of the microscope. Unable to effectively use the basic tool of psychiatric research, he felt his plan to become a professor drifting further from his reach. In July 1884 he took a position in an asylum in Lebus, a small town in Silesia. His new goal was to one day be the director of his own asylum and to continue his scientific work on the side. There was only one drawback: despite the beautiful natural surroundings, which pleased Kraepelin, the institution was far away from urban centers of science and learning.

But the job in Lebus accomplished one thing: it allowed him to finally marry. On 4 October 1884, in northern Germany, Kraepelin married his fiancée, Ina Schwabe, and brought her back to Silesia with him. For a time she acted as his assistant in experiments he conducted on the measurement of mental reactions. It was also during this period that he first tried to organize the confusing clinical presentations of his patients into categories, but this effort led him nowhere. In May 1885 Kraepelin moved to another position, in a municipal asylum in the great city of Dresden, increasing his income (somewhat) and returning to a major center of intellectual activity. He was able to continue his experimental researches in his new position, including pioneering work in "pharmacopsychology" (a term he coined).[13] But Dresden would be forever linked to misfortune. On 4 November the Kraepelins' first child, a girl, died four hours after birth due to asphyxiation by the umbilical cord. While still grieving, the Kraepelins nonetheless accepted an offer to spend Christmas with the Wundts in Leipzig.

At the age of thirty, still without the prospect of a professorship, Kraepelin toughed out the routine of the city asylum in Dresden and tried to find a way out of the dead end he found himself in. He needed the stability of the Dresden job because he was now a married man who wanted to start a family. He was once again on the verge of giving up hope of realizing his old dream of being a professor when a letter arrived in April 1886 telling him that just such a position was opening up at the University of Dorpat, a German-language university in the Russian Empire (the Estonian name of the town was Tartu). A formal offer of employment soon followed. After discussing it with his wife, he accepted. They knew it was not an ideal situation: they would be expatriates in a community of German professors among a population of Estonians, Russians, Latvians, some Germans, and a few other ethnic groups; the winters were harsh; it would be a difficult life. But the Kraepelins were still young, and it was a fresh start that could help erase the memory of the death of their first child.

The university clinic that Kraepelin now directed in a foreign country was physically and financially in distress. Tens of thousands of rubles needed to be paid to creditors. The wooden buildings were a fire hazard, and Kraepelin had fire extinguishers installed in all the rooms. He and his assistant physicians also personally installed the wiring for an electric fire alarm system. He formed a fire brigade out of the staff of physicians and nurses and had them make numerous practice drills. Although his staff was composed of Germans, the attendants spoke only Estonian or Russian, although some understood a little German; Kraepelin learned as much Russian and Estonian as he could in his spare time. As was the case in other asylums, the patients were often stricken with serious infectious diseases that needed attending.

But despite all this, Kraepelin made sure to carve out a significant amount of time for his own scientific work. He continued to conduct psychological experiments on the mental effects of factors such as fatigue, drugs (amyl nitrate, chloral hydrate, chloroform, ethyl ether, morphine, paraldehyde), and substances such as alcohol, coffee, and tea. The time measurement studies he conducted during these years demonstrating the effect of drugs on attention, memory, and language were "far ahead of his time."[14] The psychological and pharmacological experiments on mental performance were not just an effort to establish statistical norms among the mentally healthy; Kraepelin hoped they would

one day lead to objective methods to identify the various forms of insanity, and hence be used diagnostically. The study of drugs was an attempt
to produce a "model psychosis" in healthy volunteers that mimicked insanity. He had first conducted these studies in Dresden; now he brought
them to fruition in Dorpat.

He also found time to write the second (1887) and third (1889)
editions of his textbook, *Psychiatrie*. With each successive edition his increased insight into the forms of insanity became clearer. It was in Dorpat, far from the centers of medicine in Europe, that Kraepelin became
interested in the clinical conditions of catatonia and hebephrenia—two
major components of his later concept of dementia praecox—and began
to speculate on the importance of studying, over time, the course of
forms of insanity that seemed to end in terminal dementia.

Curiously it was also during his tenure in Dorpat that Kraepelin's
interest in hypnosis as a psychotherapeutic tool began to emerge, and he
became quite proficient with it. He had tinkered with hypnosis years
before, using descriptions in a book, revealing in his memoirs, "I had
already hypnotized chickens, lizards and lobsters in Hamburg in 1880."[15]
Hypnosis did not hold his attention for very long, however.

The years in Dorpat would turn out to have been a critical period
of gestation for Kraepelin. He was already thinking along lines that
would distinguish him during the next phase of his life, and he hungered for the opportunity to begin it. In March 1891 he and his family
boarded that fateful train in Riga and headed for Heidelberg.

Until he left for Munich in 1903, the place where he would live out his
life and career, the university clinic at Heidelberg would be the nexus of
an unusually productive and creative period in Kraepelin's life.[16] His experimental work in psychology and the next three editions of his textbook, each markedly revised as he achieved new insights into the nature
of the insanities, would never be matched in originality and impact by
his later work. Indeed the period from 1891 to 1899 in particular would
produce most of the major ideas that brought Kraepelin's influence to
bear on twentieth- and twenty-first-century psychiatry.

What were these ideas? And how did Kraepelin arrive at them?

The story begins much earlier, with two German psychiatrists
whose ideas Kraepelin initially rejected or misunderstood, but which

he eventually studied and admired during his Dorpat years: Karl Kahlbaum (1828–1899), who "remains as one of the great figures of nineteenth-century psychiatry,"[17] and his friend and assistant, Ewald Hecker (1843–1909). Indeed the ideas of these two men, particularly those of Kahlbaum, were essential for Kraepelin and for the later development of his concepts of dementia praecox and manic-depressive insanity.

Karl Kahlbaum was a psychiatrist who, like Kraepelin, also had dreams of becoming a university professor. To accomplish this goal he too needed to complete a *Habilitation*, a second major work of scholarship that needed to surpass his earlier work. What he produced would eventually revolutionize psychiatry once Kraepelin applied Kahlbaum's concepts in Heidelberg.

Kahlbaum's resulting book, *Die Gruppirung der psychischen Krankheiten und die Eintheilung der Seelenstörungen (The Classification of Mental Diseases and the Division of Psychic Disturbances)* was published in 1863 but was essentially ignored by the psychiatric establishment.[18] The reasons for this were easy to see: Kahlbaum had no academic standing (he was not a professor), and his ideas directly contradicted the reigning paradigm in Germany at that time: the "unitary psychosis" concept that held there was only one basic form of madness and all of the observed differences were merely stages along a continuum of this single insanity.

In direct opposition to the unitary psychosis idea, Kahlbaum proposed his own classification system (nosology) of discrete mental diseases. Because it was unnecessarily complex and the terms were unusual in construction, his classification system did not influence very many clinicians. But what did influence future generations, including Kraepelin, was the introduction of the "clinical method" from other branches of medicine to the study of mental diseases. Until that time psychiatrists who wrote textbooks on psychiatry based their collection of madnesses on cross-sectional observations of patients. In other words, they did not follow the transformation of signs and symptoms in the insane even though this was being done in other areas of medicine.

What Kahlbaum did—and this was truly remarkable—was introduce the element of *time* into psychiatry.[19] His revolutionary notion was that the only correct definitions of actual mental diseases would have to take into account their natural history of development. Cross-sectional descriptions of patients that were limited to a single time and

place could no longer be regarded as valid. Didn't the symptoms and
behaviors of insane patients change over time? Of course they did. For
Kahlbaum the most important elements were the period of life during
which the symptoms first appeared (the age of onset) and the typical
ways the signs and symptoms changed over time. Only this way of
identifying a mental disease would lead to a system of accurate diagnosis and give some hints as to the course and a probable outcome—a
prognosis—of each condition.

This linkage of diagnosis to course and outcome would become
the centerpiece of Kraepelin's later system of classifying mental
disorders.

By 1866 Kahlbaum had still not found an academic position. While
not giving up on his dream he took a position at a private asylum in Görlitz, Prussia. The following year he became its director. Hecker followed
him there to work as his assistant physician. Both had previously worked
as assistant physicians at an asylum in Allenberg. Kahlbaum would eventually own the Görlitz asylum, and Hecker would leave to set up his
own private asylum in Wiesbaden.

At this private asylum in Görlitz, far from academia and its psychiatric establishment, Kahlbaum and Hecker continued to study the
forms of insanity and produced a body of published work that, to this
day, remain classics in the history of psychiatry. With their longitudinal clinical method of psychopathology as their guiding principle, they
continued to argue that factors such as age of onset and the length of an
illness needed to be combined with careful clinical observation of signs
and symptoms. Over time, they argued, typical patterns of separate
insanities would naturally emerge from such research. And it would be
Kraepelin who would prove them right.

Throughout their years of collaboration Kahlbaum and Hecker
identified a dizzying variety of proposed insanities in this fashion. The
names they invented for many of them (but not necessarily their original descriptions) are still in use in the twenty-first century: dysthymia,
cyclothymia, catatonia, and hebephrenia. Because the latter two
formed core components of Kraepelin's later concept of dementia praecox, they require some comment.

Catatonia was a syndrome characterized by abnormal movements.
Persons manifesting catatonia could be underactive or overactive. Incessant pacing or other motor excitements, bizarre posturing, stereo-

typed movements, confusion, and even stupor could be forms of this insanity as it progressed over time. Kahlbaum had used the term *Katatonia* in lectures as early as 1868. However, the mental disease became more widely known after Kahlbaum published a monograph on the subject in 1874.[20] Kraepelin studied this work of Kahlbaum's while he was in Dorpat.

Hebephrenia (named after the Greek goddess of youth, Hebe) was a term Kahlbaum proposed in his 1863 book for a mental disease that began after puberty, but he gave few details of its signs and symptoms. In 1871 Hecker published an extensive article on hebephrenia based on a large number of cases collected by Kahlbaum as well as fourteen of his own. He vividly described seven case histories in his paper, of five males and two females, which, in accordance with Kahlbaum's method, illustrated the disease at its various stages. He also chose these cases because he had letters that the patients had written, and he quoted from them to illustrate the peculiar disorganized and tangential nature of hebephrenic speech and writing. According to Hecker:

> Hebephrenia is a disease that always erupts subsequent to the development of puberty. In all cases known to me, where the beginning of the disease is exactly dated, it manifests itself between the ages of 18 and 22. . . . This psychological process, which goes along with a range of specially marked symptoms, is rendered pathologically permanent by hebephrenia; as a result the features, which can be temporarily observed in the period of transition, press forward to an exaggerated degree leading to a distinct end stage that we call hebephrenic dementia.

Hecker argued that the natural awkwardness and emotional difficulties of boys and girls during the teenage years following puberty are "frozen" after about age eighteen. A process thereby begins that involves melancholy moods, followed by a "bizarre drive for activity," which can escalate into immature rages. Next it "usually manifests itself in senseless and aimless silly actions" and in a tendency to wander about. Bizarre ideas occur, but are fluid and not like the fixed ideas or delusions seen in other conditions. Individuals engage in "silly precocious prattle" and speak in an illogical, mixed up, and sometimes obscene manner. Thoughts and behavior become more disorganized as the final stage of dementia sets in. This terminal stage is characterized by confusion and occasional agitation, and "periodic hallucinations (namely auditory)" may occur. Hecker argued that hebephrenia was a disease that was characterized by a *rapid* progress to dementia (problems in focusing the will, attention, memory, thinking, language, and so on) that would remain permanent.[21]

Hecker insisted, "I am convinced that every psychiatrist has often encountered cases of hebephrenia and that in every asylum a considerable number of patients exist among the so-called demented," and he urged his readers to follow the method suggested by Kahlbaum and compare the "peculiarity of the end stage" with the "history in the medical records" to make the diagnosis. Because so many asylum patients suffering from paresis (later, in the twentieth century, found to be the third or end stage of syphilis) also terminated in a state of dementia, Hecker suggested that his readers follow his suggestions for distinguishing between the two conditions.[22]

The clinical method of psychopathology suggested by Kahlbaum and demonstrated in Hecker's article eventually changed the way case histories were written. The age of onset, changes in signs and symptoms over time, and the final outcome would all become features of a standard narrative used by psychiatrists that would emerge in the 1900s. But there was one problem with the nature of the evidence presented by Kahlbaum and Hecker: it was all based solely on the presentation of case history examples. Their approach was qualitative analysis, not quantitative analysis. And that's where Kraepelin made his mark.

In Heidelberg Kraepelin and his team created a "diagnosis box" in which the original diagnosis of a new patient was placed. Then, upon discharge, the final diagnosis was listed on the card and "the final interpretation of the disease was added to the original diagnosis." Realizing that even after discharge the clinical picture of the patient might still be undergoing transformation, Kraepelin made annual visits to former patients who had been transferred from his small clinic to the large state insane asylums. This system eventually became the basis of his collection of hundreds of cards on his patients (the famous *Zählkarten*), which were continually shuffled and reshuffled into groups that Kraepelin eventually identified as distinct disease forms. "The results could be seen after a couple of years. . . . I soon realized that the abnormalities at the beginning of the disease had no decisive importance compared to the course of the illness leading to the particular final state of the disease."[23] But the crucial distinction here from Kahlbaum and Hecker—and Kraepelin's major contribution—was that he had detailed, quantifiable data collected longitudinally over a period of years. No one had ever approached the identification and classification of the insanities using a structured scientific method.

This was the key to the wide acceptance of Kraepelin's classification system by psychiatrists, particularly after 1899. His proposed groupings of the insanities and their definition by typical age of onset, course, and outcome were based on *Wissenschaft,* systematic science. How could any other author compete with the (presumed) solidity of Kraepelin's methods? In an era when psychiatry strove to reestablish itself in medicine that was becoming scientific, the fact that Kraepelin's conclusions were derived from years of combining quantitative and qualitative data would eventually place the profession back in contention.

"I kept Kahlbaum and Hecker's ideas in mind and tried to collect those cases which inclined toward dementia as 'mental degeneration processes,'" Kraepelin wrote. These preliminary findings formed the basis of the classification system and terminology (nomenclature) that Kraepelin proposed for the insanities in the fourth edition of his textbook, which he had finished by September 1893. In it, for the first time, was a new disease, dementia praecox, which, Kraepelin said, "essentially corresponded with hebephrenia."[24]

In 1893 dementia praecox corresponded to only the milder forms of the illness, however, such as those described by Hecker. The severe forms had been described in a monograph in 1892 by Leon Daraszkiewicz (1866—?), a former assistant physician who had worked under Kraepelin in Dorpat.

Kraepelin was not the first to use the Latin term "dementia praecox." This distinction belongs to the German physician Heinrich Schüle (1840–1916), of the Illenau asylum in Baden. In the 1886 third edition of his textbook on clinical psychiatry, Schüle used the term "dementia praecox" to refer to hereditarily predisposed individuals who were "wrecked on the cliffs of puberty" and developed acute dementia, while others developed hebephrenia. Dementia praecox and hebephrenia were therefore terms for different conditions, one acute and one chronic. In an 1890 article by Arnold Pick (1851–1924), a professor at the German-language campus of Charles University in Prague, the argument was made that hebephrenia was a form of dementia praecox. The cases Pick had in mind were those where the psychosis began after puberty with an insidious onset and ended in a progressive dementia. So, in a sense,

Pick should get the credit for being the creator of dementia praecox. However, his paper, like Hecker's, relied upon case history material and did not have the rhetorical weight of systematic longitudinal data collected on large numbers of cases behind it. Kraepelin's did. And Schüle and Pick, in turn, had simply used the Latinized form of a French term, *démence précoce,* that had been used in 1852 and 1860 by the French alienist Bénédict-Augustin Morel (1809–1873) to describe some qualities of a small group of adolescent patients who were stuporous (a condition related to problems with the expression of the will and voluntary movement). Morel did not, as so many others later claimed (particularly in France), propose a distinct form of insanity or clinical syndrome. Kraepelin did not borrow from Morel, and may not have been aware of Morel's use of the term in its French form. But Kraepelin had cited Schüle's textbook in the 1887 second edition of his own *Psychiatrie,* and thus he knew of the term dementia praecox at least six years before he introduced it in 1893.[25]

Kraepelin was also not the first to propose that a group of disorders could be classified according to their outcome of dementia (mental weakness and permanent cognitive defect). Kahlbaum had done so with a class of illness he called "Vesania typica." The difference again, of course, was Kraepelin's structured data collection in support of such conjectures.[26]

This, then, was the state of Kraepelin's ideas about dementia praecox in 1893. Adolf Meyer had studied this fourth edition of *Psychiatrie* thoroughly at Kankakee and Worcester, and it had not moved him to become a "pupil" of Kraepelin. It would be the 1896 fifth edition of Kraepelin's textbook that would compel Meyer to introduce dementia praecox into American asylums, and the 1899 sixth edition that would convince the rest of the world of Kraepelin's value.

The years in Heidelberg would bring a bounty of good fortune to the Kraepelins. They purchased a beautiful house with a view of Heidelberg's famous castle and the Neckar Valley. Kraepelin's mother lived with them until her death, adding to the bustle of family life. And by 1898 the Kraepelins had three more healthy daughters. Life could not be better.

And there was more: Kraepelin's psychiatric clinic and its associated laboratories for experimental psychology and neuropathology—the latter headed by the pioneering Franz Nissl (1860–1919) starting in 1895—

were attracting visitors from around the world: alienists and psychologists from America, Russia, Sweden, Holland, Italy, England, France, Japan, and Turkey. Eugen Bleuler—who would create schizophrenia in 1908—visited from Switzerland. "Based on our experiences on the wards, we seemed to agree with one another on most points," Kraepelin later remembered in his *Memoirs*.[27] August Hoch, a Swiss émigré to America, trained twice under Kraepelin in Heidelberg. During his first stay, in 1894, he learned how to perform experiments involving mental measurements (charting the quantitative "ergograph," or "work-recorder") of individuals who were fatigued or under the influence of substances such as tea. He took what he learned back with him and continued his psychology experiments in the laboratory at the McLean Hospital. After his second visit, in 1897, he increasingly focused on Kraepelin's diagnostics at McLean.[28]

In the spring of 1896 thirty-year-old Adolf Meyer arrived from the Worcester Lunatic Hospital and spent six stimulating weeks with Kraepelin and his associates in the busy clinic. As he would later remember it, "The Heidelberg Clinic at that time was the center of work on 'processes.' The psychological experiment and the clinic alike dealt with processes, i.e., specific modifications of structure and function, that might be underlying specific diseases. The static, purely descriptive period had come to an end. This is what attracted me. At the same time, the form it took rather startled me." What was it that troubled Meyer? It was none other than the classification system introduced by Kraepelin in the fifth edition of *Psychiatrie,* which Meyer called "the greatest challenge that had ever come to psychiatry in the form of a text."[29]

Kraepelin was never afraid to change his opinions, and the various editions of his textbooks reflected this over the years. "I have a strong tendency to fine-hew my opinions in a pedantic way," he confessed to himself in his private "self-assessment." "I derive great pleasure from detecting new aspects under which larger groups of facts may be subsumed. . . . As a rule, I am quite aware that the generalizations gained in this way have only a passing value; and I have no difficulty in discarding views I have adhered to for years, as soon as they are refuted by experience. I am certainly receptive to new lines of thought, perhaps sometimes too much so."[30]

The historic fifth edition of *Psychiatrie* certainly proved that. Meyer was at the Heidelberg clinic in March 1896 when it appeared. The book was dedicated to the memory of Bernhard von Gudden, Kraepelin's old

chief at the asylum in Munich. The foreword to the fifth edition an-
nounced its break with the psychiatry of the past:

> What convinced me of the superiority of the clinical method of diag-
> nosis, followed here, over the traditional one, was the certainty with
> which we could predict, on the basis of our new concept of disease, the
> future course of events. Thanks to it the student can now find his way
> more easily in the difficult subject of psychiatry.[31]

The significance of Kraepelin's latest approach to psychiatry—and
it was indeed a new way of seeing the insane for the alienists who adopted it—was based on several factors.

First, he defined mental diseases according to their characteristic
patterns of age of onset, course, and outcome. Kraepelin did not create
new insanities based on a prominent symptom or group of symptoms,
thereby overthrowing two millennia of diagnostic habits by traditional
physicians, but he discarded the notion that mental diseases formed *syndromes* (a cluster of signs and symptoms that would remain consistent,
regardless of outcome). For disorders such as dementia praecox, this
meant that two patients could have the same diagnosis and yet present
very different clusters of signs and symptoms, but their outcome would
be the same: a persistent "mental weakness," "deterioration," or "defect." *Prognosis* became the organizing principle behind Kraepelin's system. For the first time an alienist could examine an insane patient and
make an informed guess about what to tell the patient or family about
the probable outcome of an illness. For dementia praecox the prognosis
was grim: incurable and permanent disability.

However, the conditions under which Kraepelin created his
prognosis-based system require some comment.

As Kraepelin's confidence in his clinical judgment increased in his
early years at the university psychiatry clinic in Heidelberg, the time
needed to make a diagnosis and prognosis decreased markedly. From
1891 to 1893 Kraepelin and his staff allowed themselves *four weeks after
admission* to render a diagnosis and prognosis. After 1893 these important opinions were rendered *during the first days after admission,* directly
after the first clinical interview. This raises several interesting questions: What was behind this increased acceleration in rendering a prognosis? Was the source of Kraepelin's confidence in clinical decision

making derived from the findings of his ongoing research? Or was the rapidity of prognosis a reflection of an administrative need to transfer patients quickly from the overcrowded, high-volume "transit station" of the clinic back to the community or to the nearby asylums in Emmendingen or Pforzheim? The historian Eric Engstrom suggests the latter, noting, "[Kraepelin] maintained that in his clinic it was common practice to submit applications for transfer immediately after the prognosis had been determined."[32] Discharges or transfers would open beds for new patients—and increase the number of case histories Kraepelin could collect for his research.

Was the concept of dementia praecox constructed *primarily* to meet institutional demands specific to the Heidelberg clinic? This interpretation suggests that prognosis-oriented diagnosis in psychiatry—which arguably began with Kraepelin in 1896—was a reflection of the triumph of institutional needs (identifying the curable from the incurable as quickly as possible to move them along a path in a system of overcrowded clinics and asylums) over the validity of scientific claims about disease specificity (the "natural" course and outcome of "real" and identifiable mental diseases). Setting aside the issue of the validity of the methods and conclusions of his research, Kraepelin's concept of dementia praecox certainly had a nonmedical function as a bureaucratic synonym or administrative flag, marking a patient as "incurable" and therefore "to be transferred to an asylum for long-term care." As we shall see, it is beyond doubt that in each institution in which it later made an appearance, rendering a diagnosis of dementia praecox did indeed serve dual medical and administrative purposes.

Second, Kraepelin claimed that he had arrived at his conclusions based on the quantitative, longitudinal study of hundreds of patients (with the data for each one kept on his *Zählkarten*). Indeed by 1896 he had already collected more than a thousand cases. Kraepelin claimed his proposals were not based on explicit appeals to "years of clinical experience" or "impressions" or credentials—although, as in any scientific enterprise, these personal factors played a role in the generation of Kraepelin's insights.

Third, he presented a thoroughly *clinical* way of looking at psychiatry in a manner that was similar to the clinical approach to diseases taken by other medical specialties. Now mental diseases were to be regarded as any other of the common medical diseases.

Fourth, he made the argument that the clinical picture of each condition, as well as its cause (etiology) and underlying pathophysiology, were all based on underlying, real "natural disease entities" (*Natürliche Krankheitseinheiten*) of an as yet unknown character. Further research on anatomy, symptomatology, and etiology would, he believed, one day converge to the point where clear scientific statements could be made about these disease entities in nature. They were specifiable, and they existed "in nature" in a reality separate from that of an individual patient or clinician. However, he believed a structured, longitudinal study of the clinical manifestations of the insanities was the logical first step to scientifically identifying differences among them. Clinical psychiatry could then shape biological research.

Fifth, his new clinical approach to mental diseases meant that clinical psychiatry could finally reject the largely unsuccessful "brain psychiatry" *(Gehirnpsychiatrie)* of those (such as Wernicke) who attempted to correlate psychiatric signs and symptoms with diseased brain cells. Kraepelin in fact often referred to such materialistic reductionist approaches as "brain mythologies." Although this grounding of German psychiatry in pathological anatomy had fused together psychiatry and neurology in the 1870s and 1880s, hence merging it with the other branches of medicine, by the late 1880s Kraepelin and others who had been influenced by the experimental psychology of Wundt protested that such an approach was sterile and one-sided. Psychological functions were ignored, not explained, by the focus on microscopic analysis. Kraepelin believed that even the most exact knowledge of brain mechanisms would not fully explain abnormal mental phenomena— something that would be possible only if the brain secreted ideas and emotions the way the kidney secretes urine. Kraepelin never lost his basic belief in the biological basis of mental diseases, or in the role of brain pathology in some of these disorders, but he did not believe the causes were necessarily, only, or originally in the brain. Potentially the entire body could be involved. Indeed, a systemic, perhaps metabolic, basis for dementia praecox would remain a lifelong speculation for Kraepein.

But what of psychological functioning? Weren't most symptoms of mental illness exaggerations or distortions of normal thinking, attention, memory, perception, and sensation? Didn't many symptoms of insanity carry an analogical resemblance to the functioning of normal persons under conditions of fatigue or intoxication? From a clinical perspective, did it really matter if point-by-point linkages between specific diseased brain cells and, say, a paranoid delusion could not be found? No. The experimental study of measurable psychological functions—the central research program of his life's work (not biological studies)—provided Kraepelin (and others) with a scientific basis for specifying mental diseases according to psychological, not biological, mechanisms. A classification system of mental diseases could thus be constructed from disease entities specified by nonbiological dimensions. This move away from neuroanatomy and toward experimental psychology was the fundamental shift in the German psychiatry of the 1890s (if short-lived), and Kraepelin was its most prominent spokesman.[33]

Sixth, his proposed classification system (nosology) not only challenged the "unitary psychosis" assumption of many psychiatrists, but it offered a persuasive argument for abandoning the widespread tendency of American asylum alienists to rely on the vague and broad "primary symptom" categories of melancholia, mania, dementia, and idiocy as the only diagnostic options.[34] Patients whom Kraepelin now defined as having a single disease, dementia praecox, could have easily fit into all four of these ancient categories. His diagnostic concepts were psychiatry's contribution to the quest for *disease specificity* that obsessed the other medical sciences.

Seventh, he introduced a broader, more comprehensive view of dementia praecox—still essentially hebephrenia, but including the full range of severe to mild cases—as part of a group of mental diseases characterized by their mental "deteriorating processes" *(Die Verblödungsprocesse),* along with two other distinct forms of insanity, catatonia and dementia paranoides. These were conditions marked by their lasting mental weakness and cognitive defect (dementia) between exacerbations of psychotic symptoms such as hallucinations, delusions, and catatonia.

Eighth, dementia praecox and the other "deteriorating processes" could be distinguished from another broad category of "constitutional mental disorders" that did *not* (usually) result in lasting cognitive defects (dementia) between flare-ups: the "periodic insanities" *(Das periodische Irresein)* and their three forms (manic, circular, and depressive). Kraepelin would later place this distinction between the "deteriorating" and "periodic" forms of insanity at the very center of his reorganization of the insanities in the 1899 sixth edition of *Psychiatrie,* creating the familiar juxtaposition between dementia praecox and manic-depressive insanity as the two great categories of the insanities.

Indeed as Meyer did in America by training alienists to collect and document facts about the patient, Kraepelin's new classification of the insanities helped to awaken alienists so that they would see patterns of meaning in their insane patients' behavior. Although William Alanson White insisted near the end of his life that "classification, then as now, had a sterilizing effect upon further inquiries into the significance and origin of symptoms," he nonetheless admitted, "When . . . Kraepelin's classification, based on a new descriptive symptomatology and the course and outcome of the disease process, came to be known, it was hailed everywhere with joy. Here was a new lease of life for all of us, a new interest in psychiatry, new points of view. The whole subject was revivified and made more alive, and the patients correspondingly became more interesting."[35]

This last phrase is worth repeating: *and the patients correspondingly became more interesting.* Once again the increased attention that patients received in countless interactions with alienists who now took a serious diagnostic interest in them may indeed have been therapeutic. Kraepelin's classification system, and his newly created mental diseases, gave American alienists something interesting to write about when, at the insistence of Meyer, they prepared their extensive notes and reports on the life history and clinical status of their patients. Daily, detailed record-keeping reflected a medical model of continuous moitoring, which was a largely symbolic expression of patient "care." However, the standard treatments for insanity—drugs, extended baths, busywork— did not change. Kraepelin and Meyer were antidotes to the slumber of learned helplessness afflicting the alienists. The patients remained inalterably insane.

What was dementia praecox in 1896?

"Dementia praecox is the name I have given to the development of a simple, fairly high-grade state of mental impairment accompanied by acute or subacute mental disturbance" was how Kraepelin introduced his new disease concept. "The course of the illness may vary."[36]

Kraepelin described, with colorful observations of the language and behavior of his patients, how the disease would progress from an initial state, where the mental faculties (attention, will, fluidity of thought) may begin to fail, though outwardly the person may still act in a relatively normal fashion, to a deterioration that may be slow or fast. Because dementia praecox in 1896 comprised the milder forms of hebephrenia described by Hecker as well as the more severe dementing forms described by Daraszkiewicz, disorganization in thought, language, and behavior—especially the inattentiveness, silliness, and fluid delusions—predominate in the later stages. In the later stages apathy, muteness, confusion, and incontinence are common. "It would seem that in most cases the disease progresses into a state of profound dementia," Kraepelin wrote. "The course of dementia praecox is generally regular and progressive. It is rare to see a substantial remission of the symptoms; at least the excitement disappears, but the mental impairment remains."[37]

These last two points—that dementia praecox nearly always progresses into a state of deterioration, mental weakness, or defect, and that this cognitive impairment does not disappear between episodes of "excitement," when delusions and hallucinations are present—would be the defining feature of this disease for years to come.

"Dementia Praecox is a very common illness. . . . Very little is known at present of the causes of the disorder," Kraepelin wrote. He goes on to say that in more than half of his cases the age of onset was between sixteen and twenty-two. The majority of the cases that began with a sudden onset and with rapid deterioration also tended to be younger. In his sample, males were three times more likely to develop dementia praecox than females. In his opinion puberty was somehow linked to the onset of the disease. He disagreed with Hecker's claim that such patients are frozen or arrested in development, instead offering the opinion that they seemed to regress. "The real nature of dementia praecox is totally obscure," Kraepelin wrote, although he offered "provisional and indefinite hypotheses" about possible biological causes and pathological processes. "What we have here is a tangible morbid process in the brain," he speculated, while acknowledging that the immediate causes might lie somewhere else in the body, perhaps as the result of a self-poisoning process or autointoxication. On the state of therapy he wrote, "Given our present ignorance of the causes of the illness, the treatment of dementia praecox offers few points for intervention."[38]

One of Adolf Meyer's greatest gifts was his ability to critique the ideas of others. His written reports offering suggestions for improving the clinical and administrative conditions in asylums display a clarity and

critical acumen that are absent in his own theoretical and methodological publications. His discussions of the published works of other
psychiatrists are also often illuminating. This was the case with the book
review of Kraepelin's fifth edition of *Psychiatrie*. Meyer was finishing it
when he wrote to his friend August Hoch in October 1896 and enthused that he was now "Kraepelinianer." While still relatively new to
the idea that he could, in good conscience, call himself a psychiatrist,
Meyer did not pull punches in his review.

He began his review by lauding the fact that Kraepelin was intellectually flexible enough to change his views from one edition of *Psychiatrie* to the next. In the fifth edition he presented "a largely clinical
way of looking at psychiatry" that "marks a complete revolution of the
views generally held." Meyer was impressed by the "interesting anam-
nestic method of following patients for years after their discharge" because the "subsequent history is of the greatest value for understanding
the clinical picture." Now, with this information, Kraepelin claims
that "typical differences can be recognized throughout between the
cases which terminate with mental defects and those which terminate
without mental deterioration." Meyer noted that the unique feature of
the fifth edition was an "emphatic plea" for the recognition of a group
of "processes of mental deterioration," of which dementia praecox was
one. This was, as Meyer well knew, classification by prognosis.[39]

After acknowledging these facts Meyer sharpened his critique. He
claimed—as he would throughout the rest of his life—that some of
Kraepelin's assertions "appear decidedly dogmatic at first sight." He
said this was due to the "didactic character of the book." Kraepelin's
comprehensive system of classification is "both the strength and weakness of Kraepelin's book." But Meyer admits that a critic of Kraepelin
would find it difficult to be to be taken seriously "unless he have as
many or more records of patients collected with the principles in view
which Kraepelin has brought forth for the first time."

Meyer did notice something in Kraepelin's definition of dementia
praecox that would have profound implications in the years ahead: "K.
makes the domain of dementia praecox and of katatonia much broader
than most alienists would do." Indeed in just three years Kraepelin
would broaden the dementia praecox concept even further, in the 1899
sixth edition. Broad diagnostic categories were like large boxes into
which alienists could fit many, many insane patients.

Meyer's main criticism, however, concerned the larger classification group that contained dementia praecox. Kraepelin had proposed—hypothetically and with "so little substantial evidence" in pathology—a class of mental diseases that were called "Diseases of Metabolism" *(Stoffwechselerkrankungen)*. A subgroup of this category were the diseases known as "deterioration processes" *(Verblödungsprocesse)*. Meyer was absolutely correct in criticizing Kraepelin on this point; it was a major leap of faith. Studies of "inner secretions" (later termed "hormones") were just getting under way in the early 1890s, but they made a major impression on Kraepelin. At this point Kraepelin considered dementia praecox to be a disorder of metabolism that resembled, in some respects, myxoedema, a thyroid gland disorder that could cause delusions and hallucinations as well as cognitive deterioration. The over- or underproduction of these internal secretions is what Kraepelin had in mind when he suggested that dementia praecox and many other mental diseases were due to autointoxication. The brain was poisoned by substances being produced in other areas of the body. Meyer would have none of it: "As long as chemistry cannot furnish more accurate data and methods, the theory of intoxication and auto-intoxication so often resorted to by Kraepelin will be a *terminus technicus* for our ignorance."

When Meyer's review was published in the *American Journal of Insanity* in late 1896 it would be the first time that dementia praecox was mentioned in print in America. Meyer noted, "The recent German text-books on mental diseases have not been the favorites of many American and English alienists." But his review, published in the journal that would reach the elite of American alienists, and the attention he would draw in New England from his reforms at Worcester, would eventually lead to Kraepelin's recognition. American alienists, like most other physicians, did not see the need to read the medical literature, nor could most read German or French. But those very few who could read German were able to read Kraepelin.

And slowly at first, almost imperceptibly, things began to change.

4

THE AMERICAN RECEPTION OF DEMENTIA PRAECOX AND MANIC DEPRESSIVE INSANITY, 1896-1905

New England was the epicenter of the Kraepelinian revolution in the classification of the insanities, and Adolf Meyer was its catalyst. Through his contacts with asylum psychiatrists in Massachusetts, Connecticut, and New Hampshire, Meyer was not only able to inspire them to adopt changes in record keeping, the structured interviewing of patients, and the holding of weekly case conferences to clinically review new cases—he was also able to convince them of the superiority of Kraepelin's new ideas in the fifth edition of *Psychiatrie*. This process took several years but proved seminal for the transformation of American psychiatry that would take place in the decades that followed.

Beginning in the autumn of 1896 Meyer trained his medical staff at the Worcester Lunatic Hospital to use Kraepelin's new classification scheme and diagnostic terms for mental diseases. In 1898 Kraepelin's categories made their appearance in a special report by Meyer, as the institution's pathologist, attached to the hospital's *Annual Report*. Other Massachusetts institutions were slower to change: in the 1899 compilation of annual statistics reported by all state asylums to the State Board of Lunacy and Charity of Massachusetts, pre-Kraepelinian categories (melancholia, mania, dementia, general paralysis, idiocy) remained the standard nomenclature.[1]

In Meyer's special report of 30 September 1898, written in a didactic style that aimed at educating state administrators about advances in psychiatry, he praised both Kahlbaum and Kraepelin. "Kraepelin was one of the first who had the courage to build a psychiatry on lines foreshadowed by Kahlbaum, and with principles derived from pure clinical observation and a view of psychiatry of his own." He then went on to reveal how Kraepelinian he still remained at this time:

> From this point of view disease concepts remain more than mere names. . . . This can be seen by a glance at the table of statistics, which contains, as it were, a curve of recoverability in the following groups: the periodic psychosis with no, or but little, deterioration after an attack; the catatonia with occasional recoveries; dementia praecox with lasting defect; and paranoic conditions and paranoia practically never curable. It goes without saying that the last word is not spoken concerning a truly medical classification of mental diseases; but in a measure, as we learn to make distinctions of practical and essential value, we shall gladly relegate the meaningless terms, mania, melancholia, etc., of our former statistics to the vocabulary of mere symptomatology.[2]

During this period of early enthusiasm for Kraepelin's classification scheme Meyer demonstrated little interest in speculations about the causes of the insanities (other than to criticize Kraepelin's autointoxication hypothesis) and no interest at all in Kraepelin's vast body of experimental research in pharmacopsychology, word associations, and the role of fatigue in the insanities. Other alienists in American asylums had indeed discovered this body of scientific work, and it was Kraepelin's experimental psychology—not his classification system— that marked his reception into American psychiatry.

Meyer's asylum therefore was not the first one touched by the work of Kraepelin. The McLean Hospital in Massachusetts had already become the first place in the United States where psychological research was conducted that was informed by Kraepelin's efforts in this area. This was due to August Hoch (1868–1919), a fellow Swiss émigré that Meyer had befriended in September 1895 during a fact-finding mission to the new McLean campus when it moved from Somerville to Waverly (now Belmont) in April 1895. The personal and intellectual lives of these two men would remain intertwined for the next twenty-four years. Both would play pivotal roles in the reframing of Kraepelin's dementia praecox into a uniquely American concept in the first decade of the 1900s.

As may be said to be true for many intimate friendships, there were both strong dissimilarities as well as congruencies in the personalities of these two men. Hoch's son-in-law, the noted twentieth-century psychiatrist Lawrence C. Kubie, remembered him as a "warm, gemütlich man—Swiss, of course, like Meyer, but totally different in personality—warm, affectionate and hospitable."[3] In his obituaries of Hoch Meyer characterized his friend as "retiring" but also as "a most genial and lovable character" who "gained the warmest affection of his patients" and "was capable of the keenest and heartiest enjoyment of friendship and social happiness with his chosen friends and his family." Like Meyer—although Meyer may not have had this opinion of himself—"Hoch was not a generalizer" nor "a philosopher," and "his first love was that of appreciation of the finer niceties of description and interpretation."[4]

August Hoch grew up in Basel. Like Meyer, his father was a minister. For a number of years Hoch's father was also superintendant of the City and University Hospital in Basel. Like Meyer, Hoch decided to emigrate to America in order to establish a new life and career outside of Europe. He did so in 1887, when he was nineteen, entering the medical school of the University of Pennsylvania. This proved to be a serendipitous choice, for it was there that he became a disciple of the renowned William Osler. And when Osler decided to leave to become the first professor of medicine at the new Johns Hopkins Medical School in Baltimore, Hoch and his friend and fellow student Charles Simon (later to become a pioneering virologist) followed him there. While working under Osler in his clinic Hoch found the time to complete his medical degree at the University of Maryland in 1890. He then worked as a neurological assistant under Osler for the next two years. It was during his tenure at Johns Hopkins that Hoch developed a specialized interest in neuropathology and nervous disorders and translated a textbook on this subject from the original German.[5]

It is at this point that Edward Cowles (1837—1919), the superintendant of the McLean Hospital, enters the story, for it was Cowles who was directly responsible for placing Hoch and Meyer into prominent positions at McLean and Worcester (respectively), from which they would introduce Kraepelin's ideas into American psychiatry.

In 1887 Cowles had taken a year's leave of absence from the McLean Asylum (as it was then called) in order to study experimental and physiological psychology under G. Stanley Hall (1844–1924) at

Johns Hopkins.[6] The two became lifelong friends, and later both were founding members of the American Psychological Association in the summer of 1892. After returning to McLean Cowles maintained his contact with the colleagues he had met there, and it was through them that he learned of the talents of August Hoch. When William Noyes (1857–1915), the physician who had been conducting physiological and psychological research at McLean since 1889, resigned, Cowles extended the offer to Hoch. In 1893 Hoch accepted the position of pathologist and assistant physician with the understanding that his primary, but not exclusive, role would be that of a researcher. To ensure that the research conducted at McLean would be of the highest quality, Cowles sent Hoch to Europe for most of 1893 and 1894, to specific laboratories where he could learn techniques associated with Cowles's own research interests. For various lengths of time Hoch studied brain anatomy under Gustav Albert Schwalbe (1844–1916) in Strassburg; correlated blood-pressure changes with mental activities in studies conducted with the Italian physiologist Angelo Mosso (1846–1910) in Turin, a noted expert on blood pressure, fear, and fatigue; learned the techniques of experimental psychology with Wilhelm Wundt and his laboratory associates in Leipzig; and then finally enjoyed a long period with Emil Kraepelin in Heidelberg, where he "studied the influence of drugs on simple psychical acts" and made clinical studies in the "pathological chemistry of autointoxication in insanity."[7] When he returned to McLean in late 1894, first for a few months in its Somerville location, then in April 1895 in its well-equipped, state-of-the-art laboratory in Waverly, Hoch initiated studies on fatigue using Mosso's ergograph (work-recorder) apparatus.

Although Hoch understood that he was sent to these European laboratories so that he could conduct research under Cowles's direction on what the superintendent believed to be the issue "of primary importance in psychiatry," that of "the fatigue question and its relation to auto-intoxication,"[8] by 1897 Hoch's new knowledge eventually led him into conflict with his chief. The seeds of this tension—which is perhaps the more appropriate way of characterizing the situation, given Hoch's generally agreeable nature—can be found not only in the personality and past experience of Cowles, but also in his views of the essential nature of the insanities, which he found difficult to relinquish even as his own institution became a primary conduit for the flow of Kraepelin's ideas in the United States.

Like many alienists of his generation, Cowles was a veteran of the Civil War. He was described by a contemporary as "a short man with a military bearing" and "a florid complexion."[9] In 1863 he received medical degrees from both the College of Physicians and Surgeons at Columbia University and Dartmouth College. Upon graduation he joined the U.S. Army Medical Corps at the rank of assistant surgeon, and in the autumn of that same year he was placed in charge of a hospital in Harrisburg, Pennsylvania, that cared for wounded Union soldiers—an exceptionally responsible position for a twenty-six-year-old recent medical school graduate. After retiring from the army in 1872 with the rank of captain, Cowles became the medical superintendent of the Boston City Hospital. His administrative and architectural reforms there became legendary. His experience in the military led him to establish firm lines in the chain of command, reducing inefficiency and negligence. In addition to instituting a training school for nurses at the hospital in 1878 (a program he would later repeat at McLean) he doubled the physical size of the hospital, renovated its heating and ventilation, and instituted other changes that eliminated the formerly large number of infections (except for surgical sepsis) that had plagued the institution. In 1879 he agreed to become the new superintendent of the small McLean Asylum in Somerville, just a few miles outside of Boston. In preparation for his new position he toured insane asylums in France and Britain in the fall of 1879; he assumed his new role in December of that year.

At McLean Cowles aggressively instituted reforms in the physical plant of the institution as well as its administrative chain of command. He also eliminated many of the barred windows, locked doors, and other practices of confinement that he deemed unfit for a hospital, and insisted on changing the name of McLean from an asylum to a hospital in 1892. From almost the beginning of his tenure at McLean he lobbied for the construction of an entirely new institution in a new location, and this dream, as has been noted, was realized in 1895. This coincided with his tenure as the president of the American Medico-Psychological Association for the year 1894–1895. It was Cowles who had helped convince the neurologist Silas Weir Mitchell to speak freely in his address the AMPA in 1894, and his sincerity with regard to the advancement of psychiatry was recognized by the alienist colleagues who elected him to lead the organization. With Cowles's national prominence and the opening of the new McLean complex and its unparalleled laboratory, the McLean Hospital was the symbolic center of the future of an American psychiatry that could be reunited with the world of general medicine.

Cowles was a decidedly visionary and driven man who was used to giving orders and having them followed. Although his talents as an administrator were unquestionably great, and, from the perspective of historical hindsight, his awareness that the path for psychiatry to reenter medicine was through physiological and psychological experimentation in the laboratory put him far ahead of his alienist contemporaries, Cowles could not change with the times. He would not be able to let go of fundamental assumptions about the nature of the insanities that he had developed by the middle of the 1880s. These views directly conflicted with those of Kraepelin and, by extension, those of Hoch and Meyer at this point in their careers.

Cowles believed in the "unitary psychosis" hypothesis: the notion that the differences among the various forms of insanity were in reality simply different stages of the development of one underlying disease process. In the 1880s he became fascinated with the popular notion proposed by the American "nerve specialist" Charles Beard that poor nutrition and the fatigue caused by the stresses of modern life led to the neurotic condition he called "neurasthenia."[10] The consulting rooms of general practitioners and specialists in nervous diseases were flooded with persons for whom the "wear and tear" on their nerves led to "nervous breakdowns" characterized by general malaise, mental weakness, depression, generalized anxiety, phobias, hypochondriacal complaints, and social withdrawal. At the small McLean Asylum, which catered to educated and affluent patients and in 1887 had a capacity for only 170 patients, Cowles and his assistant physicians saw a significant number of new admissions who seemed to exhibit the signs and symptoms of Beard's proposed syndrome.[11] Beginning around 1885 Cowles was of the opinion that neurasthenia, or neurasthenic exhaustion, constituted the first of the four stages of this unitary insanity, followed by melancholia, mania, and then a period of confusion and transition into dementia.[12] Despite a brief period of wary openness to Kraepelin's ideas in the mid-1890s, Cowles seems to have held to portions of his original unitary psychosis idea for the remainder of his life.[13]

Convinced of his theory, Cowles pressed the trustees of the asylum to give him funds to set up a laboratory that would target the physiology, biochemistry, and psychology underlying the first or prodromal stage of insanity—neurasthenia. In the context of the late 1880s this was indeed revolutionary thinking in American psychiatry, and his logic was congruent with the emerging scientific paradigms of his era. Cowles realized that a scientific understanding of the role of fatigue and nutrition in causing insanity could potentially lead not only to effective treatments for the insane, but also to prevention. Perhaps more than any other individual of his era, Cowles personified the future of an American psychiatry wed to the laboratory revolution taking place in general medicine. Near the end of his life he would be credited for inspiring "the establishment of laboratories in our institutions" and for the "*laboratory turn of mind*" in psychiatry.[14] The trustees eventually approved the funding of Cowles's laboratory, which was first established in five rooms at the Somerville campus in 1889.

When the twenty-six-year-old Hoch began work at McLean in that year he was in not only a privileged but a historic position: this laboratory for psychiatric research was the first of its kind in the United States. A Brown University professor who published an article on "psychological laboratories in America" in the *L'Année Psychologique* in 1894 described it as "the only one in America which united psychiatry and physiological psychology. In Germany there exists only one like it— that of Professor Kraepelin at Heidelberg. It attempts to combine the studies of the clinic and of neurology with those of chemistry on the one hand, and with those of psychology on the other."[15] Unlike Kraepelin's laboratory, however, the McLean Hospital and laboratories were not integrated with a university. This would not occur in America until the opening of the Henry C. Phipps Psychiatric Clinic at the Johns Hopkins University in 1913.

The new laboratory at McLean consisted of eight rooms located in a service building that also prepared food and was the site for public events.[16] The rooms were designed for pathological, physiological, and chemical studies. There was an examining room where patients could be interviewed and have their skulls measured or physically assessed for disease. A room with a hood and a ventilation shaft was where chemicals were stored and analyses done of pathological and physiological chemistry. This is where blood, urine, feces, and sputum would be analyzed, as well as any tissue specimens collected at the time of autopsy. A special apparatus room was equipped to conduct studies in physiological psychology; this is where Hoch conducted his research using Mosso's ergograph, various kymographs (for measuring blood pressure), and time-measuring devices such as the Hipp chronoscope. The other rooms included a microscope and photograph room, a dark room for photography, and a reception room for visitors. In the basement of the building were the mortuary and autopsy room. Elsewhere on the campus Cowles established a medical library that contained two thousand volumes in English, French, German, and Italian and maintained active subscriptions to forty periodicals in these languages. No other American asylum or state hospital could match the resources at McLean.

What, exactly, was Hoch doing during his early years of research at McLean? What were his findings? We know that in early 1895 he continued his ergographic studies of the effect of the caffeine in tea and co-authored a summary of these researches with Kraepelin.[17] He would not publish a description of his ergographic studies until 1901, citing his interest in the similarities in the mental weakness found in neurasthenia, dementia praecox, and the depressed phase of manic-depression as the rationale.[18] Given Hoch's careful training in Leipzig and Heidelberg, the insane subjects were compared to control groups of normal individuals. Whatever chemical and pathological analyses were conducted in an effort to correlate them with the results of experiments in the physiological psychology of fatigue were also never fully revealed.

Hoch published only three papers in English between 1896 and 1898, but none of these concerned his fatigue studies. Perhaps this was due to overwork, for Hoch was not only responsible for performing autopsies and analyzing blood, urine, feces, and sputum in the pathological laboratory but was also the sole researcher in the chemical and physiological psychology laboratories between 1895 and 1900. Or, perhaps more likely, the results may have been discouraging. This had been the case with Hoch's predecessor, William Noyes, a physician who had been hired in February 1889 as the pathologist and then was sent to Vienna and Berlin for nine months to learn experimental physiological psychology. Noyes apparently published only one paper of note during his four years in the first McLean laboratory, a study of the "knee-jerk in sleep in terminal dementia." The rest was unpublishable. "It was pioneer work, difficult and too often yielding negative results, which he modestly declined to publish, so that of much that he did there is no record."[19] The same could be said of Hoch's first five years at McLean. Although McLean's laboratories were arguably the best in American psychiatry, there was no flood of research publications in the second half of the 1890s to demonstrate to critics (such as the neurologist Silas Weir Mitchell) that anything had really changed in the sequestered world of alienists.

In January 1896 Hoch published an extensive summary of an article that had been published by Kraepelin some months earlier outlining the relevance of psychological research for psychiatry.[20] It was the first presentation of Kraepelin's experimental work in an American psychiatric journal. In this paper Hoch inserts his own advice that "the study of the first stages" of insanity in comparison to normal individuals would give the best results, and the "two factors" to be studied, "fatigue and practice," echo the views of Cowles.[21] What is significant about this essay is that the seeds of some of Hoch's later ideas about the nature of the insanities, including dementia praecox, are already evident.

Hoch expressed a view shared by Meyer at this time. Anatomical and pathological studies of the brain had yielded no insights into insanity and were unlikely to do so. "But certainly it is a mistake to think," he wrote, "as many apparently do . . . that the task of psychiatry lies solely in a pathology of the brain cortex, for we must certainly admit with Kraepelin that a pathology of the brain cortex, no matter how advanced it may be, will never give us an insight into abnormal phenomena as such." Furthermore "mental diseases have primarily a psychical side to them." Hoch again emphasized the psychological, not the organic, nature of the insanities when he summarized Kraepelin's position on "the influence which the individuality of a person has upon the development of mental disease." According to Hoch, "This he estimates to be greater than has been supposed, external influence having a smaller share than was formerly thought." Indeed "there unquestionably remain enough mental diseases in which there are no such circumscribed causes to be found at all, but in which the intrinsic peculiarities of the personality are to be made responsible for the pathological development. . . . We are dealing, not with tangible things, but with *processes*."[22] These views would form the foundation of the uniquely American conception of dementia praecox that would emerge in the first decade of the twentieth century.

In the summer of 1897 Hoch returned to Kraepelin's clinic in Heidelberg. He studied postmortem alterations in nerve cells under the direction of the noted neuropathologist Franz Nissl. Their question: Are the physical changes in the nerve cells of insane patients observed at autopsy, particularly cell shrinkage, related to the mental disease process itself, or are they artifacts of bodily death? This was a critical issue at the time, and would remain so for decades, for it called into question every abnormal finding at autopsy that others had claimed was pathological evidence that the insanities were due to brain disease. Hoch began his studies in Germany but continued the bulk of them when he returned to McLean; he published his results in October 1898. His conclusion: "Whenever we meet these alterations in our studies of the cortex of the insane, we know that they have nothing to do with the disease process of the psychosis. . . ."[23] Hoch's own experience in failing to establish such links between insanity and brain pathology mirrored that of his friend and colleague Adolf Meyer. This failure would leave a lasting impression on these two men. And they were not alone. Other frustrated neuropathologists, such as the noted Nissl and Alois Alzheimer (1864–1915), who later worked with Kraepelin in Munich, defined the territorial boundary for the new scientific psychiatry through such failures. As the historian Edward Shorter observed, "What Nissl and Alzheimer could find under their microscopes they declared 'neurology.' What they couldn't find was psychiatry."[24]

When the twenty-nine-year-old Hoch returned to McLean in the autumn of 1897 he was granted new powers within the institution by Cowles, who was then sixty. After another stint in Kraepelin's laboratory he was determined to refashion McLean along the same lines. By this time Meyer had already done so at Worcester. Hoch instituted reforms in clinical record keeping and was now the leader of the weekly case conferences for new patients attended by the medical staff and consultants. Such clinics had been a part of the routine at McLean since 1889 and were a first for American asylums. The practice was directly borrowed from German clinics. A stenographer now recorded these case conferences, and typewritten summaries were generated. But perhaps the most significant change in the newly confident Hoch was his insistence on using Kraepelin's diagnostics to classify patients. The records of the case conferences at McLean beginning at about this time reflect the collision of Kraepelinian terms such as "dementia praecox" and "circular insanity" with the older concepts of melancholia, mania, and dementia that were still dear to Cowles.[25]

Hoch also insisted on altering the focus of research that Cowles had directed him to do. As Meyer remembered it, "He returned in spirit and fact the full-fledged psychiatric leader of the staff, as well as an especially well trained histopathologist, and one deeply interested in putting the ergographic work into the service of clinical problems. Dr. Cowles never made a complete readjustment to the natural result of these developments, so that the clinical publications were retarded; but Hoch's work became more and more the clinical research with a wise perspective regarding the laboratory investigations for which we all admire him."[26]

While Cowles could not outright reject the ideas of the "Heidelberg school," acknowledging the quantitative longitudinal research the new diagnostic categories were based upon, he could not wholeheartedly accept them either. Hoch, however, had made a clear break with the past—and with Cowles. "With reference to these [mental] diseases, and in general to clinical psychiatry, I must state here that I adhere to Kraepelin's school," Hoch stridently stated in a footnote to an article he published in April 1898.[27] The generational shift in classification and nomenclature, as well as the abandonment of the unitary psychosis idea, was too disorienting for Cowles and the older alienists. At an AMPA meeting in 1899 Cowles remarked, "We who have been grounded and brought up in the teachings of our fathers have associated together or differentiated the different forms of insanity that we most commonly see, cannot drop our working knowledge of our cases. We cannot transport ourselves to a new point of view without great apparent confusion if we lose our bearings."[28] Cowles was unable—and more than unwilling—to look at the insane patients on his wards through the diagnostic kaleidoscope and risk turning it to see them crystallize into new and unfamiliar configurations.

"For the bringing of [Kraepelin's concepts and clinical methods] to us in America I wish to give here the credit due to Dr. Hoch," Cowles generously admitted to his audience, "who went from the McLean Hospital to Heidelberg in 1894 and 1897, to be a student with Dr. Kraepelin, and to Dr. Meyer, who also was there in 1896." He then described the clash of the old and the new psychiatric universes provoked by the work of Kraepelin and revealed the reluctance to give up old conceptions: "During the last three years and more, in the discussions in clinical conferences at the McLean and Worcester Hospitals the Kraepelinian propositions have been worked over and, case by case, have been tested to their acceptance, modification, or rejection. At the McLean Hospital we have been very conservative; and holding fast to that which seemed good in our observations in the past we have adopted new conceptions only as they have stood trial in their repeated application to concrete cases."[29] Later he would write, "Painstaking records, with great refinement of detail, were made in every case and discussed in the clinical conferences of the medical staff. A clear field was given for new studies; no preconceptions were allowed to obstruct them."[30]

Clearly Cowles strove to retain a modicum of American autonomy when faced with these novel conceptions from Europe. But the only "test" of Kraepelin's ideas was discussion of how well they did or did not fit an individual patient at a case conference—not structured longitudinal research. A McLean patient could be discussed at a case conference and still be labeled with the traditional symptomatic diagnoses of melancholia, mania, and dementia rather than one of Kraepelin's disease concepts, such as dementia praecox or circular insanity. Hoch and whoever else regarded themselves as followers of the Heidelberg school no doubt sat in Cowles's presence during these discussions and thought, *Yes, but Kraepelin's categories are derived from solid research, whereas the melancholia, mania, and dementia of the old alienists are not.*

In the decade that followed, clashes and misunderstandings over the merits of the traditional and Kraepelinian systems of diagnosis would be played out at case conference tables in an increasing number of American and Canadian asylums and hospitals that considered following the lead of McLean, Worcester, and other New England institutions. Many did.

But Cowles was not willing to throw out a lifetime of experience. The main thrust of his 1899 address to the AMPA was to convince his alienist colleagues that Kraepelin's new diagnostic categories could be satisfactorily placed into diagnostic schemes using the old terminology. He presented several charts detailing how this could be done, thus allowing the older American alienists who were entrenched in a lifetime of habitual diagnostic thinking about their insane patients to use the older terms as analogues to the variety of new terms coming from Heidelberg. None of the recorded discussants, including Adolf Meyer, directly criticized Cowles. After Meyer recounted how much Kraepelin's textbook helped him when he came across it, and how much his experience with

Kraepelin and the patients and staff in the Heidelberg clinic convinced him of the value of its contents, he then asked, "How can we learn this? And second, how can we carry out the work according to the rules which a better knowledge of the subject imposes upon us? . . . If we want to succeed we must bear in mind that we are doing something which has not been done before. We cannot use the old tradition as a basis in the new work, but we have to take it just as in any business enterprise, in which nobody would start without first making a close investigation."[31]

Cowles's presentation at the AMPA marked the first time that Kraepelin's diagnostics—and dementia praecox—were ever discussed at a professional meeting of American alienists.

If disagreements over Kraepelin's diagnostics weren't enough, by 1900 Hoch began to openly question the rationale behind the research conducted at McLean and elsewhere. The public airing of his views could only have been seen as a major rejection of everything Cowles had brought into being at McLean: the new hospital, the three research laboratories, and Hoch himself, whom he had twice—generously— sent for training to Europe. In a cogently argued presentation at the AMPA annual meeting in 1900 Hoch took up where Cowles left off the year before. His presentation on the clinical study of psychiatry was a de- tailed exposition of the logic of Kraepelin's methods of clinical research. The "postulated disease processes" that underlay mental disorders, he said, "can at present only [be studied] in their manifestations." And what were these manifestations? "The cause, the disease curve or course, the out- come, the symptom–picture, the pathological–anatomical changes, and finally, perhaps, such things as chemical alterations." But what Hoch said next was his strongest criticism of Cowles and the many other superinten- dents of American asylums who claimed that the mere presence of their pathology labs proved they were engaged in scientific medicine: "Only when this is carefully conducted are we prepared for studies in pathologi- cal anatomy or pathological chemistry." The argument Hoch put forth was this: let's *first* try to identify patterns in the "manifestations" that sepa- rate the various mental disorders from one another, and then and *only then* look for biological substrates.

But Hoch carried this criticism even further: "For these reasons also it seems to me that the general, otherwise very creditable, move- ment in this country towards the establishment of laboratories in insane asylums is somewhat misguided and may do a certain amount of harm. . . . The establishment of a laboratory may give us the feeling that we have sufficed all scientific needs, although the observation of the patients may be as unscientific as ever."[32]

Hoch gave voice to the central paradox that would continue to plague the psychiatric profession for many decades to come. For psychiatry to reenter the mainstream of a medical profession undergoing a "laboratory revolution," laboratory research would have to be an essential component of the psychiatry of the future. But what should be studied? Was insanity a unitary disease, or were there different disease processes behind the manifestations of different insanities? If the latter were true, as Kraepelin suggested, could they be identified and differentiated with enough precision so that distinct neuropathological, chemical, physiological, and psychological markers for each disease could be isolated? Where should a researcher focus his or her efforts?

The early role of Kraepelinian experimental psychology in American psychiatry began and ended with Hoch's efforts at McLean. Even in Germany Kraepelin's passion for experimental psychology and his belief in its relevance for psychiatry was not shared by many others. Experimental psychology would eventually prove to be a dead end in psychiatric research on both sides of the Atlantic in the early decades of the twentieth century. Physicians were reluctant to learn the experimental methods of an entirely different, nonmedical discipline, and experimental psychologists were reluctant to work with asylum patients. According to the historian Josef Brozek, "The roster of research psychologists active in laboratory investigations of psychiatric disorders between 1895 and 1910 is limited to four": Boris Sidis (1867–1923) at the New York Pathological Institute, William Otterbein Krohn (1868–1927) at the Illinois Eastern Hospital for the Insane, and Shepherd I. Franz (1874–1933) and Frederic Lyman Wells (1884–1964), both of McLean Hospital. Such efforts were short term, minimally productive, non-Kraepelinian, and largely defunct by 1910. In the 1930s some American psychologists would try again.[33] In North America the rejection of this methodological path may have been a consequence of the need of alienists to demonstrate that psychiatry was indeed a legitimate branch of medicine, and as such the style of laboratory research in psychiatry should mimic that conducted in the other medical sciences. Experimental psychology in psychiatry would therefore be regarded as irrelevant and impractical.

But was the study of the brain the way to go? No one questioned the role of the brain in producing insanity, but neuropathological studies of both the gross anatomy of the brain and its cellular conditions—the most logical approach to solving the riddle of madness—had yielded no breakthroughs. Beginning with Kraepelin's shift of focus to clinical psychiatry in the 1896 fifth edition of his textbook, doubts such as those expressed by Hoch would be repeated many times by others and would lead to a situation historians have termed "the crisis of the somatic style" or "the end of the first biological psychiatry."[34] This was certainly true in Europe. But, as we shall see, an equally fruitless biological psychiatry *not* based on the study of the brain nonetheless developed in the United States just after 1900. It was a professional necessity for alienists to do so if they wanted to have their place at the table with physicians from the other medical specialties. But not all alienists agreed with this necessity.

Of all the newly described mental diseases proposed by Kraepelin, it would be dementia praecox that would become the Archimedean point of dissension between proponents of a biological psychiatry and those who had lost their faith in the salvation promised by the laboratory.

While the Americans struggled with replacing their traditional concepts of insanity with those of Kraepelin, in Germany things were different. Whereas the Americans felt they were confronted with an either/or choice by Hoch and Meyer, Kraepelin had several prominent rivals and many more critics in his home country as well as in Austria-Hungary, France, and particularly Switzerland. The Europeans were aware of choices that insular American alienists, who could not or did not read foreign languages, did not know about. It could be said that Hoch and Meyer together acted as a conceptual and cultural filter, introducing a Kraepelinian bias at a critical point in the development of American psychiatry.

The physician and historian Silke Feldmann has argued that there were three phases in the reception of Kraepelin's classification scheme and dementia praecox concept in Germany: a phase of resistance from 1893 to 1899, a period of further criticism but consolidation of his ideas from 1899 to 1912, and the period beginning around 1912, when his ideas were generally accepted. The most influential of his critics, Alfred Hoche (1865–1943) of Freiburg, flatly rejected Kraepelin's assumption that there were specifiable natural disease entities for insanity, and his perspective would be kept alive by one of his students, Oswald Bumke (1877–1950), the man who would succeed Kraepelin at the University of Munich in April 1924.[35]

From the time he introduced dementia praecox in the 1893 fourth edition of his textbook, *Psychiatrie,* until 1898, there was no criticism of the name of the disease (a "premature," "precocious," or "earlier than expected" dementia), nor of its description. Such criticism would come later. What critics seized upon, particularly after the fifth edition of *Psychiatrie* appeared in 1896, was Kraepelin's classification scheme. As a result it spread slowly from Heidelberg, encountering significant initial resistance. Most of the criticism was directed at the groupings of proposed diseases, particularly that of catatonia as a separate disease alongside dementia praecox as progressively degenerative conditions. Some critics argued that catatonia was not a separate disease, but a collection of symptoms found across difference disease pictures; others argued against its negative prognosis.

Beginning in 1898 Kraepelin faced more direct criticism of his dementia praecox concept. The name of the disorder was criticized for being misleading due to the fact that the "dementia" in dementia praecox was not the same as that found in the senile dementia of the elderly—a fact that Kraepelin had always recognized. The term "praecox" (precocious or premature) was derided because even Kraepelin admitted that in some instances individuals in their thirties or forties could develop the disease, not just adolescents or young adults. Kraepelin's dire prognosis for the condition was also called into question—most notably, beginning in 1908, by Eugen Bleuler. Additionally his revision of the dementia praecox concept from essentially being "hebephrenia" in the 1896 fifth edition to comprising three "forms"—hebephrenic, catatonic, and paranoid—in the sixth edition of 1899 led to further skepticism. By 1903 the name of Kraepelin had become so tightly associated with the disease he created, dementia praecox, that a contemporary suggested one way to resolve the dispute over its name would be to replace it with a new one: *Morbus Kraepelini*—Kraepelin's Disease.[36]

While Hoch and Meyer were busy spreading the gospel of the fifth edition of *Psychiatrie,* Kraepelin was sorting and re-sorting his growing collection of *Zählkarten* and making new inferences from his observations of patients. He presented some of these ideas in a preliminary way in a lecture titled "The Diagnosis and Prognosis of Dementia Praecox," delivered on 27 November 1898 at a conference of southwest German psychiatrists.[37] In this lecture he introduced what would become the central fault line of the new classification scheme he would publish the following year, in the sixth edition of his textbook: that between dementia praecox and manic-depressive insanity. Indeed it is in this lecture that Kraepelin mentions manic-depressive insanity *(das manisch-depressive Irresein)* for the first time. He presented the main characteristics of the two major insanities and described how they could be differentially diagnosed, especially at the beginning of these conditions, when depression or catatonic negativism is often evident. Also, in an attempt to answer the critics who objected to the term "dementia praecox," he confessed that the name wasn't as important to him as was the group of diseases it represented and their prognosis: progressive deterioration and permanent mental weakness *(Schwachsinn).*

The sixth edition of Kraepelin's *Psychiatrie,* and no other edition of this textbook before or since, had a profound effect on psychiatry worldwide throughout the twentieth century and the early twenty-first. Since the 1970s it has been asserted that "neo-Kraepelinian" clinicians created the structure and diagnostic content of the *Diagnostic and Statistical Manual of Mental Disorders, Third Edition (DSM-III)* of 1980, and that this bias has continued in successive editions until this day, influencing both clinical practice and research.[38] Certainly the 1899 edition caught the attention of Kraepelin's contemporaries immediately after its publication, and this was especially true in America, where the new concepts of dementia praecox and manic-depressive insanity were put into use the same year this book appeared in German. At McLean there was an effort to reverse terms to "depressive-maniacal insanity" because it was observed that depressive episodes usually preceded later manic episodes (if they ever manifested at all) in the course of the illness. As early as May 1899, at a McLean case conference attended by two consulting neurologists, Hoch and his colleagues had pondered the differential diagnosis of a woman in her mid-twenties, with Hoch and the two neurologists opting for dementia praecox and another staff physician arguing for the depressive phase of "depressive-maniacal excitement." A third McLean alienist was unsure and adamantly refused to make a diagnosis. Twice.[39]

What did Kraepelin actually propose in the sixth edition of *Psychiatry*? What exactly were dementia praecox and manic-depressive insanity in 1899?

"Dementia praecox" and "manic-depressive insanities" became umbrella terms that encompassed a sizable number of older diseases known by a variety of names. Thus Kraepelin's great feat in 1899 was one of *synthesis by prognosis.* This led to two large and multiformed insanities that could, together, help clinicians make sense of at least half of the institutionalized population of insane patients in their asylums. The rest would be gathered into eleven other major groupings and split according to conditions such as paralytic insanity (general paresis or general paralysis of the insane, correctly suspected to be linked to syphilis), intoxications (due to alcohol, cocaine, and so on), insanity at the age of involution (due to aging, such as senile dementia and melancholia), paranoia, general neuroses (such as epilepsy and hysteria), psychopathic states (such as constitutional depression, compulsive insanity, impulsive insanity, contrary sexual sensibility), insanity due to exhaustion, infectious insanity (due to infectious disease such as rabies, typhoid fever, and small pox), insanity in the encephaloses, thyreogenic insanity (metabolic insanities due to thyroid dysfunction), and inhibitions of psychic development (imbecility, idiocy). But it was the two great mental diseases of dementia praecox and manic-depressive insanity that captured the attention of clinicians and dominated their discourse to this very day.

First, dementia praecox.

"Let us be permitted, for the time being," wrote Kraepelin at the outset of his chapter on dementia praecox, "to class together under the name dementia praecox a series of clinical pictures whose common characteristic is that they result in *peculiar debilities.*" He then made a cautious statement about prognosis: "Although it seems that this unfavorable outcome need not occur in all cases without exception, it is so extremely common that we would like to continue to keep to the conventional designation for the time being. Other designations, such as the Italians 'demenza primitive' or the expression 'dementia simplex' preferred by Rieger, may be more apt." So again Kraepelin signaled that he was open to renaming his proposed disease. Then he firmly stated where he believed the biological site of the illness would one day be found: "In view of the clinical and anatomical facts known so far, I cannot doubt that we are dealing here with a serious, and, as a rule, at the most only partly reversible damage to the cerebral cortex."

Kraepelin then went on to say that dementia praecox manifests in three principle groups, the hebephrenic, catatonic, and paranoid, but that these are "connected to each other by fluid transitions" over the course of a patient's illness. Thus "the diversity of the clinical pictures which we observe in dementia praecox is very great."[40] However, they are united by a common course of exacerbations of psychotic symptoms followed by a permanent mental defect between episodes and prognosis of terminal dementia. Kraepelin listed hundreds of rich examples of typical statements, actions, and expressed feelings culled from his index cards on hundreds of patients, but presented no single case history that would give flesh to a living individual (a style that future generations, particularly those who followed Meyer or Freud, would criticize as cold, impersonal, and lacking empathy for the "facts" of the "whole person"). Yet if read in their entirety throughout the chapter, Kraepelin's mosaic-like, almost poetically incongruous compilation of the expressions of dementia praecox composes tableaux of insanity that colorfully punctuate the meaning behind his clinical vocabulary. What's more, Kraepelin's exacting quotation of the utterances of dementia praecox patients resonated with readers who worked in asylums. His style of presentation seemed to capture the melodies of madness in a recognizable form, simplifying diagnosis—indeed for many making it meaningful for the first time in their careers.

What were the three forms of dementia praecox? The *hebephrenic form* corresponded to the basic description of dementia praecox in the fifth edition of his textbook. This form was described earlier in the chapter.

The *catatonic form* encompassed most of those described by Kahlbaum as "special forms of the disease," but this form was characterized by "*peculiar states of stupor or agitation with the symptoms of negativism, stereotypy and suggestibility in expressive movements and actions, which states, in most cases, end in feeblemindedness.*"[41] Depression and a long period of "nervousness" are often the start of this illness, followed by hallucinations and delusions. The following description of these by Kraepelin gives a flavor of his writing style, and such paragraphs make up most of the German text of the seventy-eight pages he devoted to dementia praecox in this edition:

> In the sky there appears a white star, pictures of saints, Christ on the cross . . . color pictures are shown on the wall; angels, devils, ghosts, wild animals, snakes and the hellhound appear in the room; flames flare up;

human heads are in the food, worms in the soup. Outside, cocks crow, chains rattle, music plays, children wail. God speaks to the patient; the devil calls his name; the whole course of his life is recounted to him. People know his thoughts, talk about him, speak of "murder and such stories." . . . There are revelations, spiritual voices, "vocal interventions," ventriloquists; when the patient thinks something, he immediately hears it being related to others. In the room there is a vapor, mephitic air, a smell of death; in the meal there is human flesh and garbage. Electric currents circulate in his body; other people's blood is pumped into the patient's head and his penis made stiff; the bed makes gestures; "large frogs crawl into the mouth through the nose and ear."[42]

The *paranoid form* essentially corresponded to the disease Kraepelin described in the fifth edition as dementia paranoides. Now he believed it was a form of dementia praecox.

In both hebephrenia and catatonia, pronounced delusions are exceedingly common. But whereas in these form they usually fade away again after a comparatively short time, as a rule, we now have to envisage a group of clinical pictures in which, *aside from the symptoms of a rapidly developing mental deficiency in which the presence of mind remains wholly intact, delusions and in most cases hallucinations constitute the most prominent disturbances for many years.*[43]

According to Kraepelin, in the paranoid form delusions of persecution ("He has been poisoned, blown up by infernal machines and killed, but for his spirit, 2000 times. . . . His whole body has been melted down") and grandiosity ("The Good Lord has shown him everything; he can eat volcanoes, carries his brain on his shoulder. . . . He owns magnificent castles in foreign parts of the world") are the most common, and the hallucinations tended to be auditory, usually of voices.[44] Although these are also part of the clinical picture of the other two forms of dementia praecox, the difference is, Kraepelin noted, that in the paranoid form they seem to be more recalcitrant and fixed.

As in the 1896 edition, Kraepelin emphasized that dementia praecox was a disease of the younger period of life, and that 60 percent of his cases begin prior to the age of twenty-five. This was especially true for the hebephrenic and catatonic forms, whereas the paranoid form had a later average age of onset. Men dominated in the hebephrenic form and women in the other two forms. As to etiology, Kraepelin could only speculate. Hereditary predisposition was found to be in the background of about 70 percent of his cases, but Kraepelin cast doubt about heredity being the strongest cause of dementia praecox. As he did in the fifth edition, he held to the speculation that a process of autointoxication was responsible for affecting the brain: "The results obtained so far with the cortex do mostly speak for the supposition of chemical damage."[45]

Manic-depressive insanity was introduced in the 1899 sixth edition, in the opinion of the psychiatrist and historian David Healy, "as a foil to dementia praecox, rather than a worked out condition in its own right. . . . Kraepelin had to have a contrasting disorder that did not lead to cognitive and clinical decline."[46] There is certainly an element of truth in this. Manic-depressive insanity encompassed all the insanities whose primary symptoms were based in mood or affect, characterized by periodic manic states, depressed states, mixed states, or varying combinations thereof, which would wax and wane over the course of a person's life but leave no or little cognitive defect between episodes. In many cases the prognosis was good, certainly better than that of dementia praecox. Thus such individuals could be functionally normal between mood episodes and retain all of their cognitive abilities (volition, attention, memory, language, and so on). Kraepelin briefly speculated that manic-depressive insanity might be caused by a metabolic autointoxication, something that might potentially be treated or cured. A precursor to this disease in the 1896 fifth edition was "periodical insanity," an alternate term used in some American asylums in the early years of the Kraepelinian revolution in that country.

Manic-depressive insanity soon became a popular—or at least uncontroversial—diagnosis in the United States. It would take at least two decades before it took hold in Britain. It was eventually welcomed by most alienists worldwide with little debate—except in Germany, where it would meet with its greatest resistance, and to a lesser extent in France, where similar concepts such as *folie circulaire* ("circular insanity") had been in use since the 1850s. The French and the Germans had a long tradition of refusing to use each other's psychiatric terms anyway.[47] Compared to the troubled history of dementia praecox, manic–depressive insanity went relatively unquestioned, unchallenged, and, until the end of the twentieth century, unresearched.[48] August Hoch called manic-depressive insanity "one of the most brilliant achievements of the Heidelberg school." Adolf Meyer concurred.[49]

It was dementia praecox that vexed American alienists.

Adolf Meyer and August Hoch, two Europeans, had brought Kraepelin's concepts and methods to the United States. Foreign-born alienists were still a rarity in American asylums. Thus it should be remembered that men of the caliber of Hoch and Meyer, with training and accents that represented the superiority of German medicine, were regarded with a certain amount of awe by insecure American alienists. Thanks to the imprimatur of the eminent Edward Cowles, who had recommended Meyer for the pathologist position at Worcester in 1895 and who had hired Hoch in 1893, by 1900 both men were regarded as rising stars among the psychiatric elite in the American Medico-Psychological Association. Their relative youth, extensive training in European laboratories, and obvious zeal for introducing administrative and clinical reforms in American asylums set them apart from their American colleagues. Since the vast majority of American alienists did not regularly read the medical literature in English, let alone in German, French, Italian, or other foreign language, and since no part of Kraepelin's textbooks had been translated into English, from 1895 to 1900 Meyer and Hoch found themselves the primary disseminators of the new clinical approach of the Heidelberg school. Although the Worcester Lunatic Hospital and the McLean Hospital were the first beachheads of the Kraepelinian invasion of America—and the first institutions where insane patients were looked at in a new way and diagnosed with dementia praecox—it is arguable that the work of alienists of another institution in New England played a greater role in spreading knowledge of this mental disease.

The Connecticut Hospital for the Insane in Middletown was one of those overcrowded state hospitals where therapeutic nihilism reigned. Like the Worcester State Hospital, the daily census in the late 1890s swelled to almost two thousand insane patients. Electric lighting, telephone service between buildings on the large campus, and other modern innovations would not be introduced until after 1900. Although a simple pathology lab for analyzing specimens taken at autopsy had first been established in 1870, it had fallen into disuse by the end of the century. The institution had sunk into a dismal limbo for both its alienists and alienated insane.

All this would begin to change within a year. Fundamental changes in the leadership and medical staff of the institution brought fresh energies and ideas into the Middletown hospital. In 1898 Charles W. Page (1845–?), an 1870 graduate of Harvard Medical School with a keen interest in both clinical and laboratory innovations, was hired as superintendent. That same year Henry Smith Noble (1845–1915) was promoted from within to become assistant superintendent. In 1899 Allen Ross Diefendorf (1871–?) was brought in as the institution's new pathologist and chief of staff. That same year "the laboratory for clinical and pathological work was established" and "proved a valuable adjunct to the scientific work of the institution."[50] With these three men came a new spirit and attitude toward clinical psychiatry, influenced in no small part by Meyer and Hoch in nearby Massachusetts institutions. Diefendorf had worked directly under Meyer in Worcester from 1896 to 1898 before moving to Middletown. According to Meyer, "Through associating himself with Dr. Diefendorf while in Middletown, Conn., [Superintendent Page] had become acquainted with the Worcester plan of daily staff conferences."[51] But the switch to Kraepelin may have already taken place at Middletown before Diefendorf's arrival. Page had introduced the discussion of Kraepelin's concepts in the state asylum at Danvers, Massachusetts, where he was superintendent before moving to Middletown.

Under the leadership of Page, beginning in autumn of 1898 the Connecticut Hospital for the Insane in Middletown was the next American asylum to totally convert to Kraepelin's system. As Page wrote in the 1900 biennial report of the activities of the institution, "It has seemed expedient to change the [statistical] table which classifies the forms of insanity to conform to the views advanced by Prof. Kraepelin of Heidelberg. . . . Its merits appear to be so superior to the old system we no longer hesitate to make the substitution in the published reports of this Hospital."[52] However, although the statistical charts explicitly state that the diagnostic categories date from "the adoption of the present classification in 1898," they were taken from both Kraepelin's 1896 fifth edition of *Psychiatrie* ("periodical insanity") and the 1899 sixth edition (dementia praecox as composed of three forms: hebephrenic, catatonic, and paranoid). This indicates that a reanalysis of the dementia praecox patients was conducted prior to publishing the

statistical tables in the autumn of 1900. When the 2,620 persons admitted during the 1898–1900 period were counted according to diagnosis, by far the largest single portion, 30.7 percent, had been given a
diagnosis of dementia praecox. The second largest category was diagnosed with another Kraepelinian disease concept, periodical insanity
(14.8 percent), followed by senile dementia (10.8 percent) and general
paresis (6.3 percent).[53]

Time and again in the decades that followed, as one American asylum after another adopted Kraepelin's classification scheme, this pattern
would be replicated. Dementia praecox would often constitute the largest number of admissions, followed by "periodical insanity" or, after
1899, "manic-depressive insanity," in statistical second place. American
institutions would find themselves flooded with the disease of dementia
praecox, just as in the nineteenth century they swelled with cases of mania, melancholia, and dementia. What happened at Middletown was
only the beginning of a wave that would engulf hundreds of thousands
of Americans throughout the first half of the twentieth century.

One further observation should be made. In Page's report there is
no equivocation or indication that Kraepelin's classification and nosology were undergoing an exploratory probationary period at Middletown, as had been the case at McLean under Cowles and at Worcester
under Meyer (as he would claim in later years, when he attempted to
assert his own intellectual autonomy from Kraepelin). The new diagnostic boxes were firmly in place at Middletown, and there was no
turning back. Except for the early reservations of Cowles, there seems
to be no evidence of any significant resistance to the adoption of Kraepelin's classification and nosology by other American superintendents
in the years that followed. In the United States only Adolf Meyer and
his closest disciples would wage a stubborn—but ultimately futile—
campaign of protest in the first decades of the twentieth century.

Henry S. Noble took over the superintendent's position at Middletown from Page in October 1901. His biography is typical for many
American physicians and alienists of the late nineteenth century. He
had learned the blacksmith's trade from his father on his family's farm
in Vermont and believed in his youth that he would live out his life in
the same manner.[54] However, as he entered his teens, other ambitions
began to surface. He became an apprentice to a country doctor in Vermont before taking up formal medical studies, earning his M.D. in

1871 from the College of Physicians and Surgeons in New York. He was a general practitioner in rural Chester, Vermont, from 1872 to the fall of 1879. In 1880 he became an alienist at the Hartford Retreat in Connecticut, and later that year secured a position as assistant physician at the state asylum in Middletown. He left Connecticut for a two-year stint as an assistant physician at the Michigan State Hospital in Kalamazoo, then returned to his post at Middletown in 1884. Like many physicians of that era he went to Europe for further training, in the summer of 1886, and after he returned he was promoted to the position of first assistant physician at Middletown. Despite his long experience in asylums, Noble was somehow able to keep an open mind about the new developments in European psychiatry that were being applied at Worcester and McLean.

In the years 1900 and 1901 the first articles devoted to dementia praecox as the main topic were published in American medical journals. For the few in the psychiatric elite who read such journals this endowed dementia praecox with a certain validity as a disease. Noble was the author of one of these signal papers.[55] These early articles are instructive, for they give us an indication as to how Kraepelin and dementia praecox were perceived in light of the current beliefs and practices of alienists. They also demonstrate the inevitable process of the didactic simplification of not only Kraepelin's methods but also the diagnostic criteria of his diseases.

"We have all been familiar, in times past, with forms of insanity developing during the early period of life and culminating in the mental wreck of the individual at a comparatively young age," Noble wrote, referring to dementia praecox interchangeably with "precocious dementia." He credits Kraepelin with introducing a concept that leads to "the understanding of the disease as a whole . . . a comprehensive picture instead of a single phase or incident, however important." Under the old classification "the emotional state of the patient was the feature which determined into what group a case should fall; the manifestation of excitement was called mania, and that of depression, melancholia. Thus, the name of a single symptom, present during a single stage, was used to designate the disease." As the illness progressed and "dementia arrived," the diagnosis was simply changed from mania or melancholia to dementia. "We see, therefore, that the term precocious dementia covers many cases that we formerly knew as manias and mel-

ancholias, and likewise the terminal states of dementia which follow. . . . The same may be said of the insanities of masturbation, adolescence, etc." Much of the remainder of the paper summarizes
information taken from Kraepelin's sixth edition regarding the role of
heredity, sex differences, and defining characteristics of the hebephrenic, catatonic, and paranoid forms of dementia praecox. In referring to
Kraepelin's acknowledgment that 15 to 18 percent of the admissions to
his Heidelberg clinic were cases of dementia praecox, Noble omi-
nously reveals, "Our observations at the Connecticut Hospital for the
Insane during the past year compels us to believe that, in Connecticut
at least, the disease is considerably more frequent." He puts the figure
at 24 percent of all admissions. Noting that "the next in frequency was
Periodical Insanity in its various forms" in the previous fiscal year, he
attached great importance to the fact that 46 percent of all admissions
were due to these two disease forms.[56]

Two things immediately strike the reader of Noble's paper. The
first is that he does not regard the fact as troubling that he is finding
more dementia praecox at his institution than Kraepelin is finding at
his. He believes he understands Kraepelin's diagnostic concepts and that
he and his medical staff are applying them correctly. Exactly how they
are doing this is left unsaid. Noble instead alludes to possible demographic differences between Heidelberg and Middletown. Second, he is
equally untroubled by the fact that, prior to introducing Kraepelin's classification into Middletown, the diagnoses of mania and melancholia
made up 50 percent (and often more) of the admissions. Dementia praecox and periodical insanity (later manic-depressive illness) simply took
their place in the statistical tables of that asylum. Half of the madness in
an asylum could be accounted for by either of two terms. Where Kraepelin's terms seemed to have an advantage—perhaps the only advantage
over the older terms—is that they implied something about prognosis.

This had two advantages to American alienists toiling away in asylums, one humane and one inhumane. First, both patients and their
family members could be told something about the future. Would the
patient get better? A diagnosis of manic-depressive insanity would give
qualified hope. Second, and this is the shadow that dementia praecox
would cast over the next century, Kraepelin's dire prognosis for as
much as a quarter to a half of the institutionalized insane rationalized
their nontreatment, mistreatment, and failure to improve. From the

political perspective of asylum management, dementia praecox could be a useful construct.[57]

Noble concludes his article with a short table that compares and contrasts dementia praecox with periodical insanity so that his colleagues can make the proper differential diagnosis. He compares their different "prodromes" ("headache, insomnia, change of disposition" for dementia praecox; "lacking" for periodical insanity), onset (gradual versus sudden), psychomotor condition ("depression without retardation" versus "depression with retardation"), emotional attitude ("variable" versus "tolerably uniform"), consciousness ("clear" versus "disturbed"), course and final result ("progressive deterioration" versus "little deterioration"), and prognosis ("unfavorable" versus "favorable").[58] Given the fact that Kraepelin's writings had not been translated into English, and his ideas about these two diseases had not yet appeared in English-language psychiatric or neurological textbooks, simplifications such as Noble's may have been the only source of information for those few physicians and alienists eager to apply the latest medical concepts from Germany.

It would be Noble's colleague at Middletown, Allan Ross Diefendorf, who would do more than anyone else to bring Kraepelin's actual words to American alienists. Diefendorf was born into a family whose Dutch ancestors landed on American soil in the 1750s, and he and his siblings were raised in upstate New York. Diefendorf went to Yale University as an undergraduate and graduated from Yale Medical School in 1896. After graduation he was one of Adolf Meyer's junior assistant physicians at the Worcester Lunatic Hospital. By 1898 he had become second in command to Meyer. At Worcester he learned the extensive interviewing and record-keeping techniques demanded by Meyer, presided over daily case conferences, and conducted neuropathological work, including "the preparation of a valuable study of serial sections of the brain with complete isolation of the optic system in one hemisphere." He also—"on his own initiative," according to Meyer—began translating and adapting Kraepelin's textbook into English.[59] After a brief stint in the laboratory department of the Boston City Hospital in 1899 he accepted the pathologist and chief of staff position at Middletown. He also became a lecturer at Yale Medical School. While at Middletown he produced the first book-length translations of Emil Kraepelin's *Psychiatrie* into English, with translations of the 1899 sixth edition appearing in 1902 and the 1904 seventh edition appearing in 1907.[60] Diefendorf's translations became the primary vector for the spread of Kraepelin's concepts among American alienists who bothered to read the medical literature. Books, not journal articles, were far more likely to find their way into even the most rural or hopeless of the asylums.

Thus, with the efforts of Page, Noble, and Diefendorf at the Connecticut Hospital for the Insane at Middletown during the years 1898 to 1902, we see how Kraepelin and his disease slipped from the interpretive grasp of Hoch and Meyer and began a new, independent journey of transformation. Patients were now diagnosed by alienists who had never met Kraepelin, nor were these alienists supervised by anyone who had done so. Diefendorf's translation of Kraepelin's textbook allowed interested American physicians who could not read German to challenge the authority of Hoch and Meyer as the anointed interpreters of its contents.[61] New American "experts" on Kraepelin who had never been to Heidelberg ventured to summarize and explain his ideas in print, in lectures, and in their own asylums. Some were not even alienists.

Indeed neurologists were among the first American revisionists of dementia praecox. In a lengthy lecture to the American Neurological Association in June 1901 the Philadelphia neurologist Francis X. Dercum acknowledged his debt to Hecker, Kahlbaum, and Kraepelin, but admitted, "I can only briefly state my own interpretation [of dementia praecox]." Dercum criticized Kraepelin's concept as too limited because it did not include the whole class of paranoid, chronic, "systematized delusional insanity" that is often found in "mature adult life." He objected to "the absurdity of regarding as insanities of pubescence, cases beginning at thirty-five or forty-five years of age or later."[62] Another neurologist, speaking to the Philadelphia Neurological Society in December 1900, criticized Kraepelin for rendering "hebephrenia, the first described of all types of adolescent insanity," as now "the least definite of them," a mere undefined "group of the unclassified members of dementia praecox."[63] When compared to their neurologist colleagues during these early years of Kraepelin's reception, American alienists tended to accept, simplify, and apply, not criticize. That of course would come soon enough.

The first indication that dementia praecox had spread from the reservoir of New England asylums to the American heartland came in 1900. Gershom H. Hill (1846—?), superintendent of the Iowa Hospital for the Insane in Independence, presented a summary of Kraepelin's views on dementia praecox in May 1900 in Richmond, Virginia, at the annual meeting of the American Medico-Psychological Association. It was the first time in the history of American psychiatry that dementia praecox was the main subject of discussion at these annual meetings of the psychiatric elite. Hill published three almost identical versions of his presentation on dementia praecox in American medical journals—another first.[64] Why the first publications in the American medical literature devoted to dementia praecox should have come from an alienist in Iowa, who had never even trained in Europe, rather than Hoch, Meyer, or their associates remains a mystery.

Hill was born in Clayton County, Iowa. As a youth he worked on the farm of J. B. Grinnell, the founder of a town and a college of that name. A story that he told throughout his life ended up in a thumbnail biographical sketch by an Iowa historian: "One night in June, 1861, young Hill drove a wagon load of escaping slaves from Grinnell's house, which was a station on the 'underground railroad,' to Marengo, on their way to Canada and freedom."[65] In 1863 he briefly taught primary school, and in the summer of 1864 served in the Union Army in Tennessee during the Civil War. Later he went to Chicago and in 1874 earned his medical degree at Rush Medical College. The following year he took a position as assistant physician at the state asylum in Independence, Iowa, and in 1881 was elevated to superintendent. There is nothing in Hill's background to indicate his reception to the new ideas coming from Heidelberg, but he may have had contact with Adolf Meyer. In a statement made in 1901 Hill indicated that he may have been applying Meyer's procedures for more intensive record keeping, as well as those for integrating the pathology laboratory with the clinical work on the wards, as early as the autumn of 1898.[66] In another paper published that year he stated that he had six physicians on staff and that they met daily for an hour-long case conference. "In our attempts to study mental derangements scientifically we are using the method of Kraepelin as our guide. There are a few hospitals in New England in which insanity is now studied in the same manner. . . . We look at the outset for the prognosis."[67]

Hill's AMPA presentation in May 1900 was an unremarkable and superficial sketch of Kraepelin's basic ideas about dementia praecox and its three forms. His talk followed one on the issue of primary dementia, a diagnosis for permanent mental weakness or cognitive defect of relatively recent onset found in those who were not yet "senile" (a condition that was then called "senile dementia" or "terminal dementia"). Similarities between primary dementia and the new dementia praecox were noted by Hill. What *was* remarkable, however, were some of the comments made by some prominent alienists in his audience.

"I believe the Kraepelin system of classification will eventually prevail," predicted Charles W. Page from the Connecticut Hospital for the Insane at Middletown.

> Since the adoption of the Kraepelin system, a year ago, every new case is made the subject of a clinic before the full staff, meetings for that purpose being held daily, and the various assistants alternating in taking charge of the clinic. After a year's work according to this method of study and classification, these gentlemen have found a fresh interest in the study of insanity, and more satisfaction than ever before in classifying mental diseases. All consider the Kraepelin system a great advance over previous methods, both as regards classification, general management and clearness of the distinction between the several forms of mental affection.[68]

Here again in Page's statement is an admission that the adoption of Kraepelin's system made the patients more interesting to the alienists; the temptation is to interpret its impact mostly as an antidote to the learned helplessness that afflicted so many American alienists in asylums across the country. The patients were more creatively classified, and certainly more attention was now being paid to them, but traditional asylum therapeutics remained the same.

Perhaps the most revealing comment came from the superintendent of the City Asylum in St. Louis, Edward C. Runge. His confession should be considered carefully; it was probably echoed by most asylum alienists as one institution after another adopted Kraepelin for their classification of the insanities. "I personally have not the time to work out any new schemes," he said, "either as to classification or scientific research. In going through the wards there are many cases which puzzle us, and we do not know how to classify them. I have found dementia praecox a very comfortable, I may say vulgarly, dumping ground."[69]

In the first five years of the new century Kraepelin's classification marched through both asylums and, eventually, general hospitals. The classification of diseases was not only a problem for psychiatry; it was also a pressing issue in general medicine. Nomenclature was an issue as well, for physicians were wont to use a fluid variety of diagnostic terms for identical conditions. In 1903 Bellevue Hospital in New York City attempted to resolve this issue by adopting a uniform system of classification and nomenclature of diseases and other medical conditions as part of an effort to improve record keeping. The Bellevue system was eventually adopted by many large general hospitals in the northeastern United States and had an impact nationally. Because Bellevue had long maintained a reception pavilion (acute ward) for insanity cases, the new uniform classification scheme included psychiatric diagnoses. Among them were Kraepelin's diseases: dementia praecox (in its three forms) and manic-depressive insanity.[70]

Of all the asylums and state hospitals in the United States that converted to Kraepelin, the Manhattan State Hospital on Ward's Island was perhaps the biggest prize. It was the flagship institution of the entire New York State system and, since December 1902, was the site of the laboratories of the Pathological Institute of the New York State Hospitals. In 1904 the Manhattan State Hospital became the first in the state system to adopt a new diagnostic classification scheme for its statistics. As I discuss in a later chapter, Adolf Meyer, by then the director of the Pathological Institute, reluctantly played a key role in this development.

The conditions on Ward's Island were nightmarish. Until they were consolidated into one hospital in 1905, Manhattan State Hospital was divided into branches, West and East, each with its own superintendent (E. C. Dent and A. E. Macdonald, respectively) and separate annual reports. Overcrowding had swelled the combined census of these two complexes to almost four thousand insane patients. The buildings could not contain this crush of humanity. Since 1901 hundreds of patients had lived in tents in year-round "camps" (named A, B, C, D, and so on). A large ferry named *The Wanderer* brought new patients from the reception pavilion at Bellevue Hospital across the East River in Manhattan. "[Sixty] or 70 new patients might be brought at one crossing," remembered an alienist who was there. "They were representative of many races, and exhibited a vast variety of clinical states."[71] For transport across the river they were most likely heavily drugged. Bellevue was continually urged to funnel new patients to other institutions, such as the newer state hospital in Central Islip, Long Island.

The annual report of the consolidated institution for the year 1 October 1904 to 30 September 1905 is a vivid illustration of American psychiatry in transition.[72] As had the Manhattan State Hospital in its previous, separate annual reports, all of the other state hospitals submitted statistical tables using non-Kraepelinian terms as diagnoses for the 1904–5 fiscal year.[73] But now, at Manhattan State, separate diagnostic boxes were presented for dementia praecox (148 cases), dementia praecox (paranoid) (55 cases), dementia praecox (hebephrenic) (14 cases), dementia praecox (katatonic) (12 cases), and dementia praecox (allied) (24 cases). The report separated the 232 cases of the various forms of dementia praecox from the additional 24 mystery cases that were believed to be "allied to dementia praecox." In a year in which there were 810 new admissions, dementia praecox replaced the previous year's "mania" as by far the most prevalent disease diagnosed by the alienists at Manhattan State, swallowing up 29 percent of all new admissions.

"This grouping [dementia praecox] is by far the most comprehensive in our nosology," noted Superintendant E. C. Dent in his report. The disease was "a retrogressive developmental psychosis for which we as yet have no acceptable pathological anatomical basis. It is reeking with the stigmata and transmissions of many generations. . . . Having an unfavorable prognosis, it is undesirable and clearly prejudicial to make a diagnosis in many cases, unless the diagnostic features are clearly established."[74] This reference to the intergeneration transmission of "stigmata" indicates that Dent believed Kraepelin's disease was due to hereditary degeneration.

Manic depressive insanity was the second most commonly diagnosed mental disease in the first year of its use as a category of madness. Like dementia praecox, it was separated into various forms: manic depressive insanity (40 cases), manic depressive insanity (depressive type) (13 cases), manic depressive insanity (manic type) (32 cases), manic depressive insanity (mixed type) (2 cases), and manic depressive insanity (allied) (22 cases). This diagnosis comprised 87 cases, with an additional 22 that were thought might be "allied" to it. Manic depressive insanity was thus found in 11 percent of all new admissions. "A large percentage of our recoveries is drawn from this type of insanity," the author of the report admitted.[75] The next two most commonly diagnosed conditions were "Paranoic Conditions" (77 cases, or 9.5 percent of the total), and "Alcoholic Psychoses" (68 cases, or 8 percent of the total).

These statistics fit a pattern that had been repeating itself in American asylums and state hospitals since 1898: the first year that Kraepelinian diagnoses appeared in the statistical tables of an asylum's annual report dementia praecox and manic-depressive insanity were often the two most prevalent diseases observed in new admissions, sometimes together constituting more than 50 percent of the total. This pattern of ranking persisted in American state hospitals until well into the twentieth century.[76] In the case of the Manhattan State Hospital during 1904–5, a full 40 percent of new admissions had either dementia praecox or manic-depressive insanity.

Why did institutions make the decision to adopt the new classifications from Kraepelin? Institutions followed the conversions of superintendents, individual by individual. It should be emphasized that such decisions were made by the superintendents for a variety of reasons. Perhaps there was a genuine scientific interest in the latest trends of German psychiatry. Perhaps it was the desire to emulate respected figures and institutions, such as Cowles at McLean and Meyer at Worcester. Perhaps it was a reflection of the growing professionalization of psychiatry, an indication that some superintendents and assistant physicians "began to care more for the approval and esteem of their disciplinary colleagues than they did for the ordinary standards of success in the society that surrounded them . . . not simply a transfer of scientific data and laboratory techniques [from Germany] but of values and attitudes as well."[77] Perhaps, as may have been the case in the New York State system, they felt they had no choice due to pressure from more powerful state officials.

But once a superintendent converted (with or without administrative coercion from above), the medical staff had to follow. And they were not pleased or impressed. "Oh, this is a new fad," said some alienists in the New York system. Others said, "This is just the method of Kraepelin and in a few years we'll have another one."[78] Comments like these indicate that, at the level of the assistant physician, the grand ideas of the American psychiatric elite were taken with a grain of salt. The average asylum alienist used these categories because they were told to by their bosses; it was just a new part of their job, that's all.

Once these new diagnostic boxes were learned, however, it was found that dementia praecox could be applied to just about any new insane patient, especially the young ones. It became a useful, even preferred, diagnosis.

In 1905 Clarence B. Farrar (1874–1969), then an assistant physician and director of the Laboratory of the Sheppard and Enoch Pratt Hospital in Baltimore, compared annual report statistics from nine northeastern asylums and state hospitals, documenting the familiar pattern in a series of graphs for four of the seven institutions in his sample that had converted to Kraepelin between 1896 and 1905. "The diagnosis has had the ill-fortune to be a popular one," Farrar observed in his article. "The tendency among adherents of a new school to out-Herod Herod is in part responsible for the unusual hypertrophy which the new disease concept first undergoes."[79] How the alienists were making such determinations is anyone's guess. But perhaps it didn't matter. Jules Christian (1840–1907) of Alsace, a French expert on hebephrenia, certainly didn't think so: "A mistaken diagnosis is really of little importance, in either case the only thing that can be done is to render their existence as pleasant as possible."[80]

Perhaps valid methods for applying Kraepelin's disease categories could be followed only in small clinics, such the one in Heidelberg, with a daily census no greater than 120 patients who were serviced by four to six highly trained and motivated physicians. Kraepelin insisted on a careful (if, by 1893, an increasingly rapid) diagnostic process, including follow-up studies, which required an intellectual focus and time commitment that harried American alienists swimming in a cauldron of thousands of insane patients simply did not have. More likely than not most patients admitted to large institutions were rapidly interviewed and instantly diagnosed based on only one or two diagnostic features they were told had been identified by Kraepelin. There was "a tendency to consider an actual study of the patient's condition sufficient if it yields a few shabby facts thought to be needed for a lofty diagnosis of 'manic-depressive insanity' or of 'dementia praecox.'"[81] Whereas American alienists may have mastered the new terms of disease, it is unreasonable to think that most changed their daily style of making snap clinical judgments. Still, institutional size may not have been the most important variable driving the phantom epidemic of dementia praecox; after all, in 1901 Kraepelin himself, together with his Heidelberg associates, diagnosed 51 percent of the new admissions to their clinic with this disease.[82] However, the question remains: What were the textual sources—if any—of the American alienists' diagnostic criteria? Whether the alienists were using single-page, typewritten outlines of Kraepelin's classification scheme (the most likely situation), Kraepelin's own texts in German (the least likely situation), Diefendorf's translations, journal articles by American and British interpreters or translations from German or French authorities, or the chapters on dementia praecox and manic-depressive insanity found in textbooks such as that by Stewart Paton—a 1905 work that is regarded as the first "modern" textbook in American psychiatry—is unknown.[83] What *is* known is that after yet another year in which dementia praecox admissions flooded the Manhattan State Hospital, one of its exasperated assistant physicians would ask, "Is dementia praecox the new peril in psychiatry?"[84]

5

THE LOST BIOLOGICAL PSYCHIATRY

In the year 1895 no one in the United States suffered from the disease of dementia praecox. By 1905 the number of people who had been given such a diagnosis could be counted in the thousands. Simply put, in 1895 it did not exist; in 1905, for many Americans, it did.

Historians of medicine and sociologists of science have long been intrigued by the genesis and development of scientific "facts." This has been particularly true for concepts in the biological sciences relating to disease and health.[1] Repeatedly in the history of medicine—and especially in the history of psychiatry—there are moments separated by what the French sociologist of science Georges Canguilhem called "discontinuities," discernable conceptual and social breaks (sometimes interpreted at the time as break*throughs*) in which new sciences appear to spring from nothing, develop rapidly, and expand the social distance between the experts who possess such novel scientific knowledge and those less expert, who then must translate such claims to new "truth" into simplifications of thought and language for the purpose of communicating them to those with no expertise whatsoever.

The year 1896 marked just such a discontinuity in the history of psychiatry. Following the publication of the fifth edition of *Psychiatrie* in 1896, Emil Kraepelin and his colleagues in Heidelberg introduced a new vision of mental disease into medical discourse, both in print and in person. They also created new mental diseases and new methods for diagnosing them. By the autumn of 1896 there were very personal, face-to-face transmissions of this expert knowledge from Adolf Meyer to primarily uneducated or undereducated persons in extreme states of distress and alienation who were, in all likelihood, incarcerated against their will in a lunatic hospital in Worcester, Massachusetts. Thousands of similar conversations would take place in other American asylums in the years that followed. Dementia praecox descended from the medical elites of Germany into the lowest social strata of everyday American life with railroad speed.

What were these patients told about their illness? Certainly they were told the name of their disease, an ominous and unfamiliar pair of words that, just by their sound, indicated the gravity of the situation. Perhaps they were told of its prognosis. Certainly family members and friends were informed of its incurability. Possibly they were told they had inherited it, that they were the end products of a tainted family line, or that some unknown disease process in their body had sent poisons to their brain. We will never know how such conversations were conducted nor fully understand the emotional effect such physician-patient interactions had on the insane and their families.[2]

In truth these few details about dementia praecox probably reflected the extent of the knowledge of most American alienists about this affliction in 1905. For many struggling to learn the new terms, Kraepelinian classification seemed more like a demand than a method. For those convinced their wards reeked with the human filth of hereditary degeneration, the diagnosis of dementia praecox was a morality more than a theory.

The importance of this first victory in the Kraepelinian revolution—the acceptance of a new classification by prognosis and a new nomenclature—was only the first step in making dementia praecox a "real" disease, a scientific "fact." Physicians told patients they were sick and there was a name for their disease; that alone was a powerful enough dynamic in making dementia praecox real. Certainly *insanity* was real, as real as sin or error or bad blood. And it was real because it was biological. That was the common belief in 1905. Even the widespread condition of "nervousness," or neurasthenia, which was not considered insanity, was presumed to be a biological response to stress, poor nutrition, and toxins. But if insanity was not a unitary psychosis, a single spectrum of madness, this would mean that each of Kraepelin's diseases must have something biologically unique about them, something that distinguishes them from each other and from sanity. Hooking the dementia praecox concept to a set of biological findings, whether through clinical observations made of patients in the examining room, findings at autopsy, or discoveries in the laboratory, was the second necessary agenda in making it a scientific fact. From a historical perspective, the reception of a new disease concept is not only evidenced by its use by physicians and its appearance in publications, but also when it frames laboratory research, when it becomes an object to study. That is the path to disease specification.

But where to look? What to study? What was relevant? What was irrelevant? This is where theory, but also serendipity, came in.

Before the laboratory came the clinic. Observations made during the physical examination of the insane patient by the doctor were considered highly relevant to the insanity itself. The general physique of the patient, the size and shape of the head and the ears, the color and texture of the skin, the behavior of the eyes, body odor, the pulse and blood pressure—all of these signs were significant to the alienist or neurologist of the late nineteenth century and early twentieth. For many physicians abnormal physical traits were interpreted as stigmata of hereditary degeneration and supported the belief widely held, even by Emil Kraepelin, that heredity at least played a role in the predisposition to insanity, if not causing it directly. But such features of the patient's condition were routinely reported by alienists for a larger purpose: they might one day be found to be biological markers of madness. In the case of dementia praecox, a cluster of physical signs that any doctor could easily observe in the examining room became part of the biological concept of the disease, making it a real phenomenon that could be seen by anyone with medical knowledge. This was of particular importance to many alienists and older physicians of that era who had never conducted laboratory research, did not understand laboratory research, and did not trust it. The use of the five senses in the ancient doctor-patient dyad extended to a diagnosis of dementia praecox as much as it did to a diagnosis of asthma.

In 1899 Kraepelin described a series of observations in the physical field that set the pattern for such discussions of dementia praecox

by American alienists, neurologists, and other physicians in the first decade of the twentieth century. Many case histories would mention
whether each sign was present or not upon examination as they followed
Kraepelin's biological template. After first describing some instances of
convulsive-like "fits" that some of his patients had just prior to the first
onset of their symptoms, Kraepelin provided a summary of physical signs
that could be followed by any physician in private practice or in a clinic
attempting to verify (that is, make a "scientific fact" of) dementia praecox in a person who was also exhibiting psychotic symptoms:

> The tendon reflexes are generally heightened, often very greatly; in
> many cases there is also increased mechanical excitability of the muscles
> and nerves. The pupils are frequently strikingly dilated, particularly in
> the states of excitement; now and then, distinct but changing pupillary
> difference is observed, and also restlessness of the eyeball. Also com-
> mon are vasomotor disturbances, cyanosis, localized edema and dermo-
> graphia in all gradations; in certain cases there is strong perspiration.
> Salivation appears to be increased in many cases. . . . Cardiac activity is
> subject to great variations, now slowed down, more often slightly ac-
> celerated, often also weak and irregular. The body temperature is
> mostly low; I once saw it go down to 33.8 C. Menstruation tends to
> cease or become irregular.[3]

It is clear from passages like these that when a patient with dementia praecox came under the physician's gaze, Kraepelin's disease was
not simply a disease of the brain. The psychic symptoms—lasting cognitive defects, delusions, hallucinations, and so on—certainly implicated
the cerebral cortex of the brain in the disease process. But many of the
physical signs—abnormalities in reflex responses, eye movement and
pupil activity, and heart rate—pointed elsewhere: to the brain stem, sub-
cortical structures, and especially to the peripheral nervous system, particularly the involuntary or autonomic division that in Kraepelin's day
was often referred to as the "vegetative" nervous system. Dementia praecox was not just a central nervous system disease; it was systemic and
involved other nerves and organs in the body. Remember that Kraepelin
had observed similar abnormal responses of the autonomic nervous system when he had conducted his experimental studies of artificially induced psychoses when his subjects were under the influence of drugs or
other chemicals. For example, the behavior of the pupils of the eyes in

artificially induced psychoses and in dementia praecox were of great significance to him. This earlier work in experimental pharmacopsychology would provide an analogical bridge—the effect of chemicals on the functioning of both the central and vegetative nervous systems—to his later dementia praecox concept.

In the 1896 fifth edition of *Psychiatrie* Kraepelin had included dementia praecox as one of many "Metabolic Diseases" *(Die Stoffwechselerkrankungen)*, along with dementia paralytica (general paresis or paralysis, later proven to be due to tertiary syphilis), myxodematous insanity and cretinism (both caused by thyroid dysfunction), and two diseases that would later become part of the dementia praecox concept, katatonia and dementia paranoides. As was noted earlier, in 1896 Adolf Meyer had correctly criticized this diagnosis by presumed etiology as baseless. Dementia praecox was removed from any such grouping of metabolic disorders in the 1899 sixth edition, but Kraepelin was not willing to let go of the cognitive connection. It survived in his description of a set of physical signs pointing to a metabolic (endocrine) disturbance that, in his mind, kept his causal speculation in contention. He wrote:

> I very often observed diffused enlargement of the thyroid gland, occasionally the disappearance of such enlargements immediately prior to the first appearance of the symptoms, and also repeated rapid changes in the size of the gland during the development of the illness. In single cases there was exophthalmus and trembling. Finally, we and the patients' relatives were quite often struck by the myxedematous thickenings of the skin, particularly in the face. Unfortunately, these findings cannot be further utilized for the time being, owing to the frequency of cretinistic traces in our country. Anemic conditions seem to be very common. Sugar was found in the urine once, and once there was polyuria.[4]

Such observations of the presentation of the physical symptoms of dementia praecox in the clinic were an important aspect of the "biological psychiatry" of the early twentieth century.

Following the first American publications concerning dementia praecox, in 1900 and 1901, which essentially summarized Kraepelin's diagnosis by prognosis and included brief descriptions of the three forms of the disease, the next wave of publications came from physicians who reported one or more case histories of persons they had diagnosed with dementia praecox. The earliest American contributions were a series published by William Rush Dunton Jr. (1868–1966), an assistant physician at the Sheppard and Enoch Pratt Hospital in Towson, Maryland, near Baltimore. Like the Connecticut Hospital for the Insane in Middletown, this was an influential locus for the reframing of dementia praecox in America. In these early years Dunton worked at Sheppard Pratt with Stewart Paton, Clarence B. Farrar, Francis Barnes, and William Burgess Cornell, all of whom made contributions to the American medical literature on dementia praecox between 1902 and 1912.

Dunton came from a distinguished medical family. He was a distant nephew of Benjamin Rush, a signer of the Declaration of Independence and a man regarded as the first true alienist in the United States. Dunton graduated from the University of Pennsylvania Medical School in 1893 and then went to Johns Hopkins, where he received further training. He left Hopkins to become an assistant at the Sheppard Asylum, a precursor to the Hospital. Although he is remembered for his pioneering efforts during World War I to institute occupational therapy in asylums, his early publications on dementia praecox are also noteworthy, for they were the first of their kind in American medical journals.

In 1902 Dunton published a paper based on cases of dementia praecox he had encountered while working in the neurological clinic of the Johns Hopkins Dispensary. He argued that neurologists were better situated than asylum alienists to make scientific observations about dementia praecox: "The physicians in general practice and the neurologist have a much better opportunity to observe the early symptoms of mental trouble than the alienist, and it is toward the former that we should look for an increase of our knowledge." In his article he described the cases of three female patients (ages seventeen, twenty-one, and thirty-three) whom he believed presented with signs and symptoms consistent with the beginning stage of the illness. "Certain symptoms which I have observed seem to me to be of no little diagnostic importance in differentiating neurasthenia with depression from the initial stage of dementia praecox. . . . There is a symptom noted by Kraepelin, but not emphasized by him, which I have seen exhibited in a very pronounced manner in a number of cases. . . . This is the mechanical irritability of the facial nerve which when present and associated with mental aberration is of diagnostic value."[5]

In the young woman in his first case example Dunton noticed a series of signs that corresponded with others that Kraepelin had observed and reported in his textbooks: "a sallow complexion," anemia, "dermatographia," and an irregular pulse. In the second case there was "psychomotor retardation, a slight reaction on tapping over the facial nerve, active reflexes, occasional auditory hallucinations, and a mild degree of dementia." In addition to the facial nerve reaction, which he elicited by gently tapping the cheeks of his patients with a percussion hammer, he argued, "[The] psycho-motor retardation [is] of value from a diagnostic standpoint. It has been present in every case of dementia praecox that I have seen." Continuing to follow Kraepelin as a guide he added, "The increase in the reflexes is most important as a means of diagnosis. In every case of dementia praecox I have seen, the knee-jerks and other tendon reflexes have been exaggerated. The superficial reflexes are also increased." In his third brief case example no physical signs are detailed; instead Dunton uses the described behavior as an illustration of "negativism": "silly, purposeless resistance to every external impulse."[6] He followed these articles with two publications detailing the autopsy findings of two patients with dementia praecox—also a first in the American literature.[7]

A few years later Dunton published a short communication in which he backed off from his early enthusiasm for the mechanical irritability of the facial nerve as a diagnostic sign of dementia praecox. What had seemed a serendipitous scientific finding about the illness had faded in significance over time. "It must be remembered that the physical signs of dementia praecox are multiform and it is usually a mistake to give undue prominence to any one symptom, which mistake I believed I made in my paper."[8] Other authors alerted physicians to look for the cyanosis in the hands of dementia praecox patients as a way of distinguishing them from manic-depressive patients, or to be aware of a series of eye symptoms unique to the disease that would confirm an early diagnosis of dementia praecox.[9]

Dunton's pioneering publications give us a useful perspective on how American physicians were interpreting dementia praecox as a legitimate, real disease. In them Dunton made four points. First, dementia praecox was a biological disease that affected both the central (brain function) and peripheral (reflexes) nervous systems. Second, any physician, but especially neurologists, could confirm a diagnosis of dementia praecox in an insane person through a physical examination that could be done in any private practice office or clinic, and without the need for any laboratory analyses of the blood, sputum, urine, or feces. Third, autopsy findings, including those for the gross anatomy of the brain as well as the condition at the cellular level, did not yield signs of pathology in two persons with dementia praecox he had examined. Fourth, a point he made at the end of his second autopsy report when he again found nothing neurologically remarkable, "in dementia praecox we are dealing with a degenerative psychosis, probably of autotoxic origin, and of slow course," which is "probably emanating from the reproductive organs."[10]

After the battles to win acceptance of Kraepelin's classification system and nomenclature it was inevitable that the issue of *etiology* would surface. In the first decade of the twentieth century etiology would replace classification and nomenclature as the flashpoint in debates about Kraepelin's disease. Criticism of these latter issues would not entirely go away, but the attention of the psychiatric elite who published in medical journals did markedly shift to etiology.

In 1896 Kraepelin had introduced a method of diagnosing mental diseases that was not based on *just* the signs and symptoms of the patient at first presentation, nor did it depend on diagnosis through presumed cause (hereditary degeneration, masturbation insanity, puerperal insanity, "metabolic diseases," and so on). Kraepelin had dethroned etiology. According to him, knowledge of the cause was often irrelevant to understanding course and outcome. He had found an intellectual path around the sink hole of speculation about causes. But he himself was not immune from such musings. In every edition of his textbook, for every one of the "functional" psychoses (those for which no biological cause was known), he could not resist the temptation to devote a few sentences to possible causes. And for both dementia praecox and manic–depressive insanity, he believed that autointoxication, some sort of self-poisoning process in the body, would one day be found to be at the root of these diseases.

With the return of etiology as a concern, in the new century the psychiatric elite divided into two camps that were characterized as the "mind twist men" (those who held to psychogenic theories) and the "brain spot men" (those who held to brain disease theories).[11] Historians of psychiatry have likewise portrayed this period in this dualistic fashion (as we have seen with such designations as "the crisis of the somatic style" or "the end of the first biological psychiatry"). But neither somaticism nor biological psychiatry disappeared. In truth, when the literature of the era is examined carefully an argument can be made that a vibrant and quite dominant biological paradigm for understanding mental diseases between the 1890s and the 1930s existed as a third option: autointoxication.

Autointoxication theories informed theories of etiology, course, signs and symptoms, prevention, therapeutics, and even cure. Because neither one's heredity nor one's brain disease could be "fixed" or "corrected" in any way by alienists, neurologists, or surgeons, autointoxication theories opened a creative field of possibilities for speculation and, most important, laboratory research. And such laboratory research in psychiatry, despite its abject failure, did more to enhance psychiatry's image as a medical science worthy of rejoining the American medical profession in the early twentieth century than did the dwindling number of postmortem studies of the brain anatomy of the insane. Autointoxication therefore was a significant scientific and cultural force in the "lost biological psychiatry" in histories of early twentieth-century American medicine.

To fully understand Kraepelin's conception of dementia praecox, and those who adopted it, we must first understand the medical world in which he lived and worked. The cognitive categories of that era shaped the thoughts, feelings, and behaviors of its actors. It was an era energized by the laboratory revolution in medicine and the resulting rise of bacteriology in the 1870s, endocrinology in the 1890s, and serology and immunology in the first decade of the twentieth century. Each of these new medical sciences played a role in framing the various theories of autointoxication. Autointoxication had the potential to be a unifying theory in medicine that could link these emerging medical sciences with older ones such as physiology, pathology, gynecology, neurology, and even surgery. American psychiatry reentered mainstream medicine in part through the adoption of these theories. They were highly regarded in their time, but vanished by the mid-1930s.[12]

Among the learned elites of medicine, if not among the majority of practicing physicians, by 1880 the germ theory of disease and the new medical science of Louis Pasteur of France and Robert Koch of Germany, bacteriology, offered a novel and potentially fruitful paradigm for comprehending the causes of illness.[13] Following the replicable laboratory demonstration that bacteria, or microbes, were involved in processes such as putrefaction, fermentation, and infection, it was a natural analogical leap to hypothesize that they were involved in the etiology and pathophysiology of many, if not most, diseases. The applicability of the germ theory of disease to the study of insanity was suggested in the American literature as early as 1874 by Theodore Deeke, the pathologist of the New York State Lunatic Asylum in Utica.[14]

By the late 1880s it was argued that diseases were not caused by microbes acting directly, but by the toxins they produced. Poisonous ptomaines (the products of proteins formed in putrefaction), or "toxalbumins," were formed that could be circulated by the body's bloodstream and potentially produce a wide variety of diseases affecting every organ. The excitement generated by this idea in the medical world and popular culture of the late nineteenth century and early twentieth can be compared to the perceived promise of molecular genetics research and its hypothesis of genes as a unifying explanatory principle in the medical world and popular culture of the late twentieth century and early twenty-first.

In the original, classical autointoxication theory, the intestines were most often cited as the locus of this systemic self-poisoning process, with the kidneys and the liver assuming lesser importance in theoretical speculation. The terms "intestinal autointoxication" and "gastrointestinal autointoxication" were those most often used in the literature of that era. In later years this variant of autointoxication theory would be called "focal infection" or "focal sepsis." Beginning around 1900 the teeth, gums, and tonsils were increasingly cited as the original source of the pathogens that would spread throughout the body and infect various organs and tissues.

A second variant of autointoxication theory arose in the 1890s, when endocrinology began to emerge out of physiology as a distinct discipline of clinical and research medicine. The French physiologist and neurologist C.-E. Brown-Sequard (1817–1894) and his assistant Arsene d'Arsonval (1851–1940) published an article in April 1891 in which they proposed that disease could result from the lack of production of "internal secretions" in animal tissues; this newly posited pathogenic mechanism was incorporated into autointoxication theory.[15] The work of the British physiologist George Redmayne Murray (1865–1939), who in

1891 discovered the cure of myxoedema by the subcutaneous injection of thyroid extract, particularly intrigued Kraepelin. By 1900 the over- or underproduction of "internal secretions" in the organs of the body were posited as the cause of a wide variety of diseases, both physical and mental. It was this "interstitial" or "metabolic autointoxication" theory that influenced most biological psychiatrists in the first three decades of the twentieth century.

The disease theory of autointoxication first appeared in the German medical literature. Hermann Senator (1834–1911), a clinical professor of medicine at Berlin University in Prussia, had speculated as early as 1868 that "self-infection" *(Selbstinfektion)* arising in the intestines could be a source of disease elsewhere in the body. Later he argued that mental disturbances could be caused by this process, claiming that the acute delirium of diabetic coma may have its origin in *Selbstinfektion*.[16]

However, it was the work of French physicians that fueled the rapid expansion of this theory to all categories of disease, including mental disorders. Autointoxication theory rose to international prominence in medicine after the 1887 publication of *Leçons sur les auto-intoxications dans les maladies* by Charles Jacques Bouchard (1837–1915), an early student of Charcot's and an eminent professor of pathology at the University of Paris.[17] For both Senator and Bouchard, the founders of autointoxication theory, the disease-causing poisons were the products of putrefactive processes in the intestines. Although these putrefactive processes are a normal part of the digestive process, under certain conditions (such as fecal stasis) the overproduction of these toxins could not be filtered by the liver or kidneys and, as they entered other organs, disease would result. Bouchard's vision of the inner life of the human body is dramatic: "I have said that the organism, in its normal, as in its pathological state, is a receptacle and a laboratory of poisons. . . . Man is in this way constantly living under the chance of being poisoned; he is always working toward his own destruction; he makes continual attempts at suicide by intoxication."[18]

It is not until 1893, however, that we find the first indications that autointoxication theory is being seriously discussed as a possible etiology for mental disorders. On 1 August of that year, at the fourth session of the French Congress of Psychological Medicine held in La Rochelle, the *rapporteurs* François-Andre Chevalier-Lavaure, a physician from Aix-en-Provence, and Emmanuel Regis, a physician from Bordeaux, drew attention to the value of autointoxication as a possible organic cause of madness by organizing and leading a panel titled "Auto-intoxication in Mental Disease." This topic had been the subject of Chevalier-Lavaure's doctoral dissertation in 1890. In their presentation they argued that it was difficult to distinguish between cases of autoin-toxication and those of infection from sources outside the body, but that a clear diagnostic distinction should be made between "infectious' insanity"(mental disturbances following acute infectious diseases, such as meningio-encephalitis) and "visceral insanity," which is "associated with disease of the internal organs" and is "also very probably due to autointoxication."[19]

When Bouchard's book first appeared in English in January 1894 Thomas Oliver noted in his translator's preface, "The part played by auto-intoxication in mental diseases is attracting attention."[20] In 1895 extensions of autointoxication theory to psychiatry were offered in the German medical literature by D. E. Jacobson of Copenhagen and in the American medical literature by Albert E. Sterne of Indianapolis and the neurologist Francis X. Dercum of Philadelphia.[21] Even Julius von Wagner-Jauregg (1857–1940), who would later win a Nobel Prize for his therapy for neurosyphilis, speculated that disturbed mental states may be caused by the influence of intestinal toxins on brain cells.[22] The gastrointestinal tract continued to be the most often cited etiologic locus of "autointoxication psychoses" in psychiatric circles.[23]

The rise of the bacteriological paradigm after 1880 had initiated and fueled autointoxication theory. Between 1890 and 1905, the year the English physiologist Ernest Starling (1866–1927) first proposed the modern concept of the hormone, advances in the understanding of metabolic processes and the endocrine system added a new endogenous etiological hypothesis: metabolic or "interstitial autointoxication" due to the over- or underproduction of internal secretions in the organs with ducts (liver, pancreas, and kidney), those without ducts (thyroid, adre-nals, pituitary), and especially the sex glands (gonads). Prior to World War I there was considerable confusion in the emerging discipline of endocrinology regarding the nature of hormones and their similarities to enzymes, general metabolites, toxins, antitoxins, and vitamins. Some researchers proposed that several of these latter substances, when imbal-anced in the body, could be the agents of autointoxication. Although what neurologists identified and treated (unsuccessfully) as "trophoneu-roses" in the 1880s and 1890s would be treated successfully by 1910 with animal gland extracts administered by internists and endocrinologists, there was room for speculation about the role of hormones (and other substances) in the cause of other mental diseases. American psychiatrists and neurologists played a strong role in the multidisciplinary Association for the Study of Internal Secretions, which was founded in 1917. The Endocrine Society (as it was later called) "immediately became a major force in American medicine, almost a separate therapeutic sect," keeping alive, for a time, autointoxication theories of dementia praecox.[24] The 1920s held the promise of a conceptual realignment of the mental diseases, with much interest in the development of an "endocrine psychiatry."

Emil Kraepelin would remain convinced for the last thirty years of his life that a systemic, metabolic autointoxication was the most plausible cause of dementia praecox. For a man who admitted he often liked to revise his ideas, absolutely nothing could shake him from this core belief.

What exactly did Kraepelin say about the causes of dementia praecox? In the general discussion of the causes of the insanities that opened the 1896 fifth edition of *Psychiatrie* Kraepelin noted that many of the characteristic signs of glandular and metabolic disorders appear during the development of mental deterioration, especially in dementia praecox.[25] Later in this book, in his very first detailed description of dementia praecox in a chapter titled "Die Stoffwechselerkrankungen," he stated that he had "serious objections" to the point of view that dementia praecox is caused by "inadequate constitutional faculties" or "hereditary degeneration [*erblischen Entartung*]." Instead he offered an alternative hypothesis: "I consider it more likely that what we have here is a tangible morbid process in the brain [*einen greifbaren Krankheitsvorgang im Gehirne*]. Only in this way does the quick descent into severe dementia become at all comprehensible." He admitted the failure of neuropathological studies to find any characteristic cellular pathology in dementia praecox, but attributed this to an inadequate effort to search for such morbid changes.

What then caused this "tangible morbid process in the brain," if not heredity? Kraepelin is clear on this point: "In light of our current experience, I would assume that we are dealing here with an autointoxication [*Selbstvergiftung*], whose immediate causes lie somewhere in the body."

However, he makes a major departure from classic autointoxication theory by rejecting the intestines as the source of toxins. Instead he finds the *locus morbi* in the gonads: "If we consider the tendency for the illness to strike at the age when sexual development is still taking place, then it is not out of the question for there to be a connection between the illness and some processes taking place in the sexual organs. These are, of course, only provisional and very indefinite hypotheses."[26]

Critics of the autointoxication theory of dementia praecox, such as Adolf Meyer, had little impact on Kraepelin; he remained convinced. In the 1899 sixth edition of his textbook he continued to make the argument that the sex glands are the source of the toxins that poison the brain and produce dementia praecox. In that edition, however, his claims were more textured: "In view of the close connection for the disease with the developmental age, with menstrual disorders and reproduction, and in view of the absence of any recognizable external cause, the most obvious thing to think of is probably an *autointoxication* which could possibly be in some close or distant connection with processes in the genital organs." To support this speculation he referenced the 1895 review article on this subject by D. E. Jacobson. However, Kraepelin tempered his earlier dismissal of the role of heredity in the cause of dementia praecox: "The frequency of hereditary disposition to mental disturbances and their physical and mental symptoms would only signify a lowered resistance to the actual cause of the disease."[27]

In the third volume of the 1913 eighth edition of *Psychiatrie* Kraepelin cautiously asserted that it was still too early to make etiological conclusions about dementia praecox, but that it generally might be said that "a number of facts [*eine Reihe von Tatsachen*]" about dementia praecox suggest "an autointoxication as a resulting of a metabolic disturbance might be probable to some extent [*einer Selbstvergiftung infolge einer Stoffwechselstorung bis zu einem gewissen Grade wahrscheinlich*]."[28] As an ailing Kraepelin prepared the ninth edition with his colleague Johannes Lange (1891–1938) in the last months of his life (he died on 4 October 1926), the final words he wrote on dementia praecox were concerned with an a systemic, quite possibly autotoxic, etiology: "We also have to search for the most likely origins of the illness in the processes which originate in the body itself. . . . Certainly heredity and predispositions play a considerable, perhaps even a decisive role, but we don't know at which point the influence takes hold."[29] Due to his final illness Kraepelin could not complete the chapter on dementia praecox in this last edition of *Psychiatrie;* Lange did. It appeared in print the year after Kraepelin's death.

What has been missing in the current scholarship on Kraepelin is a discussion of this key component of his medical cognition: the belief that dementia praecox was due to an endogenous process of chronic *autointoxication* that led to a "self-poisoning [*Selbstvergiftung*]" of the body and, eventually, the brain. Scholars who continue to cite only the fatalism of heredity or degeneration keep missing the point: in Kraepelin's view the true origin of dementia praecox was not to be found in the cells of the central nervous system, nor (entirely) in the shadowy ancestral chambers of the germplasm, *but active and alive elsewhere, perhaps everywhere, in the present body.* Furthermore if dementia praecox was directly caused by proximal rather than distal biological processes, it was a potentially *preventable* and *treatable* disease. Kraepelin held out no hope for complete cures, but, at least for a time, he believed that the prevention of dementia praecox and the development of rational therapies were possible if only the mysterious mechanisms of the self-poisoning process could be discovered.

Kraepelin's autotoxic etiology of dementia praecox commandingly framed the cognitive categories of some of his prominent European peers. Rather than proposing a strong alternative hypothesis of the biological causes of dementia praecox, they followed Kraepelin's lead. For example, several prominent German and Swiss psychiatrists who made contributions to the understanding of dementia praecox in the early twentieth century also suspected an autotoxin might be its cause. Wilhelm Weygandt (1870–1939), an associate of Kraepelin's in Heidelberg who is best remembered for a monograph he published on the nature of "mixed states" in manic-depressive insanity, wrote in 1907, "Dementia praecox, in particular, is more and more regarded as an illness based on some metabolic disturbance. . . . I should like to put forward a tentative explanation of dementia praecox of my own. . . . I would suggest that so far as the organic side is concerned the most plausible concept is one of autotoxic damage affecting genetically predisposed brains."[30] In this same article Weygant was critical of the illogic of the chimerical psychoanalytic and autointoxication theory of dementia praecox put forth by Carl Gustav Jung (1875–1961) in his famous 1907 monograph on the subject, *Über die Psychologie der Dementia Praecox: Ein Versuch.* Jung proposed that a "complex" created by an intensely emotional event might lead to the production of a biological "hypothetic X, metabolic toxin(?)."[31] The persistence of the complex, which could be removed through psychoanalysis, produced a chronic autointoxication that acted on the brain to produce dementia praecox. However, even Jung admitted in his monograph that the autotoxic process might be primary and therefore, by implication, probably unaffected by psychotherapy. Jung's chief, Eugen Bleuler, also held to a variant of this chimerical theory of the etiology of dementia praecox, claiming that the fundamental symptoms of the disease had biological origins, but the secondary or accessory symptoms were psychogenic. Unlike Jung, Bleuler did not believe that a traumatically caused "complex" (a split-off portion of consciousness that consisted of thoughts, feelings, and images clustered around a central theme or motif) could cause dementia praecox. Despite his short-lived infatuation with Freud and his disagreement with Kraepelin on issues such as prognosis, Bleuler made it clear in his classic *Dementia Praecox, oder die Gruppe der Schizophrenien* (1911) how influential Kraepelin's etiologic hypothesis remained in his thinking: "As long as the real disease process is unknown to us, we cannot exclude the possibility that various types of auto-intoxication or infections may lead to the same symptomatic picture."[32]

Before Kraepelin's autotoxic disease had arrived on American soil, others had already prepared the ground. Dementia praecox took root in American medicine in part because laboratory research in the psychiatry of the 1890s was thoroughly framed by autointoxication theory. It was a good fit for the dominant biological paradigm adopted by those alienists and neurologists who sought the disease specification of the insanities in line with that of other diseases (such as tuberculosis) that were the objects of study in the laboratory movement in general medicine. Neurasthenia, a non-insane condition, was largely under the professional jurisdiction of neurologists. Still it was the first condition to be specifically studied in asylum laboratories, but after 1904 or so it would retreat to its natural habitat in the outpatient consulting rooms of nerve specialists. In dementia praecox, an asylum insanity largely under the jurisdiction of alienists, American psychiatry had finally found an object to study in the laboratory that would prove to the larger world of scientific medicine that it too was a true medical science.

In the 1890s there were only two respected centers of laboratory research in American psychiatry. As noted in the previous chapter, the first was the McLean Asylum, where Edward Cowles had initiated a research program in 1889 into the "fatigue question" in neurasthenia, which he viewed as a potentially prepsychotic condition that could morph into insanity, and its relation to autointoxication. This was the reason for Cowles's addition of a chemistry laboratory to the pathology and experimental psychology labs at McLean. Autointoxication research continued at that institution even after Cowles retired in 1903.[33]

The second, and much grander, center of laboratory research in psychiatry was the New York State Pathological Laboratory. It had been set up in 1895 in New York City as "a central pathology laboratory to service all the state mental hospitals."[34] But with the appointment of Ira Van Gieson (1866–1913) in 1896 as its new director, the name was changed to the New York State Pathological Institute and the focus of its activities changed to that of basic research in a number of disciplines. Van Gieson, who specialized in histological studies of the nervous system as well as pathology and cellular biology, sought out experts in physical anthropology, comparative neurology, bacteriology, pathology, biochemistry, and psychology (the "psycho-motor phenomena" that paralleled biological processes). Philosophical training was a desired prerequisite for candidates. Separate departments were established for each of these disciplines. The creation of such an institute was due entirely to efforts of the visionary Van Gieson. For many years he had lobbied New York state medical officials and politicians for its establishment. Although the dream lasted only until 1899, when state funds were cut off for basic research and his extraordinary team of experts had to be disbanded, Van Gieson stayed on until 1901.[35] He would be replaced by Adolf Meyer—and the fundamental vision of what psychiatric research at the Institute should entail would change radically.

Van Gieson was a firm believer in the essential toxic basis of mental diseases.[36] "The majority of the diseases of the nervous system (including diseases of the mind) are to be led back to one form or another of 'poisoning,'" he argued in 1897.[37] The familiar vectors posited by European autointoxication theory were their source: metabolic imbalances or bacterial infections within the body, or toxic substances that had been ingested or absorbed from without. The effects on the brain and the rest of the nervous system were merely the final chapter in the mechanistic narrative of mental disease.

Although Kraepelin and his associates (including August Hoch) had explored hypotheses derived from autointoxication theory in their research, it was Cowles and Van Gieson who pioneered this approach in the United States. And it was at McLean, under Cowles, that we find the first such evidence that dementia praecox became an object of laboratory research.

In September 1900 Cowles hired Otto Folin (1867–1934) to direct research in the chemistry laboratory at McLean, thus releasing August Hoch from his responsibilities for an area of research that was not his main interest or area of particular expertise. Folin, who was born in a small village in Sweden, was a physiological chemist who had received his doctorate from the University of Chicago in 1898. After a stint in 1899 as a professor of analytical chemistry at West Virginia University in Morgantown he came to the attention of Cowles. When he arrived in October 1900 funds were provided for him to bring along a young assistant, Phillip Schaffer, and to reequip the chemistry lab with state-of-the-art instruments ordered from Germany. Folin had no prior interest in insanity, but the opportunity to conduct research using the latest equipment and methods of his discipline held a certain promise for his main interest: the intermediary stages of protein metabolism. The foundational research he would do in this area at McLean would be recognized for its originality in the years to come, and it led to his appointment as a professor of biological chemistry at Harvard University in 1907.

But the same problems faced by other laboratory researchers became Folin's puzzle: What aspect of the biology of the insane should be analyzed? And how? As he recalled in autobiographical notes from 1924 that were found among his personal papers after his death, "It was hopeless to try to find deviations from the normal in the metabolism of the insane without far more exact knowledge of the human waste products than was available. My immediate and comprehensive problem became, therefore, the chemistry of the urine."[38]

According to Folin's assistant, Phillip Schaffer, the first plan at McLean was "to search for clues to possible abnormality of metabolism among mentally disturbed patients. The first effort, soon abandoned, was a study of the toxicity of normal urines versus that of mentally disturbed patients by intravenous injection of urine and its known constituents in rabbits." There were no unusual findings in the urine using this approach. "The second effort was more extensive and somewhat more successful, but the clue was not appreciated and an opportunity may have been missed." And what was this missed opportunity?

> In the course of prolonged study of metabolic discrepancies as revealed by analysis of the urines of normal and disturbed persons [reported in long papers published in 1904], a case was encountered of a patient having a remarkable daily cycle in mental state and a corresponding alternation in amount of urinary excretion of inorganic phosphate; the data were published in the *American Journal of Physiology* in 1902 (over the protest of the editor, W. T. Porter). Years later the paper was cited as of interest to psychiatrists, and the wide role of phosphate in many metabolic reactions gradually came to be appreciated. In that later development Folin had no part.[39]

The unique patient with correlated mental and physical cycles that was the subject of the 1902 article was diagnosed with manic-depressive insanity at McLean, but when August Hoch and another colleague autopsied the body in January 1904 it was found to be a case of general paralysis.[40]

When Folin's research was finally published in 1904, charts reporting the results of the analysis of the urine of sixty-seven insane patients indicated their general physical condition as well as their diagnosis, including the three forms of dementia praecox as well as cases of manic-depressive insanity. Among the normal subjects used as controls and identified by initials in the first of the two published reports were members of the McLean medical staff, including Hoch (Aug. H.) and E. Stanley Abbot (E. S. A.). However, Folin and his associates reported, "The investigations have so far failed to show any characteristic metabolism peculiarities corresponding to the different psychiatrical groups of cases."[41]

Folin's final conclusion about his years of metabolism studies of the insane was that "they teach very little that is tangible concerning mental diseases": "It is not claimed that such characteristic abnormal metabolism may not exist, but simply that the experiments recorded in the literature are insufficient to demonstrate this fact."[42]

The 1904 publication of Folin's research provided American psychiatry with the prestige it needed in its efforts to prove to the rest of the medical community that it could henceforth be regarded as a modern medical discipline. Indeed especially after Folin achieved fame as an innovative biochemist in the years that followed his tenure at McLean, these studies were cited for decades as proof, especially to neurologists, that things had changed in the world of the alienists. On the other hand, Folin's results were used as ammunition for those among the psychiatric elite who would oppose autointoxication theory in psychiatry, such as those holding to psychogenic or neuropathological hypotheses about the causes of mental disease. As one observer put it in 1944, "The publications of Folin's studies constituted a solid and enduring contribution to scientific research in psychiatry. His findings were negative and therefore disappointing, but they tended to check the more rash speculations on the metabolic etiology of the psychoses, and on metabolic theories of their therapy."[43]

But metabolic studies of dementia praecox continued. In fact in 1904 the first study published in the American medical literature in which a group of dementia praecox patients were specifically targeted for investigation also involved metabolism.[44] Before Folin's publications had appeared, Eugene McCampbell, a bacteriologist who had assumed a position as assistant pathologist at the Columbus State Hospital in Ohio, began a study of the urine of two normal persons and five patients diagnosed with dementia praecox. McCampbell added a note at the end of his article indicating that he had contacted Folin after seeing the latter's publications, admitting his own equipment and methods were inferior to those used at McLean. As in Folin's study, the biochemical results were not remarkable.

Thus by 1904 it was clear that some American researchers had accepted dementia praecox as a biological disease process with a presumed autotoxic basis. The previous year a noted Scottish psychiatrist, Lewis C. Bruce, had published a clinical and experimental study of the katatonic form of dementia praecox and had concluded, "Katatonia is an acute toxic disease."[45] In the English-speaking medical worlds on both sides of the Atlantic dementia praecox had become a legitimate object of biological research, a scientific "fact" worthy of laboratory study. But these early negative results in the American literature called into question the methods researchers had employed. In both instances metabolic processes were studied by the analysis of urine.[46] Future investigations would focus on other bodily fluids and physiological processes.

Not counting the articles on neuropathology that began appearing again around 1910, or the contributions of the Chicago bacteriologist and surgeon Bayard Taylor Holmes and his associates (a singular story discussed in a later chapter), between 1904 and 1920 at least thirty-six biological studies of dementia praecox, most involving laboratory analyses, appeared in the American medical literature. Most either explicitly or implicitly were based on hypotheses generated from late nineteenth-century autointoxication theories, now reframed as biochemical, immunological, or endocrinological studies. These included studies of the blood, the thyroid gland, cerebrospinal fluid, brain chemistry, the ductless glands, lymph node abnormalities, the thymus and pituitary glands, optic neuritis and abnormal ocular reactions, the saliva, the fundus oculi, and the "simian" shape and movement of the hands, and review articles of the evidence for autointoxication or "endocrinopathy" in dementia praecox.[47] Through the publication of these laboratory studies of dementia praecox in journals such as the *American Journal of Physiology, Archives of Internal Medicine, Journal of the American Medical Association, Journal of Experimental Medicine, Ophthalmology,* and the *Journal of Laboratory and Clinical Medicine,* American psychiatry strove—with limited success—to reenter the mainstream of general medicine.

The vast majority of other articles published during this time were clinical in nature, usually an idiosyncratic mixture of personal opinion and bedside observations of a patient or two with only perfunctory references to Kraepelin. What is striking about the hundreds of both clinical and laboratory research articles on dementia praecox published in English-language (mostly American) journals between 1900 and 1930 is how *absent* Kraepelin seems to be; only a handful of North American authors demonstrated evidence of actually having *read* Kraepelin (most usually parroting the same thumbnail summaries of his ideas from previous authors), and fewer still (perhaps only Adolf Meyer, August Hoch, A. A. Brill, George Kirby, C. K. Clarke, Bernard Sachs, E. E. Southard, Smith Ely Jelliffe, F. X. Dercum, and G. Alder Blumer) dared to offer a few lines of an informed *critique* of *some aspect* of Kraepelin's dementia praecox concept. Reading the medical literature of this era one might very well get the impression that, other than his nomenclature and autotoxic hypotheses, Kraepelin had very little to do with Kraepelin's disease in America. And yet it is beyond doubt that something called dementia praecox, certainly without many of the subtleties and complexities of Kraepelin's original creations of 1896 and especially 1899, was accepted as a specified disease by most American alienists.

"The alienists who at the present time deny the existence of the clinical form of insanity known as dementia praecox are very few," William Rush Dunton Jr. observed in May 1907.[48] As Dunton himself knew, dementia praecox was a real disease that presented with physical signs and was based on an autotoxic process that could be studied in the laboratory. The role played by the publication of these clinical opinion pieces and laboratory research reports in the reification of Kraepelin's disease in America should not be underestimated. Such reification had first been tried with neurasthenia, the only original American disease concept (all the rest were imports from Europe), but that disease was regarded by many as the first stage of a unitary psychosis, or a condition that could lead to insanity if left untreated, not a discrete form of insanity per se. Neurasthenia did, however, open the door to autointoxication theories in psychiatry. Whereas the laboratory study of neurasthenia by Cowles and Hoch at McLean had quickly reached an unpublishable dead end by 1900, with Kraepelin's dementia praecox modern psychiatry now had a new and potentially more viable biological object of its own to study in the laboratory.

Not all American alienists were happy with autointoxication theories. Adolf Meyer was the earliest and most critical, having outright dismissed the autotoxic theory of the etiology of Kraepelin's disease in his 1896 review of the fifth edition of *Psychiatrie*. But the main problem that would plague proponents of autointoxication theory was stated succinctly by a homeopathic alienist, R. O. Woodman: "Autotoxic theories as to the cause are in general favor but lack evidence as to what the toxins are."[49] Indeed beginning with Folin's studies at McLean, one published study after another rendered either negative results, uninterpretable positive results, or unreplicable results. Charles Macfie Campbell (1876–1943), an associate physician who worked under Meyer on Ward's Island in New York City, made it clear that he thought autointoxication research was a waste of time: "That this hypothesis, so vague as to be worthless, should be formulated at all in the present state of our knowledge shows that the attitude of the individual in the matter is apt to be determined by general principles rather than by any adequate body of observations. In the absence of the latter, surely it would be better to forego any hypothesis rather than to adopt one which is apt to give an undue bias to clinical investigations."[50]

A middle ground was occupied by William Alanson White, superintendent of the government Hospital for the Insane in Washington, D.C. He believed some of the positive findings in autointoxication research were valid. However, he astutely recognized that they implied nothing about the cause (etiology) of dementia praecox, but perhaps instead said something about its pathophysiology: "Now it seems to me . . . that these changes which are found in the secretions are the results of disturbed tissue metabolism due to the disease and not indicative of the presence of toxins which are to be regarded as causative factors."[51]

As with Kraepelin, such criticisms did not change the mind of one of the earliest and most vocal proponents of the autotoxic theory of dementia praecox, the eminent Philadelphia neurologist Francis X. Dercum. Although he consistently proposed changing the boundaries of Kraepelin's disease, including widening the inclusion criteria and reformulating its subtypes, Dercum was in complete agreement with Kraepelin about its cause: "When we recall the known role which infections and intoxications play in the production of delirium, confusion, and stupor, it is certainly not going too far to infer that dementia praecox is probably due to a toxin—a toxin which at first calls forth by its action upon the cortical neurones hallucinations and their dependent delusions, and later on, in given cases, brings their destruction."[52]

Dercum was not alone. The autointoxication theory of dementia praecox would live on for several more decades. While most hoped for a serendipitous discovery of a cause of Kraepelin's disease, more sophisticated investigators settled for hints of its pathophysiology. Some, such as Roy Hoskins, the director of the Memorial Foundation for Neuro-Endocrine Research at the Worcester State Hospital from the late 1920s to the late 1940s, would continue to explore possible endocrinological hypotheses.[53]

What kept hope alive for so many laboratory researchers in psychiatry was the story of syphilis.

No event was more thrilling to alienists and neurologists than the May 1906 announcement of the development of the serodiagnostic Wasserman reaction test for syphilis.[54] Then in 1913 researchers demonstrated

the correlation of positive Wasserman reactions with the presence of
the bacterium *Treponema pallidum* in the brain tissue of mentally disordered persons diagnosed with general paralysis. Thus a familiar disease
of the asylum, also known as paresis or dementia paralytica, had submitted its secrets in the laboratory.

But the success story of the development of the blood test for
syphilis would prove to be an elusive model for dementia praecox researchers to emulate. The identification in 1905 of the spiral organism
that caused syphilis gave researchers a clear basis for developing the
Wasserman blood test and the later redefinition of general paralysis of
the insane as neurosyphilis. Its clinical syndrome, cellular pathology,
and etiology were tightly linked in less than a decade. Asylum alienists
were unclear about the exact parameters of the clinical syndromes con-
fronting them, and not knowing how to operationally define mental
illnesses such as dementia praecox or manic-depressive insanity except
as vaguely "organic" or "biological," most laboratory researchers simply applied methods inspired by the latest conceptual or technological
innovations in the various medical sciences and hoped there would be
a serendipitous payoff in the search for the etiology, pathophysiology,
and eventually treatment of the insanities.

For asylum alienists, neurologists, and laboratory researchers intrigued by the stories blood may reveal, there were at least four questions that needed to be addressed: Is the blood of diseased persons different from the blood of healthy ones? Can specific diseases be diagnosed
by specific changes in the blood? Is the cause of madness in the blood
itself? In other words, is "mad" blood "bad" blood (the question of *etiology*)? Are differences in the blood of the insane merely clues to the hidden causes of madness that are to be found elsewhere in the body (the
question of *pathophysiology*)?

The development of the Wasserman reaction test for neurosyphilis in 1906 was a turning point for biological psychiatry. For the first
time there was a blood test for madness—at least for one variety of
madness. Could such serodiagnostic tests for the other insanities be
developed? Could one serologic test be developed that could differentially diagnose the major forms of insanity, dementia praecox and
manic-depressive illness?

But if dementia praecox researchers were to replicate the victorious
story of neurosyphilis, the ultimate question they had to answer was

this: How does one define *dementia praecox* and set up a *blood test,* so that after *some experience* almost any research worker will be able to demonstrate a *relation between them* to a degree that is adequate in practice?[55]

Soon the spirits of American alienists would be raised again, indeed *twice* in a few short years, by news of more miracles of German medicine.

In 1909 two German researchers from Eppendorf created a minor sensation when they injected patients with cobra venom and found that all of the dementia praecox patients, and a portion of the manic-depressive subjects, invariably reacted to the toxin, whereas other psychiatric patients and normals did not. The study was reported in the *New York Times* on 1 August 1909, but with the caution "Its efficiency is doubted here."[56] The excitement over the "Much–Holzmann psycho-reaction" was over almost as soon as it had begun: "Unfortunately the original claims have not been substantiated, and it is definitely known that as a diagnostic measure the Much–Holzmann test is of little value."[57] Although the "Much–Holzmann psycho-reaction" was quickly discredited by other researchers, it was the first promising differential diagnostic immunoserologic finding for dementia praecox and manic-depressive insanity.

In May 1913, at the annual meeting of the German Psychiatrists Association in Breslau, a presentation of experimental research findings by August Fauser (1856–1938), a psychiatrist from Stuttgart, created an international sensation that would capture the imagination of medical researchers for the next several years. Fauser reported that he had used a recently invented immunodiagnostic test in an examination of the blood of 250 psychiatric patients and found that it could differentially diagnose dementia praecox from other psychiatric disorders. Furthermore Fauser claimed that this blood test could also differentiate normal controls from persons suffering from severe mental disorders.[58] His stunning announcement of the discovery of a blood test for madness held out the promise that psychiatry would now share in the success of other medical sciences that had been revolutionized by laboratory studies in bacteriology, endocrinology, and serology. This remarkable new immunoserodiagnostic tool was known as the Abderhalden defensive ferments reaction test, originally developed in 1909 by the Swiss biochemist Emil Abderhalden (1877–1950) as a purported method of diagnosing pregnancy. Abderhalden continually refined his procedure and central concept—that of the "defensive fer-ments," the *Schutzfermente* or *Abwehrfermente*—and a 1912 book on his discovery went through two more editions by 1914.[59] The third edi-tion of 1913 included a bibliography of more than four hundred pub-lished studies using his serodiagnostic technique.

In a lecture on 27 October 1912 in Halle at a congress of German psychiatrists and neurologists, Abderhalden himself had suggested that his new blood test might be applied to the study of nervous and mental disorders.[60] Fauser, under the direct guidance of Abderhalden, carried out this research plan and published a short research report on his find-ings on 26 December 1912. The story somehow found its way into the *New York Times* on 22 February 1913 before Fauser had a chance to fully present his findings to his colleagues.[61] It was Fauser's presenta-tion at the May 1913 meeting of the German Psychiatrists Association that caught the medical world's attention. For a very brief but exciting period in the history of psychiatry, many researchers in Europe and North America believed that psychiatry now had the equivalent of the Wasserman reaction test for dementia praecox.

Fauser's claim to have found a blood test that could differentially diagnose dementia praecox from other psychiatric illness and from healthy persons was, for a time, internationally accepted as valid because of the congruence of his specific findings with the etiological specula-tions of Emil Kraepelin. As noted earlier, Kraepelin rejected notions prevalent in medicine at the time that bodily autointoxications primar-ily arose from the intestines, instead proposing that dementia praecox was caused by a metabolic disturbance originating in the sex glands.

One of the major claims of Abderhalden's defensive ferments reaction test was that it could identify diseased internal organs in the body through a reaction of hypothesized "defensive ferments" *(die Abwehrfermente)* in the blood of a patient when it came into contact with tissue from correspond-ing human organs taken from a cadaver. Abderhalden's assumption was that debris from a diseased organ, toxalbumins, would end up in the bloodstream. Because such material was poisonous to the blood and not excreted through the kidneys, the blood produced "defensive ferments," or enzymes, which dissolved this debris, catabolizing it and making it into a peptone and amino acid. Specific defensive ferments would be pro-duced in the blood only when coming into contact with tissue from spe-cific organs, and this process could be experimentally replicated in a test tube outside of a living body. An experimental reaction indicating the creation of defensive ferments in the blood in response to contact with corresponding tissue would result in a bright violet color. Such a color would confirm which organ in a patient's body was diseased.

Thus Fauser found that defensive ferments in the blood of all persons with severe mental disorders caused a reaction against tissue from the cerebral cortex, thereby supporting Kraepelin's contention that dementia praecox is caused by a tangible morbid process in the brain. Fauser further corroborated Kraepelin when he reported that he found defensive ferments reacted against sex gland tissue only in the blood of persons with dementia praecox and not in those diagnosed as manic-depressive, hysteric, or with purely degenerative insanity. The serum of male patients reacted only with testicular tissue, and the serum of female patients only with ovarian tissue.

Fauser's report, and subsequent research publications from his clinic, immediately inspired replication efforts around the world. The most notable of these was a study conducted with the blood of 106 psychiatric patients at the Sheppard and Enoch Pratt Hospital by the noted virologist Charles E. Simon.[62] In an article published in the 30 May 1914 issue of the *Journal of the American Medical Association* Simon provided a critical review of the work of Fauser and subsequent researchers who did not confirm Fauser's findings, pointing out possible flaws in their use of Abderhalden's complex methodology as a reason for conflicting results. In Simon's own study the sex gland reaction was found in nearly all dementia praecox patients, but he directly rejected Fauser's claim that such a reaction is exclusive to dementia praecox. Simon also directly accused Fauser of manipulating his data to achieve the expected outcome. According to Simon:

> In surveying the literature just outlined, one cannot help being impressed . . . by the wonderful apparent uniformity of the results reported by Fauser, and . . . by the total lack of uniformity of those obtained by others. . . . The thought naturally suggests itself that two factors may have been operative to this end, namely that Fauser was carried away by his enthusiasm and allowed himself to be influenced unduly in the direction of his own wishes, and that [others] lacked complete control of the technic. As a matter of fact, there is good ground for the belief that both factors were operative.[63]

Despite an acute awareness of the chaos in the medical literature on what Simon renamed the "Abderhalden-Fauser Reaction," he insisted on the reality of Abderhalden's proposed defensive ferments and on the method for detecting them: "It is my firm conviction that . . . Abderhalden's basic work in this field should be viewed as one of the most important contributions to modern experimental science."[64]

Charles E. Simon never again mentioned the "Abderhalden-Fauser Reaction" in any subsequent publications—and for a very good reason. In the four months before Simon's paper appeared in print, a series of devastating critiques of Abderhalden's defensive ferments reaction test began to appear in German medical journals. Serious criticisms of Abderhalden's methods and even the validity of the defensive ferments continued in English-language journals.[65]

With the wisdom of hindsight at our disposal, all of us know why the Abderhalden defensive ferments reaction test did not revolutionize biological psychiatry: Abderhalden's defensive ferments simply do not exist. They never did. All of the reports of positive results with the Abderhalden reaction test were based on error—if not worse.[66]

But surely the hundreds of published experimental reports of positive findings using Abderhalden's test were not fraudulent? There is of course another explanation: human fallibility. Because the reaction depended on the researcher's ability to perceive a particular color, the method was not quantitative; instead it was highly subjective. Some researchers saw the color all the time, some saw the color some of the time, and some never saw it no matter how carefully they followed Abderhalden's procedures. The story of the rise and fall of Abderhalden's blood test is more akin to a social psychology experiment on perceptual bias and the consensual nature of reality rather than fraud perpetuated on a massive international scale. August Fauser and his colleagues in Stuttgart clearly saw the color every time it fit their preconceptions about the locus of the diseased organs in dementia praecox. Because of this highly subjective element the hundreds of experimental reports often wildly conflicted in their results. Charles Simon was therefore correct in his suspicion of experimental bias on the part of Fauser, but failed to discern the essential weakness in Abderhalden's method. By 1917 it was clear to most of the world that Abderhalden's defensive ferments did not exist and that the method purported to detect them was flawed. In 1920 Jacques Loeb could write to a biochemist colleague, "Nobody speaks of the Abderhalden reaction any more in the United States and I am very much surprised to see that in his journal Abderhalden still continues that myth."[67] However, scientific articles reporting the use of Abderhalden's test continued to appear in German publications for several more decades.

Despite the general rejection of Abderhalden's defensive ferments and the test purporting to detect them, a minority of physicians in the United States continued to believe in them and in their promise to revolutionize biological psychiatry. These physicians were Albert Sterne of Indianapolis, Bayard Taylor Holmes of Chicago, and Henry A. Cotton of Trenton. What united these men in their continued advocacy of Abderhalden and his test was their strong belief in the autointoxication and focal infection theories of the cause of dementia praecox and other mental disorders. For two of these men, Holmes and Cotton, we shall see in a later chapter that these beliefs rationalized some quite radical experimental treatments for Kraepelin's disease.

The growing number of American asylums and state hospitals with functioning pathology labs after 1900 led to an increase in the number of autopsies performed on the insane. As we have seen, the two reports by William Rush Dunton Jr. were the first published postmortem analyses of the brains of insane persons characterized as special in some way only by virtue of their Kraepelinian diagnosis.[68] Because neuropathologists and their students could not gain access to large numbers of human brains for didactic or research purposes in general hospitals— families tended to shun autopsies of their loved ones—they soon discovered that insane hospitals could meet their scientific needs. Large numbers of neglected, forgotten persons died in asylums (mostly from infectious diseases) and could be dissected without family interference. Asylum epidemics of diphtheria, typhoid fever, and dysentery were a serendipitous boon to pathologists who happened to be in the right place at the right time. Such was the case following a dysentery epidemic in 1908 at the Danvers Insane Hospital in Hawthorne, Massachusetts.[69]

The leading pathologist at Danvers, Elmer Ernest Southard (1876–1920), split his time between the asylum and Harvard Medical School. Since January 1906 he had been making these trips to Danvers several times a week to collect pathological specimens for the purpose of

amassing as large a comparison group as possible for research and analysis. When the dysentery epidemic exploded in July, August, and September 1908 he and two of his laboratory colleagues were diverted
from their neuropathological work and instead focused on the intestinal lesions caused by the Shiga bacillus (first identified in Japan in
1900) that had been determined to be the cause of the outbreak. Of the
thirty-six patients who had died from dysentery, Southard and his colleagues autopsied sixteen. Out of this experience grew an interest in
the internal bacilli of the colon and how they might migrate into the
blood and cerebrospinal fluid—and therefore perhaps even affect the
functioning of the nervous system. In the years after the epidemic
Southard and two colleagues, Frederick P. Gay (1874–1939), a bacteriologist who had been on staff at Danvers from 1906 to 1907, and Myrtelle Moore Canavan (1879–1953), who had worked at Danvers since
the summer of 1907, continued to compile and analyze data on more
than a hundred asylum cases in which such colon bacilli were detected
in these fluids at autopsy. They argued that these bacilli had migrated
while the patients were still alive and were not postmortem artifacts.

With Canavan, who would become a lifelong collaborator, Southard published four papers that implicated a path of transmission from
minor tears in the colon wall to the mesenteric lymph nodes, and from
there into the blood and spinal fluid, where access to the brain and spinal cord were possible. Southard and Canavan were cautious in their
conclusions—no attempt was made to place their findings in any grander
theory of disease. But what they had done—quite without intending to
do so, as Gay admitted decades later—was to provide "a concrete basis
for the somewhat mythical condition known as 'autointoxication.'"[70]

Although a neuropathologist, after 1910 Southard would rise in
prominence in psychiatry. Between 1910 and 1920 he was the only
true public adversary of Adolf Meyer, who by that time had become
the most powerful psychiatrist in the United States through his ability
to place his associates and students in jobs and by virtue of his position
as head the new Henry C. Phipps Psychiatric Clinic at Johns Hopkins.
Until his untimely death, Southard would single-handedly become the
only American neuropathologist to follow in the tradition of Franz
Nissl and Alois Alzheimer in Kraepelin's clinics in Heidelberg and
then, after 1903, in Munich. Like the Germans, Southard set his sights
on big game: finding and identifying the disease process in the brains
of persons suffering from dementia praecox.

Southard rose rapidly in the academic and scientific worlds. As an undergraduate he had been a devoted disciple of his Harvard College professors Josiah Royce and William James, attending seminars with Royce on subjects such as the "morphology of concepts." He visited the leading European centers of neurological and psychiatric research, including a period with Kraepelin, Nissl, and Alzheimer in Heidelberg in 1902. After blazing through Harvard Medical School he was appointed its first Bullard Professor of Neuropathology in 1909. This would be enough for any man, but Southard took on additional responsibilities as the first pathologist to the State Board of Insanity of the Commonwealth of Massachusetts (starting 1 May 1909) and became the first chief of the Boston Psychopathic Hospital when it opened as a department of the Boston State Hospital. As Adolf Meyer would do in the large system of New York state hospitals between 1902 and 1910, Southard's analogously powerful position as the statewide pathologist allowed him to personally train all physicians in the state hospital system in Massachusetts by having them cycle through the Boston Psychopathic Hospital between 1912 and 1919 (his last year of regency there). As state pathologist, Southard had supercustodial authority over seventeen public institutions, twenty-two private hospitals, and fourteen thousand patients. Meyer assumed responsibility for thirteen state hospitals and almost twice as many patients in May 1902, when he took command of the New York Pathological Institute in New York City.

New York and Massachusetts were the states that dominated the American mental disease professions of alienists and neurologists between 1880 and 1930. Meyer and Southard were state officials who wielded considerable power within their domains. Like Meyer, Southard was the apex of a professional patronage network, the father of many psychiatrists' careers. Southard's influence on the intellectual tenor of American psychiatry during these years, and for a time thereafter, was second only to Meyer's in the United States. By all accounts, he was one of the most remarkable physicians in early twentieth-century American medicine.

Southard (his intimates called him "Ernie") was remembered by his contemporaries in metaphors more appropriate for a comet than a man. Perhaps this has to do with his sudden death at the age of forty-three on 8 February 1920 from influenza that quickly transformed into fatal pneumonia. His biographer, former colleague, and life-long friend, Frederick Gay, collected numerous memoirs from Southard's associates attesting to his boundless energy, his sanguine temperament, his humor, his love of wordplay, his scintillating intellect, his power to inspire others, and his polymathic creativity. He exhibited an "Edisonian habit of sleeplessness," often arriving at work in the morning after playing chess all night, sometimes competing in contests of "blind chess," in which his extraordinary powers of visualization and spatial cognition enabled him to play as many as six games simultaneously. He was enthralled by the aesthetics of Cubist art, particularly that of Marcel Duchamp.[71] He wrote poetry and was intrigued by the Vedic philosophy and spirituality of India. Complex concepts were like mind candy to him, his craving for them never sated.

L. Vernon Briggs, an associate of Southard's who would later write a history of the Boston Psychopathic Hospital, claimed, "He himself said that most people fell within one of the classifications of mental disease, and he felt himself to be of the manic-depressive type. We seldom saw the depressive side of him though it was undoubtedly there; ordinarily he appeared carried away with enthusiasm about his latest interest—and everything worthwhile interested him." Gay, whose biography of Southard is occasionally spiced with details not often found in such medical hagiographies, reported that his beloved friend "had no hesitation in classifying himself temperamentally . . . as actually hypomanic." "He was forever 'starting things,' and he has been accused of not finishing them," Gay observed, and the wide range of topics explored in his neuropathological studies, his writings on psychiatric classification and nomenclature, psychiatric social work, and mental hygiene attest to his wandering intellectual interests.[72] He read French and German fluently and published thick, comprehensive review articles of the latest psychiatric literature in these languages, including critical reviews of the books on dementia praecox by Emil Kraepelin and Eugene Bleuler.[73] But the flashes of brilliance in the three books and 179 published articles he left behind never compensated for one basic fact: today he is not remembered for any single medical or scientific breakthrough. However, it is clear from the testimonies of his colleagues and from his literary remains that he believed his greatest accomplishment might very well come from his work on dementia praecox.

By poking fun at the schism in psychiatry between the "mind twist men" and the "brain spot men," and denying a strictly functional or a strictly organic interpretation of mental disease, Southard believed that science was best served by investigating dementia praecox from complementary angles of approach: *both* the clinical and the anatomical, *both* the psychopathological and the neuropathological.[74] As for Southard himself, his position on the mind-body problem was always uppermost in his philosophical mind: "I wish . . . to say personally neither parallelism nor interactionism seems to me safe ground and that some kind of identity hypothesis for all the operations concerned would be better consonant with my views."[75]

Southard wrote of beginning his neuropathological study of dementia praecox in 1910, "It seemed to me that very probably the brains of dementia praecox patients would be found to be normal." He was surprised to find evidence to the contrary. As he expanded his series of dementia praecox subjects he continued to find diffuse structural abnormalities in most cases, but many fewer in cases of manic-depressive insanity or normal controls (by which he meant all of the normal brains he had autopsied and analyzed in his career, not a structured match of characteristics common to all groups compared in a given study). He judiciously did not overinterpret his findings to argue that dementia praecox was definitively found to be an organic disease in etiology, nor did he claim to have discovered a definitive characteristic cellular pathology for it. He professed the need to keep an open mind about the matter and often argued that his findings were provisional.[76] The cognitive categories that guided his personal approach to understanding mental disease were *structure* and *function,* and he understood the two to be intertwined: "Structure is in the main the spatial aspect of facts and events, function in the main the temporal aspect of the same facts."[77] But according to one colleague who knew him well, "Southard's conclusion regarding dementia praecox was that it is in some sense structural. Manic depressive he regarded as more likely a metabolic disturbance."[78]

Southard was regarded as the leading neuropathologist of his generation in the United States, and his findings were difficult to ignore, even by the most ardent psychogenicists. But he did have critics from his own field of pathology, particularly Clarence O. Cheney, a former pathologist at the Manhattan State Hospital who had risen to the position of assistant director of the New York Psychiatric Institute. After reviewing Southard's publications on dementia praecox, Cheney confessed he was unable "after intensive effort to follow him in his kaleidoscopic changes from fact to fancy."[79]

However, Southard's own colleagues marveled at the way he could glance at a fresh human brain and instantly see its uniqueness in a manner similar to the way he could glance at a chess board and see the possibilities inherent in its implicated structure. "While to most of us brains are as alike as Chinamen, he seemed to possess something of the 'photographic mind' which instantly detects slight peculiarities," reported one colleague. "I still retain a vivid memory of seeing him at his task of examining brains and of noting how unhesitatingly, in the course of the rapid inspection, he pointed out small variations, and how confidently, as he ran his fingertips over the fresh surface, he dictated his impression of differences in resistance."[80]

Southard's acute sensitivity to neural tissue in an era of technological simplicity led to a creative interpretation about the neuropathology of dementia praecox; because almost every part of the brain in persons with Kraepelin's disease had been found to have abnormalities in one study or another, this might be evidence in support of an "embryonic"—or to use a twenty-first-century term, neurodevelopmental—origin for the disease.[81]

Dementia praecox was the subject of thirteen publications by Southard between 1908 and 1919, ten of which were either reports of neuropathological studies of the brains of persons with dementia praecox or comparisons with the brains of persons with manic-depressive illness and those of normal individuals.[82] His conclusions are difficult to summarize with specificity; he did indeed claim to find subtle abnormalities in the gross anatomy of the brain, its structural layers, and at the cellular level, but the findings were diffuse and not consistent in every dementia praecox brain. In February 1919, near the end of his life, he admitted in a lecture to the Boston Society of Psychiatry and Neurology, "For the present neither the anatomy nor the microscopy of cases of so-called Dementia Praecox indicates with more than probability the existence of an entity."[83] Thus it once again appeared that the nosological and biological boundaries of Kraepelin's disease would remain elusive as it completed its second decade of existence.

One of the most extraordinary research projects in American psychiatry in the first two decades of the twentieth century—a story heretofore untold—involved a collaboration of the superintendent Charles

Whitney Page and Southard at the Danvers State Hospital. Upon re-assuming his former position as superintendant in 1903 after an equally innovative stint at the Connecticut State Hospital in Middletown (1898–1903), Page aggressively took steps to transform Danvers into a dual-purpose institution, serving both clinical and research goals. He eliminated the case books and replaced them with a system of individual case records (including preprinted loose-leaf forms), formally adopted Kraepelin's 1899 classification scheme (as he had at Middletown), and, most intriguingly, created a catalog of cards for each patient admitted since 1879. The project took considerable effort but was complete by the time Page retired from Danvers in 1910.[84] On the front of the card was the case number, demographic information about the patient, and the diagnosis; on the back was a list of the prominent symptoms displayed by the patient. Unlike Kraepelin's index cards, no information about course or outcome were collected. Page's primary interest, indeed his passion, was to create a comprehensive "index of symptoms" that could be used as the backbone of future psychopathological and neuropathological research in psychiatry. The card catalog was cross-indexed by symptom and by diagnosis. For example, by searching "Hallucination," with the subset "Auditory," one could identify all the patients who had such a symptom. The same would be true if searching for all those who had been given the diagnosis "Dementia Praecox." By 1914 at least seventeen thousand patients—every admission since 1879—had been included in the Danvers index of symptoms.[85]

Southard was introduced to the Danvers index of symptoms after assuming his part-time position as assistant physician and pathologist in January 1906. He replaced Albert Moore Barrett (1871–1936), who had trained with Kraepelin in 1900 during his tenure as pathologist at Danvers (1898–1906). Barrett, who had trained with Gershom S. Hill and Adolf Meyer in the 1890s, left Danvers to become the director of the new psychopathic ward of the University of Michigan Hospital along with an appointment as associate professor of neuropathology (1906) and professor of psychiatry and nervous disorders (1907). The University of Michigan Hospital psychopathic ward in Ann Arbor was the first institution in the United States to mimic the German university clinic model, although the Henry C. Phipps Psychiatric Clinic would be the first freestanding clinic associated with a medical school (1913). Barrett turned the psychopathic ward into a one-man research project in the decades to come, interpreting psychiatric research narrowly along neuropathological lines.[86]

During the three and a half years of his formal staff appointment, which ended in May 1909, Southard received Page's blessing to conduct any manner of research that he wished. Southard did so, collaborating in neuropathological, bacteriological, and epidemiological work on a variety of medical issues with the talented group of young researchers he was able to attract to Danvers. Either alone or with his Danvers collaborators Southard published no fewer than thirty-four papers during his four-year association with the state hospital. Under Page and Southard, between 1903 and 1909 the Danvers State Hospital was arguably the most productive and creative center of multidisciplinary psychiatric medical research in the United States, perhaps not to be rivaled until the years of the New York Psychiatric Institute under George H. Kirby in the 1920s.

Why was the Danvers "index of symptoms" project significant in the history of psychiatry? Because it was the only true American rival to Kraepelin's clinical research program conducted at his Heidelberg and Munich university clinics. The gigantic Danvers database *could* have been the foundation of the creation of an entirely new American classification system of mental diseases. But it was not. A follow-up study component *could* have been added to the ongoing data collection in order to replicate Kraepelin's longitudinal methodology and challenge his claims regarding course and outcome, but this also did not transpire. European concepts were reflexively absorbed, not challenged, in American psychiatry a century ago. Furthermore the veracity of scientific claims were still too firmly predicated on the reputation and integrity of the scientist making them—in this case Kraepelin, an icon of "superior" German medicine—not on the methods used to arrive at his conclusions. Whereas such social factors still unquestionably play a role in the acceptance of scientific claims today, in the American medicine and (particularly) psychiatry of the early twentieth century they trumped debate over methodology. Other than the research program of Eugen Bleuler and Carl Jung in Zurich, whose focus was narrower, no one in Germany, the United States, or anywhere else in that era attempted to replicate the exact research methods of Kraepelin. At least none did so on the scale necessary to determine whether the classification of mental diseases that would dominate the next century of psychiatry had any validity.

Instead Southard, a neuropathologist, correctly viewed the symptom index as a rich source of clinical information to correlate with anatomical findings recorded at autopsy. Thus instead of the creation of new insanities, the material was used to extend the clinical-anatomical method that had transformed medicine in the nineteenth century to a large series of cases in order to find correlations between specific symptoms of insanity and brain pathology. Southard and his colleague H. W. Mitchell published the first such studies using the symptom index in 1908, attempting to link autopsy findings with melancholia and "delusions of negation" in one study, and with age of onset of insanity in another. By 1914 Southard could correlate symptoms from the Danvers index with approximately one thousand autopsy records. He used the Danvers database to correlate symptoms from the index with autopsy findings in several later studies published between 1913 and 1916.[87] Harold I. Gosline, a pathologist at the Worcester State Hospital in Massachusetts, created his own index of symptoms of approximately 500 of 1,200 autopsied cases in 1915 and 1916, but the project was abandoned when he moved on to other employment.[88]

After leaving Danvers in 1909 Southard used his position as state pathologist to allocate State Board of Insanity funds to hire staff to continue the index of symptoms project at Danvers under his direct supervision. He also authorized additional funds to create a modern, entirely new index "based upon the accredited or classical symptoms found in the works of Kraepelin, Wernicke, Ziehen, as well as of Janet and Freud and of English and American writers."[89] His goal was to introduce the new index of symptoms into all Massachusetts institutions, standardizing research throughout the state. But by 1914 the statewide index project had been abandoned—like so many projects in Southard's life—and he instead made revisions to the checklist of symptoms in use at Danvers, incorporating new ideas for symptoms from the latest German, French, and English psychiatric literature. Among these were the inclusion of the "Wernickean trilogy" of classes of delusions: "autopsychic" (delusions that arise from having false impressions of oneself), "allopsychic" (delusions arising from false impressions of the environment), and "somatopsychic" (delusions arising from a distorted experience of one's own body).

Because the institutionalized patients of that era are hard to characterize—a diagnosis of dementia praecox, for example, tells us next to nothing about the nature of the illness of a person in the past—the twenty most frequent symptoms recorded from seventeen thousand admissions to Danvers between 1879 and 1914 provide us with a window into their lives. These, then, were the most likely behaviors and symptoms to lead to involuntary commitment to an asylum in that era:

Psychomotor excitement (6,903 cases)
Delusions, allopsychic (6,844)
Dementia (5,841)
Hallucinations, auditory (5,428)
Motor restlessness (5,428)
Depression (5,015)
Delusions, autopsychic (4,897)
Insomnia (4,354)
Incoherence (4,130)
Amnesia (3,422)
Violence (3,244)
Hallucinations, visual (3,186)
Irritability (2,714)
Defective judgment (2,596)
Disorientation (2,419)
Destructiveness (2,362)
Confusion (2,120)
Resistiveness (2,051)
Delusions, somatic (1,829)
Sicchasia (refusal of food) (1,597)

According to Southard, the first ten symptoms "occur in 10 per cent of *all* cases of mental disease, of whatever nature." Furthermore these twenty symptoms would occur in "20 per cent of any series of cases."[90] But what did these terms actually refer to? In 1914 Southard admitted that there were a "number of weaknesses in [his] system," complaining specifically about "the indiscriminate use of the terms 'dementia' and 'the demented' (there seem to be approximately as many dements with intact-looking brains as with damaged brains), and the omission of specific statements embodying endeavor to analyze *attention*," as well as "the very important lack of unanimity as to what 'psychomotor excitement' and 'motor restlessness' severally mean."[91] Statements such as these are reminders of the challenges inherent in writing histories of psychiatry.

The institutionalized patient of the early twentieth-century was as difficult to characterize by the psychiatrists of that era as for the historians of
our own.

After more than a decade of using the Danvers index of symptoms
for correlational clinical-anatomical work, in 1918 Southard proposed
that the database might be useful for constructing a classification of
mental disease allowing for a deductive "diagnosis by exclusion."[92]
However, he made no real effort to do so. By 1922 similar symptom
indexes were created at the Rhode Island State Hospital at Howard and
at McLean Hospital in Massachusetts. At McLean S. M. Bunker said
that the system of index card files was valuable in part because "it ac-
cepts Kraepelinian terms at their face value, thereby laying a fair basis
for criticism of the whole Kraepelinian school."[93] But no challenge to
Kraepelinian classification ever emerged from this effort.

More than any of his contemporaries, Southard was uniquely
poised to become the American Kraepelin. Whether he would have
become so—had he lived—is an intriguing question.

When his father died in 1910 Southard had the brain removed and preserved for later study. He left instructions for his own brain, and that of
his mother if he died first, to be removed and preserved in the same
fashion. Southard's mother died in 1921, a year after her son. When her
brain became available for a comparative study, it was the task of
Southard's cherished collaborator, Myrtelle M. Canavan, to do the
postmortem examinations of the family. In her published pathological
analysis of the three brains Canavan recorded a rather cryptic summary
of Southard's last days:

> The last year of his life was fraught with singular difficulties producing
> considerable mental discomfort, resulting in an edgy spirit of unrest. To
> compensate he worked feverishly at writing, skimmed the library for
> the stimulation of novel facts, poured over word studies, and became
> worried over facts he had hitherto neglected as unimportant. In the fall
> of 1919 he visited the Georgia State Sanitarium at Milledgeville and
> came home talking much of religion, of God, and of the simplicity of
> Blacks. At times he said, "I shall not live long, I must hurry; I must get
> lots of others busy."[94]

Canavan's medical examination from an "endocrinological stand-point" was conducted in December 1919, and she interpreted Southard's escalating difficulties as consistent with "a persistent thymic state."[95] Around the time of Christmas 1919, according to Canavan, he spoke of one of his many great unfinished tasks as "his hope to put together all his ideas on Dementia Praecox for review and refutation of the criticisms of his 1910 studies on the subject."[96] This was not to be.

6

Nobody denied that dementia praecox was *real*. It was just that there were few points of agreement about what it actually *was*. After almost a decade in American asylums, dementia praecox seemed to become more prevalent and less understood with each passing year.

"To strain a classification to such an extent that 40 per cent of the admissions of a hospital for the insane can be included under the heading 'dementia praecox' is certainly adding little to science, but rather tending to befuddle the whole subject," complained the Canadian alienist C. K. Clarke.[1] Others were alarmed as well.

In 1904, for the first time, we see American alienists and neurologists daring to question the validity of Kraepelin's disease. The backlash against Kraepelin's concept in the United States was characterized by several dimensions, some of which were issues that had already been raised by Kraepelin's critics in Germany.[2] However, the sense of urgency expressed in the American medical literature of 1905–1907 certainly indicates that some members of the psychiatric elite believed they were in the midst of a crisis.

If a moment in time can be identified for the beginning of this backlash, it would be the day Bernard Sachs (1858–1944) delivered a presentation on dementia praecox at the annual meeting of the American Neurological Association in September 1904. Sachs was a prominent New York City neurologist in private practice who would be remembered through the disease that carries his name, Tay-Sachs disease. He was highly regarded by the community of alienists and, like the neurologist Silas Weir Mitchell before him, was invited to address the American Medico-Psychological Association's annual meeting in 1897. In this address he singled out Adolf Meyer by name as an innovator in psychiatry, which did much to boost Meyer's reputation.[3]

Sachs argued that Kraepelin's definition of dementia praecox was "broad enough to embrace almost every form of psychic derangement in the young" and that based on his experience in private practice and in institutions such overdiagnosis was unfounded: "I can state with confidence that there is a great temptation to diagnosticate a vast majority of the cases of mental diseases in youthful individuals as cases of dementia praecox. . . . It is against these tendencies of the day that I consider it fair to enter a strong protest." In this practice "many alienists have evidently exceeded the intentions of Kraepelin himself." Because the diagnosis carried a prognosis of incurability and terminal dementia, Sachs correctly identified the danger of labeling young persons with this term when the actual long-term outcome of their illness—and their lives— was not yet known: "In this present day conception of dementia praecox, the very term implies a grave and, I believe, a far too grave prognosis in many of the cases so labeled. . . . Making the diagnosis of dementia praecox puts the stamp of an incurable malady upon persons who may be sufficiently alert to be useful to themselves and others for a long period of years and in that sense does them distinct injustice."[4]

The issue that Sachs and others had raised—dementia—cut to the heart of the problem with Kraepelin's term and concept. What was it? Was it the same as the dementia found in elderly persons (senile dementia)? How was Kraepelin defining this term?

As the psychiatrist and historian German E. Berrios has documented, the concept of dementia had undergone a narrowing process throughout the nineteenth century. In the early decades the term referred to "psychosocial incompetence" characterized by problems in memory, attention, and behavior (stuporous states known as "acute dementia") as well as hallucinations and delusions, but dementia was not linked to old age or the notion that it was irreversible. By 1900, however, the dementia concept was undergoing a process completed by 1915 or so in which it was defined as cognitive impairment (not psychosocial incompetence) without delusions and hallucinations, and it was irreversible. The three categories of dementia commonly recognized by physicians in 1900 were senile (the dementia of old age), arteriosclerotic (a "hardening" of the arteries of the brain that cut off the exchange of oxygen and glucose and destroy brain cells), and "vesanic dementia" (an 1840s term for the cognitive disorientation following bouts of insanity, which in some cases was thought to be recoverable, a condition called "pseudodementia" in the 1880s). Kraepelin's use of the term did not fit any of these three categories, Berrios argued. The cognitive defect in dementia praecox was not reversible between periods of florid insanity—indeed this was the central defining feature of Kraepelin's concept. Berrios proposed that this mismatch with the evolving concept of dementia in general medicine and neurology may be one of the reasons why dementia praecox was later "hidden" under a different name, schizophrenia.[5]

This was the thread taken up in an insightful critique of Kraepelin's use of the term "dementia" in 1906 by G. Alder Blumer, the medical superintendent of Butler Hospital in Providence, Rhode Island. Butler Hospital was a small elite institution that resembled McLean Hospital in Massachusetts. In his article Blumer carefully examined the recent seventh edition of *Psychiatrie* (1904) and sharply noted, "Kraepelin . . . seems studiously to avoid references to, or discussion of, the simple term *Dementia*. . . . The word appears rarely and one looks in vain for an analysis or a characterization of the condition." Blumer correctly noted that the German word *Blödsinn* was translated as "dementia" in English and that Kraepelin used this term to refer to senile dementia ("der Alterblödsinn"). However, Blumer observed, "in the description of *Dementia praecox,* the terminal state is never referred to as *dementia* but as *Verblödung, Schwachsinn* or *Defekt,*" three German words translated as "deterioration process," "mental weakness," and "defect," respectively. The "dementia" of dementia praecox existed only in its name. Because Kraepelin always held the door open to the possibility of rare cases of "complete recovery" in his chapters on dementia praecox, Blumer argued that Kraepelin's definition was "a generic one, including all forms of acquired permanent weak-mindedness or defect . . . and even *temporary* mental disturbance may fall under this appellation."[6]

Blumer had indeed identified a major weakness in Kraepelin's disease concept: the vagueness of his definition of the term "dementia" and its incongruities with the three metaphors he used for the end state of the illness. With so many similarities to the "vesanic" or "pseudodementia" concept, Kraepelin's other major disease concept, manic-depressive insanity, could theoretically be described as manifesting periods of dementia too. The confusion of American alienists over the proper application of Kraepelin's diagnostic terms may have been caused in part by their confusion about what he meant by dementia.

Another dimension of the backlash was cultural. Anglo-American alienists began to express prejudices against the German origin of the classification system they were being pressured to adopt. "I cannot understand why continental thought should set the pace for the rest of the world, more especially for this country," wrote J. T. W. Rowe, an alienist at the Manhattan State Hospital. "We are still influenced and guided by the dictation of foreign savants and writers, and we are asked to bolt unquestioningly the conclusions they have derived from sometimes very limited fields of observation. It is high time we made our own the predominating statistics in this country, and stood by them."[7] In 1909 the Canadian alienist C. K. Clarke reported, "I have been belaboured privately and publicly because I have adopted German methods of investigation, and German systems of classification, instead of showing a delightful imperialistic spirit of patriotism, which must in its narrowness select British models as its best. As science is international, or . . . without nationality, I am free to confess that I shall willingly accept a South Sea Island method if it is better than the one we have."[8]

Yet another dimension of this backlash—or "awakening," depending on one's perspective[9]—was the subtle beginning of the reframing of dementia praecox into a psychogenic condition. Adolf Meyer led this movement and would soon be joined by August Hoch and others influenced by the psychoanalytic ideas of Sigmund Freud (1856–1939) and, perhaps even more important, Carl Gustav Jung (1875–1961). For the Meyerians it would be a backlash against autointoxication theories and the prognostic fatalism of Kraepelin's disease. In reality this turn of mentality was more literary than clinical, an internecine conflict that played out on paper and at conferences. For the vast majority of assistant physicians in asylums between 1903 and the 1920s, psychogenic theories were irrelevant, if known at all. And most persons diagnosed with dementia praecox continued to struggle through their daily reality of elusive alienists and asylum therapeutics (sedative drugs, baths, and diversions). Our present perception of a historical discontinuity was not the preoccupation of the people of the past.

But before the unhappy members of the American psychiatric elite could get around to creating a nativist conception of dementia praecox, or at least a name change, it escaped from the pages of medical texts and through the apertures of asylums into the collective consciousness of the American public. And once the spirit—or demon—was out of the bottle, it was impossible to put it back in or summon it by a different name. At least for a while.

As described in the introduction to this book, dementia praecox first came to the attention of the wider American public (except for those who had the diagnosis or knew someone with it) through an article about the murder trial of Harry K. Thaw published in the *New York Times* on 5 March 1907. This was the first time Kraepelin's disease had appeared in the pages of that newspaper. After this point the term would appear in the *New York Times* for the next half-century in reports about purported medical breakthroughs, mental hygiene concerns about prevention, professional meetings in which the disease was discussed, and, perhaps most important, in the coverage of later trials in which dementia praecox was used as part of an insanity defense.[10] Dementia praecox had entered the courts and the culture.

The first Thaw trial in 1907 (which ended in a hung jury) was a media event of the first magnitude, just as the 1881–1882 trial of Charles Guiteau, the assassin of President James A. Garfield, had been a quarter-century before. The historian Charles E. Rosenberg argued that the Guiteau proceedings "was the most celebrated American 'insanity trial' of the nineteenth century, and perhaps only the Harry K. Thaw and Leopold-Loeb cases in the twentieth century rival it in prominence."[11] Daily, almost verbatim, reports of the testimony of the medical experts for both the prosecution and the defense were published in the *New York Times* and quoted liberally in newspapers across the United States. It is almost certain that somewhere, in some courtroom in the country, an alienist acting as an expert witness had offered "dementia praecox" as a possible or probable diagnosis of a defendant, but the newspaper coverage of the Thaw trial made Kraepelin's disease a psychiatric celebrity in its own right.

Shortly after Thaw murdered Stanford White in New York City on the night of 25 June 1906, Thaw's family retained Allan McLane Hamilton (1848–1919), the leading forensic alienist of his era.[12] Hamilton, the grandson of Alexander Hamilton, was a tall and distinguished-looking man who was a fixture in the New York society scene. He interviewed Thaw on four occasions in his jail cell and wrote a report for Thaw's attorneys in which he diagnosed Thaw with "dementia praecox of a paranoid type, a form of insanity from which recovery is very rare." During the trial Hamilton said it was a form of insanity from which "only two percent" might recover.[13] This did not please Thaw's family, who of course wanted their experts to testify that Harry was temporarily insane at the time of the murder, not chronically insane.

The Thaw family of Pittsburgh—whose fortune at the time was estimated to be approximately $800 million (in 2008 dollars)—also hired numerous other distinguished alienists and neurologists to be expert witnesses. These included Charles G. Wagner, the superintendent of the state hospital in Binghamton, New York; William Alanson White, the superintendent of the government Hospital for the Insane in Washington, D.C.; Smith Ely Jelliffe, a prominent New York City neurologist; Charles W. Pilgrim (like White and Wagner, a future president of the American Psychiatric Association); Graeme Hammond, a noted neurologist; and Britton Evans, the superintendent of the state asylum in Morris Plains, New Jersey, who was a published expert on forensic issues.[14] Expert witnesses for the prosecution included Allan Ross Diefendorf from the state hospital in Middletown, Connecticut; William Mabon, the superintendent of the Manhattan State Hospital; William Pritchard of the New York Polyclinic Hospital; and Albert Warren Ferris of the New York College of Physicians and Surgeons.

As with the Guiteau trial of the nineteenth century, the expert testimony of these alienists and neurologists proved to be an embarrassing spectacle for the profession of psychiatry. Because there was no uniform system for the classification of mental disorders in 1907, nor any consensus as to nomenclature, numerous possible diagnoses were offered by both the prosecution and the defense witnesses. Only White and Jelliffe refused to offer a diagnosis, but they did testify that at the time of the murder Thaw was insane in the sense that he could not distinguish between right and wrong. In 1907 "insanity" was both a medical and a legal term, and it would not be until the 1920s, in part through the efforts of psychiatrists such as White and Jelliffe, that psychiatry would separate itself from the term "insanity" and its legal interpretation in favor of its own vocabulary for a range of discrete mental diseases.[15]

A good deal of the mockery of the alienists in the press came from a statement made by Britton Evans about his observations of Thaw: "I observed a nervous agitation and restlessness, such as comes from a severe brain storm, and is common in persons who have recently gone through an explosive or fulminating condition of mental unsoundness." "Brain storm" became part of the American vocabulary, lampooned in newspapers and made into music. (Within a few months after Evans's statement in court, sheet music for a song entitled *Brain-Storm Rag* appeared in stores.)[16] When the alienist Charles Wagner was cross-examined by the prosecutor, according to the *New York Times* on 5 March 1907, "he found it difficult to classify the form of insanity which Thaw is alleged to have suffered from at the time of the shooting. He said that there were symptoms of dementia praecox, of progressive insanity, and the insanity of adolescence."[17] On 20 March the newspaper quoted Wagner as saying Thaw exhibited "some symptoms" of manic-depressive insanity and some of dement praecox.[18] Unlike the "brain storm" theory, neither of these references to Kraepelin's disease provoked any reaction.

Dementia praecox may have remained an obscure shadow in the collective consciousness of Americans for years to come if it was not for the fact that both the defense attorney, Delphin Delmas, and the prosecutor, William Travers Jerome, invoked a caricature of it during their closing arguments. Delmas did so as a way to mock the opinions of Allan Lane Hamilton and Charles Wagner. The defense had argued that Thaw was not guilty because he was justified in murdering White due to the "unwritten law" that a man can commit murder to protect the honor of one's wife, family, or home. Thaw was protecting the honor of his wife, the actress Evelyn Nesbit, who had been seduced by White a few years before Thaw had married her. Delmas did not directly appeal to an insanity defense for Thaw, but instead offered the mock diagnosis *dementia Americana* during his closing remarks:

> The learned alienists have left the matter in an uncertain condition, because they have not classified the insanity under which the defendant was laboring at that time. Gentlemen, I care not whether you give that

insanity a name or not. It is a species of insanity which, though it may be unknown to those learned alienists, is perfectly familiar to every man who has a family, and to the history of jurisprudence in these United States. It is a species of insanity which has been recognized in every Court, in every State in this Union, from the Canadian border to the Gulf of Texas. It is that species of insanity which, if you desire to give it a name, I will ask you to label it *dementia Americana*.[19]

Jerome, the prosecuting attorney, sealed the fate of "dementia Americana" by referring to it multiple times during his own closing argument, granting the term, and its obvious reference to dementia praecox, lasting notoriety. It no doubt embarrassed alienists about the nature of their own profession. For some the embarrassment must have deepened when the newly elected Charles G. Hill gave his presidential address to the American Medico-Psychological Association on 7 May 1907 and blindly regarded the terms of ridicule that emerged from the Thaw trial as legitimate clinical concepts: "Though our classifications are so numerous that there is little room for addition . . . they are so imperfect and incomplete that leading alienists publicly differ as to the category in which to place certain groups of symptoms, and occasionally find it necessary to coin new terms to describe them, such as Brain-Storms or Dementia Americana. With all of our complex divisions and subdivisions how often does it occur to us in admitting a patient undoubtedly insane, that we are at a loss to know under what classification to place him."[20] Hill obviously was clueless. He had not followed all the details of the Thaw trial and did not know that attorneys, not alienists, had coined "dementia Americana." It is clear from his remarks that he felt the need to defend the right of alienists to create new diagnostic terms on an as-needed basis to classify difficult cases. Such was the state of American psychiatry in 1907.

In the second, and brief, Thaw trial in 1908, all three alienists for the defense agreed on a single diagnosis for Thaw: manic-depressive insanity. The prosecution did not prolong the proceedings and Thaw was sent off to an institution for the criminally insane. Once again another of Kraepelin's new disease concepts was given national exposure due to newspaper reports of the trial. However, the 1908 trial was not the spectacle that the first trial had been.

The Thaw trials are important in the story of dementia praecox in America not only because their publicity gave wide exposure to Kraepelin's two new, great insanities, but also because they demonstrate that attorneys and judges now had to join alienists in the struggle to comprehend a new language for madness. Whereas a legal concept of insanity was congruent with a general medical acceptance—in practice if not always in textbook theory—of a "unitary psychosis" notion by alienists, the introduction of Kraepelinian classification to the United States after 1896 brought with it a very different concept: the claim of disease specificity. It was inevitable that psychiatry would eventually have to embrace such an assertion if the profession was to be regarded in the courts as a modern branch of medicine. The Guiteau and Thaw trials had exposed the lack of anything resembling a scientific consensus about diagnosis in the profession of alienists. But differential diagnosis of the insanities using a classification system based on prognosis had profound implications for the ways an insanity defense could be argued and judicial decisions rendered in the courts. The Thaw trials were the first major flashpoints between law and medicine wrought by Kraepelin's diseases of poor prognosis (dementia praecox and its dire chronicity) and good prognosis (manic-depression and its periodic episodes of temporary insanity between long periods of lucid sanity). Should a criminal found insane, even if a murderer, be committed to an asylum for life, or merely until the periodic episodes of temporary insanity subsided? Were there now different types of temporary insanity (single-episode crimes of passion, a disease marked by multiple episodes)? The new insanity concepts from Germany raised new judicial questions.

The tension between legal and medical conceptions of insanity fueled by Kraepelinian classification contributed to a fundamental split between the two professions. When the literary focus on disease specificity in American psychiatry took hold by 1910, matters became correspondingly complex. "*Insanity* (a legal conception) has been supplanted by the *insanities* (a medical conception)," wrote E. E. Southard in 1910. "And *the insanities* now grow, divide, multiply and die in the periodical literature quite after the fashion of disease entities in general."[21]

In order for the judicial system to stay current, revisions in the area of law known as medical jurisprudence needed to be made. The first inclusion of dementia praecox in an American legal textbook was in the chapter on the subject in the 1905 fifth edition of *Wharton and Stille's Medical Jurisprudence*.[22] This book was considered to be the standard text in medical jurisprudence a century ago. Dementia praecox also makes its first appearance in a second highly regarded text of that era, John J. Reese's *Medical Jurisprudence and Toxicology*, in its 1911 eighth edition.[23] However, while Kraepelin's concepts made inroads into psychiatry, the path through the legal system was much slower. As late as 1918 an author of an article in the *Michigan Law Review* remarked, "Dementia praecox is the form of insanity which is most favored by the medical profession at this time. . . . While doubtless Kraepelin's work was of substantial value in the study of mental disease, the law should not be severely criticized if it does not at once drop all learning from medical science which preceded Kraepelin, and regard dementia praecox as the last word on the this subject." The author then recommends the continued value of a "well regarded" work on medical jurisprudence from 1898 that does not mention dementia praecox.[24]

Harry Thaw endured a series of insanity hearings after incarceration, including one in 1912 in which William Alanson White declared he was now a "normal and sane person." At this trial Adolf Meyer was characterized as his "principal alienist," perhaps indicating that Meyer had been retained by Thaw's family as his private consulting physician. According to the newspaper report, Meyer "reluctantly" offered the court a diagnosis of "constitutional inferiority."[25] This, as we shall see, reflected his new view of the place where psychopathology began: the unique circumstances of the individual personality.

Adolf Meyer had worked long and hard at the Worcester Insane Hospital in Massachusetts teaching his physicians how to conduct mental status interviews, take patient histories, examine patients physically, participate in daily clinical staff meetings, integrate observations on the ward with pathological findings at autopsy, use Kraepelinian diagnostic concepts, and record this information in great detail. *Exceptionally* great detail.

To Meyer this was the "Worcester plan" for conducting psychiatric research. Everyone—the pathologist, the assistant physicians, the interns, the nurses, and attendants on the wards—everyone was involved in research, as if the entire insane hospital was one big laboratory. It took him four years to transform the daily operation of Worcester: "Only about 1900 had I obtained an organization which seemed to be adequate to the task."[26] But to him, and apparently to the medical staff, who may have felt their duties had some future importance, it was worth the effort. What no doubt seemed like endless, seemingly purposeless paperwork and administrative headaches to some was scientific research to Meyer. This point cannot be stressed enough, for it is the essence of what Meyer meant by "research." Research was bureaucratic in its nature, not biological. Research meant administrative procedures and daily staff meetings and extensive data collection of the minutiae of patients' lives without any quantitative analysis or even publication. Laboratory work served only as a secondary and supportive source of "facts" about a "whole" individual. Basic or foundational laboratory research was of even less importance because it was impersonal and not clearly linked to identifiable patients. Individual patients were "experiments of life," and it might take years of data collection on a single person to draw any "firm" conclusions about that individual. Every clinical opinion about a patient was tentative—had enough facts been collected to make a generalization about that human being? Clinical judgments were made—they had to be for administrative purposes—but they were merely hypotheses in a constant process of being tested through more data collection. In later years Meyer would have the audacity to call this vision of psychiatric research "psychobiology."

Meyer would take this model to the large New York state system of hospitals after being appointed director of the Pathology Institute in May 1902. It would take him far longer in New York to achieve even modest goals; in 1903 there were approximately twenty-five thousand insane patients in thirteen New York state hospitals. But one thing was clear: the original vision of Ira Van Gieson for a multidisciplinary institute devoted to basic research in psychiatry would not be reinstated under Meyer. But research on a reduced scale did continue.

One of the first things Meyer did at the Pathology Institute was establish three separate research departments. The first was the clinical division, headed by George H. Kirby (1875–1935), who had formerly worked under Meyer as an assistant physician in Worcester. Kirby was given a twenty-bed ward in the Verplanck building of the Manhattan State Hospital to conduct psychiatric research. The chemical and histological departments were headed by two holdovers from the Van Gieson era: Phoebus A. Levine and the pathologist Charles B. Dunlap. Levine had conducted much of the autointoxication research at the Institute. By 1908 both the chemical lab and its work were closed down.

Meyer summoned all the superintendents of state hospitals in New York for a series of training sessions at the Institute on Ward's Island in the first week of December 1902. This would become a yearly ritual.

In a long lecture he gave to the superintendents he made his priorities clear: given the evil of "poor administration and poor nursing of the patients" on the one hand, and "poor medical care" on the other, he said that "poor medical work is the lesser evil." "Nature" would help the patients, but "nature cannot do anything against poor nursing."[27] The new mission of the Institute was to be primarily educational, to provide the administrators and the staff with training specific to their jobs in hospitals for the insane. The training for the physicians would be designed to make up for the deficiencies of medical schools, since most offered no training in psychiatry. He sent the superintendents back to their hospitals with typewritten instructions on how to interview insane patients. In the latter half of 1903 Meyer visited every institution in the state, often staying for two weeks, and made the alienists present written case summaries of patients so that he could assess their level of sophistication. It is to his credit that by the time he left the Institute in 1910 the state hospitals in New York were the best in the United States from an administrative and clinical perspective.[28]

Meyer knew he had to find a way to wake up the alienists and spark an interest in their insane patients. Because there was nothing new that could be done to treat or cure insanity, he focused on curing the alienists of their ignorance and lassitude. Training was the cure. And when it took hold it had a cascading effect on the institution as a whole: "It has not been difficult to see that wherever there was at least one member of the staff well enough informed on these issues . . . a sound interest in the patients naturally increased," and this "carried the physicians to do twice and three times the amount of work with interest and satisfaction."[29]

The one clinical issue that Meyer thought was relatively unimportant was the diagnostic classification of patients. "My first advice was to let classification rest or to give it a secondary place," he wrote in his annual report for 1903. Instead he instructed his alienists to simply "collect the facts . . . and to group them according to their merit."[30] Ultimately Meyer's method was no method. He would continue this practice at the Henry C. Phipps Psychiatric Clinic at Johns Hopkins from 1913 to the end of his life. At a small clinic under his sole command he could get away with this elusive charade. But in New York he soon learned that the large insane hospitals under his leadership needed some sort of structure for classifying their tens of thousands of patients. So instead of introducing Kraepelin's, he made up his own.

Gone was the enthusiasm of his early days in Worcester for Kraepelin's disease concepts, as well as his admiration of the fact that Kraepelin had claimed they were derived from long-term quantitative and
qualitative research. Nowhere to be seen were the thirteen classes of insanities that Kraepelin proposed in the 1899 sixth edition of his textbook. Instead, when the superintendant-pupils were summoned to their
headmaster's office on Ward's Island in December 1903 they were given
a typewritten sheet of paper and told to use the classifications on it to
generate their annual statistical tables. These were, simply: 1. Imbecility
and idiocy; 2. Epilepsy with insanity; 3. General paralysis; 4. Senile insanity; 5. Alcoholic insanity; 6. Other psychoses; and 7. Not insane.[31]
The thinness of this classification system, and the absence of any trace of
two great insanities, dementia praecox and manic-depressive insanity,
marked a fundamental turn away from Kraepelin. But it would not last.

The annual reports of all New York institutions for the 1903-1904
fiscal year used the old mania, melancholia, and dementia categories, but
for the 1904-1905 annual reports all except Manhattan State Hospital
used Meyer's skeletal classification scheme. Needless to say, the category
of "Other psychoses" was the largest in each hospital by many hundreds
of patients. Patients were told they were insane but not given anything
resembling a medical diagnosis—and they wanted one. Something must
have happened by the autumn of 1904, perhaps complaints from physicians and family members that reached the ears of higher state officials,
because an even newer classification hastily put in place at the Manhattan State Hospital meant Meyer had been forced to rethink things.

In his 30 September 1905 annual report to the State Commission
in Lunacy he described a "movement for a change in statistics," duti-
fully reporting, "A strong effort has been made this year to harmonize
the official statistical returns with the newer developments of medical
and psychiatric interests." Meyer's distaste for classification systems is
clear from reading this document. The tone was didactic but defensive.
He was critical of Kraepelin in particular. Meyer told state officials that
his ideal system would be for physicians to collect all the necessary facts
about a patient and come to a conclusion based on "independent
thought." Incredibly he admitted, "I should by far prefer to give every
hospital the right to make its own diagnostic tables for what they are
worth." This time around, Meyer proposed a revised classification
with three major groupings corresponding to the organic psychoses
(those with a known biological cause, such as definite brain diseases, or

those that are toxic or autotoxic), another to the functional psychoses (those without known biological causes), included in which were dementia praecox and "manic-depressive states," and finally a class devoted to the "recognized neuroses" (neurasthenia, psychasthenia, epilepsy, and hysteria) and to those conditions due to "make-up" ("constitutional inferiority and abnormal make-up, with or without outbreaks," and idiocy and imbecility).[32]

"The claim that the practitioner and the family want a diagnosis is a matter not of medicine but of professional habits," Meyer claimed in the conclusion of his report, making his antipathy plain to the state officials who, in all likelihood, were pressuring him to put a more elaborate classification in place.[33] There is no doubt that he considered these "professional habits" bad ones.

This revised classification scheme was the one put into place at the Manhattan State Hospital on Ward's Island and appeared in its annual report for 1904–1905. As we have seen, what resulted from the adoption of this classification scheme is exactly what Meyer feared: an institution almost half-filled with the diseases created by Emil Kraepelin. It would not be until the annual reports ending 30 September 1909 were submitted that it became clear that all state hospitals had finally been forced to use a single uniform classification system—a first for any state in the country. But it had been earlier, by the fiscal year ending in 1907, that all of the state hospitals included both dementia praecox and manic-depressive insanity in their statistical tables regardless of classification scheme—and with the predicted effect. For example, in places like the state hospital in Rochester, New York, dementia praecox would make up "50% of the permanent population of the hospital." Whereas before 30 September 1904 there had never been a single case of dementia praecox recorded in the state hospitals of New York, by 30 September 1913 there were 16,299 such cases.[34] Meyer's reluctant decision to infect the patients of the state hospitals of New York with Kraepelin's disease would haunt him until he could escape to his small clinic at Johns Hopkins. When he finally did so in 1913, he made sure he did not carry this plague with him.

Adolf Meyer's rise to such prominence in the largest system of state hospitals in the United States certainly made him conscious of the fact that he was arguably the most powerful man in American psychiatry. This may very well have been a factor in his attempts to get out from under the shadow of Emil Kraepelin and put forth original theoretical ideas of his own. This is not to say that he lost any respect for Kraepelin or his work. Indeed he would continue to recommend to members of his junior staff that they go to Munich and gain some experience working with Kraepelin. One such individual was George Kirby, the head of his clinical research department at the Institute.

Kirby was born and raised in North Carolina. His father was a physician and, for a time, the superintendent of the state hospital in Goldsboro, near Raleigh. Kirby graduated from the University of North Carolina in 1896 and moved to New York to attend medical school at the Long Island College Hospital, finishing his medical degree in 1899. Having developed an interest in the insane while working with his father during the summers when he was not attending medical school, Kirby wrote a letter to Meyer in September 1899 asking for a position. Meyer interviewed and hired him, and Kirby became perhaps Meyer's closest disciple during the period they worked together at the Worcester Insane Hospital, 1899–1902. When Meyer moved to his new position at the Institute he brought Kirby with him. Kirby was conscientious, trustworthy, and in awe of Meyer's intellect and Old World charm.

With Meyer's encouragement Kirby left his post at the Institute in January 1906 and went to Munich for several months of study with Kraepelin, and then for a shorter period in Zurich with Jung. Jung was pioneering the use of the word association test with his institutionalized patients, and Kirby was one of the many American alienists (such as the neurologist Frederick Peterson, A. A. Brill, and August Hoch) who studied with him for varying periods of time to learn the technique. Kirby returned to the United States in July 1906.

Kirby was not fluent in German and had great difficulty in conversing with Kraepelin when they first met. Kirby wanted to get to work right away in the clinic, but in a letter to Meyer he complained that Kraepelin told him that "for work in the laboratory or clinic one must have an exact knowledge of the language and also be familiar with the literature." Kraepelin told Kirby to go to the library and sit and read the first volume of *Psychologische Arbeiten,* the journal Kraepelin published that contained the reports of the experimental work done by him and his associates. This did not please Kirby. For the following

week he bought tickets for the postgraduate program lectures by Alzheimer on "brain and soul" and "the anatomy of the cortex," Kraepelin on "forensic psychiatry," and several two-hour clinics with Kraepelin and medical students in the psychiatric clinic.[35] The Munich
clinic had one hundred beds for patients and six full-time physician-
researchers tending to them. In addition there were numerous German
medical school students as well as students and physicians from around
the world, including many Americans, paying for postgraduate training. The Munich clinic was the best of its kind in the world.

It should be remembered that, other than his summers in his father's state hospital in North Carolina, the only experience or true
training Kirby had ever received in psychiatry was with Meyer in
Worcester. By the time Kirby had arrived in late 1900, Meyer had already reformed the hospital to a point that it was unlike any other in
America. The emphasis was on the exacting documentation of all clinical encounters. This model would be carried by them to New York.
Kirby assumed that Meyer had simply transplanted the typical procedures and practices of German psychiatry to America. By the end of
February, when Kirby's ability to speak and understand German had
improved, he became more aware of what was happening around him.
And the experience was not what he had expected:

> I feel some that they do not make such comprehensive record as we do.
> One is struck by the *absence* of note taking. K. makes the rounds, talks
> with each patient and not a word is recorded! The records are of course
> written in a script with the exception of a short abstract (type written)
> and this K. seems to depend on mainly at the clinical presentations. The
> clinics are conducted in what I suppose is the classical way—the patient
> is brought in and two students are called down to make the examina-
> tion and then a diagnosis! After this K. reads the summary and makes
> some remarks. It all goes pretty easy and only occasionally is there any
> doubt about a case. The symptoms are run over in catalogue style and I
> have been quite disappointed in not hearing finer analyses.[36]

When Kirby returned he published a short but interesting report
on Kraepelin's clinic and the varieties of research that were under way
under his direction. Among these were studies of the cerebrospinal
fluid, psychological experiments on fatigue, and an examination of the

unusual pupil reactions in the eyes of dementia praecox patients. He also commented on Kraepelin's methods of treatment in the Munich clinic. Unlike the experience of patients in all American institutions, German patients in Kraepelin's clinic were not heavily drugged:

> The Kraepelinian school has been criticized for a lack of interest in treatment. Indeed one quickly observes that drugs are rarely prescribed and then only to meet definite physical conditions; on the other hand hydrotherapy is carried out in the clinic probably more extensively than in any other institution in the world. Tubs suitable for the continuous bath have been liberally provided, there being no less than eighteen available for this purpose. There appears to be no contraindication to the continuous bath; all forms of excitements and agitations are favorably influenced—manic attacks, delirious alcoholics, anxiety psychoses, and excited general paralytics are treated by this method. No drug sedatives or restraint of any kind are used.[37]

Other than learning the experimental methods of the word association technique, Kirby had another reason for visiting Jung at the Burghölzli mental hospital in Zurich after his time with Kraepelin. By 1906 Jung was already interested in Freud's theories and treatments and was using psychoanalysis as an interpretive guide for his clinical and experimental work. Kirby had learned about Freud and Jung from Meyer. As part of his ongoing courses for physicians at Manhattan State Hospital, Meyer had been discussing Freud's work in his classes as early as 1905. Abraham Arden Brill (1874—1948), who later became America's first Freudian analyst as well as the driving force behind the psychoanalytic movement in New York, first learned about Freud's ideas from a class he took with Meyer. At the time Brill was a neurologist at the Central Islip State Hospital on Long Island. Kirby had become so smitten with the psychoanalytic interpretation of symptoms that another physician who was at the Manhattan State Hospital at the time recalled, "Kirby, the Clinical Director, as well as Dr. Macfie Campbell . . . encouraged the Freudian approach consistently."[38]

As the historian John Gach has observed, "In the first decade of the twentieth century the New York State System became the chief conduit through which psychoanalytic teaching flowed to America. . . . One can infer the extent to which psychoanalysis had infiltrated the staff at Ward's Island [in this first decade] from the fact that of the fifteen founding members of the New York Psychoanalytic Society in February 1911, ten were or had been associated with the Manhattan State Hospital."[39]

But Meyer never became a disciple of Freud or Jung, nor did he ever use psychoanalytic techniques in his treatment of patients. Meyer can be generously characterized as "eclectic," but in truth he was temperamentally unsuited to follow any other man or his ideas. The only problem was he didn't have many original ones of his own.

In 1903 Meyer began to present papers and publish articles putting forth a view of human nature that he would regard as his most original contribution to psychiatry. For more than a decade he had been quite creative as a reformer of American institutions for the insane. But he had published no textbook of psychiatry—indeed no books of any sort—and his power was institutionally based and limited to his reputation in America. He was not recognized internationally for any intellectual contributions. His name was not associated with any new discoveries about mental disease, nor with any syndrome, nor with any theory of insanity. Meyer knew this—but Kraepelin was hard to top. Where were the holes in Kraepelin's work? Meyer believed he had found a major one.

Kraepelin primarily focused on the course of a disease *once it had already begun* and its outcome. As with the question of etiology, Kraepelin had little to say about *and did not systematically research* the premorbid personalities of persons diagnosed with dementia praecox or manic-depressive insanity, the two functional psychoses whose causes were unknown. Kraepelin did report anecdotes about signs and symptoms exhibited by his patients prior to admission, but in most cases he did not observe these directly. He regarded these as the milder, prodromal indications that the disease process had started, and he considered them to be part of the course of the disease. Although he admitted that in many cases of dementia praecox there were numerous anecdotal reports from family members and friends that some patients were odd or eccentric even in childhood, he knew he could not study the past in a scientific manner. Even when questioned about the timing and nature of the onset of physical diseases such as diabetes, for example, the typical patient was an unreliable witness and the recollections of family members and friends were often no better. Plus, anecdotes about subtle personality changes, subjective changes in thought and mood, or other events in a patient's distant past were not often verifiable. Only those phenomena under the researcher's direct gaze, or that of his colleagues, yielded scientific information about the manifestations of the underlying disease process. Observations could be made, noted on cards, cataloged, and followed up after the patient was discharged.

Meyer, on the other hand, held to a different concept of what constituted scientific research in psychiatry. He valued induction: the unit of study was the individual case. He deliberately avoided structured or quantitative analyses of his considerable mass of case material for the purpose of drawing generalizations. Such deductive exercises created artificial abstractions—such as diagnostic categories—that smothered the richness of the experiential details of an individual life. By 1900 quantitative (and statistical) methods had increasingly come into vogue in American medicine and the social sciences as tools for testing and rejecting theories. But Meyer viscerally resisted this falsifying impulse in science, believing that each theory of psychopathology was flawed but also contained a "perspective" or kernel of truth that threw light on the lived experience of individuals. Although he lapsed from his own scientific ideals and engaged in speculative proposals for his own quasi-diagnostic "reaction types" (based only on his general philosophical impression from his data collection of individual cases, not from structured or quantitative analyses of his case histories), *it is clear that by at least 1903 he had fundamentally repudiated the demand for disease specificity in psychiatry.* By doing so Meyer turned his back not only on Kraepelin, but also on the modernizing impulse in an increasingly rationalized and laboratory-driven general medicine.

Because of Meyer's extraordinary influence in the United States, particularly between 1902 and 1940, his reluctance to create a common scientific language about the insanities encouraged conceptual confusion and compromised communication in American psychiatry. Meyer *consciously* derationalized the profession, pulling it in a direction opposite that of the historical trajectories of the other branches of medicine. He would of course write and speak of dementia praecox, schizophrenia, and manic-depression, or of any other diagnostic term in existence, as if they were factual entities. But it is clear he did so reluctantly, always redefining them according to his own criteria, later

even renaming them. He refused to impose boundaries on them, re-
sisting any effort that encouraged disease specificity by keeping diagnostic concepts fluid, tentative, and vague. In print or in person it was
difficult to understand Meyer with any clarity. Although he apparently
believed he was operating from the best philosophical principles of
American pragmatism (he had known John Dewey in Chicago), his
clinical eclecticism was a scientific swamp for an American psychiatry
struggling to catch up with early twentieth-century general medicine.

Meyer's rejection of the specification of mental diseases also kept
alive (by default, and implicit in everyday clinical practice) the old notion of a unitary psychosis, a single fluid spectrum of madness rather
than discrete disease-like insanities. Any neurosis could blossom into a
psychosis, any shy child into a case of dementia praecox. Any malady
could transform into any other one—there were no rules of order.
Such a continuum would later appeal to those influenced by psychoanalysis and would shadow American psychiatry until the last quarter
of the twentieth century. What would be termed "neo-Kraepelinian"
in American psychiatry in the 1970s was in part a reassertion of the
principle of disease specificity after decades of erosion by Meyerians
and Freudians. From the perspective of his medical cognition, Meyer's
personal vision of psychiatry was a throwback, a branch of medicine
that had more similarities to the traditional practice of medicine of the
mid-nineteenth century—with its emphasis on the individual, restoring natural balances, and on proximal, external, and visible causes—
than the modern research-based, rationalized, disease-specified medicine of his own era (a vision for psychiatry promoted by Kraepelin).

The case history method located the roots of insanity in the unique
life circumstances of the individual, each individual being a "type" of
one, not an example within a category of mental disease. With his obsession for recording every reported aspect of the patient's life, Meyer
believed in the veracity of his case histories. History was a *Wissenschaft,*
a systematic collection and structured study and interpretation of information. Meyer, and many who would follow his lead, such as August
Hoch, Smith Ely Jelliffe, and of course the later proponents of psychoanalysis, believed in the scientific soundness of the case history method.
Despite the serious logical flaw of generalizing inferences about human
nature drawn from one or a few individual case histories, many did so.
Under Meyer's influence a detailed case history filled with as much in-

formation as possible about the life of a patient *before the moment he or she was admitted to a hospital for treatment* would soon become more important than the study of the signs and symptoms, course, and outcome of a patient in an institution once he or she was clearly sick. Indeed, if the assumption of disease entities were dropped there would be no reason to study the "course" of illness.

From Meyer's perspective this was the hole in Kraepelin's method. A detailed case history could provide clues to the cause of the illness. Perhaps it could even conclusively identify etiology. It could provide a reconstruction of the patient's premorbid personality. And most important, if there were certain typical abnormal personality patterns that could be linked to the onset of dementia praecox or manic-depressive insanity later in life, perhaps, just perhaps, these could be identified in young people and some sort of intervention (prophylaxis) could be administered to keep them out of the asylums and state hospitals.

Meyer turned the gaze of some influential members of the American psychiatric elite *backward* in time. Retrospection through narratives of the reconstructed life histories of patients became the only scientific data necessary for discovering the causes of not only the psychoses, but also the neuroses. When the powerful Adolf Meyer shifted his gaze to the period in a patient's life before the manifestations of insanity were evident, others turned their heads as well. Conducting longitudinal studies of course and outcome, such as those carried out by Kraepelin, seemed to lose their relevance—so American alienists did not try. Meyer started this process in 1903 and to a large extent opened the door for the related methods and causal assumptions of psychoanalysis. Within just a few years a uniquely American concept of dementia praecox would emerge, one that was uncoupled from biology and the disappointing failures of laboratory research, a condition based on *psychogenesis*.

To put in another way: for Kraepelin and most other psychiatrists, for a new disease concept to become a scientific fact, to become "real," at some point in the future a nosological term and its diagnostic criteria had to be coupled with biological data. In 1896 Kraepelin had explicitly separated his diagnostic concepts from any specific linkage to brain anatomy or biology—but this was understood to be a necessary first step that would precede, *indeed make possible* such a linkage in the future. Experimental psychology was his preferred research paradigm for guiding and shaping later clinical and biological research, but this laboratory approach held no interest for Meyer. The physiological signs of dementia praecox that any physician could observe during a physical examination, the findings at autopsy, and ongoing laboratory research were all part of the separate but necessary secondary agenda in the process of making Kraepelin's disease a scientific fact. Beginning in 1903 the Meyerians and the Freudians eliminated the necessity of this secondary agenda. The importance of what would be referred to as the patient's "constitution," the physiological state of an individual that may or may not be due to heredity, was never denied. It was just set aside. Biology was dethroned in favor of a new secondary agenda: history.

At the time there was an undeniable logic to this new approach. Except in the instance of the discovery of the Wasserman reaction for syphilis in 1906, biological research in psychiatry had consistently failed. Kraepelin himself had decoupled dementia praecox and manic-depressive illness from biology and defined them in terms of course and prognosis. And no one, certainly not Kraepelin, had ever attempted to systematically document the traumas, insecurities, sexual preoccupations, disappointments, obsessions, and relationships of persons diagnosed with dementia praecox or manic-depressive insanity. After all, these were very new disease concepts. New ground could be broken with a historical research agenda. Could something scientifically useful be found if this was done? Could the environment be as important a factor as past personal experiences? There were many such questions to be answered.

Perhaps, just perhaps, a new nosology of personality types or character types could be identified as precursors to Kraepelin's concepts. A new classification and nomenclature could then emerge *as a prior but parallel scheme,* a new spectrum that would place the units of study—now typological variations of the prepsychotic personality—to a point further back in time from Kraepelin's, whose framework was valid only *after* dementia praecox had been observed in its incipient, irreversible state.

The psychogenesis of the functional psychoses, dementia praecox and manic-depressive insanity, was a bold turn of mind. It spread quickly between 1903 and the Freudianized 1920s among important members of the American psychiatric elite, as evidenced in their literary discourses. It was based as much on curiosity as capitulation, however. By the mid-1920s almost half of the population of most state hospitals and asylums were filled with people with these Kraepelinian diagnoses, and they were becoming more chronic and financially burdensome to state governments. How did they get this way? No one knew. What could be done for them? Nothing now—they were too far gone. But *something* had to be done, at least for the sake of those who would end up in asylums in future generations. *Save the children.* Prevention and treatment, two issues at the forefront of the rising, pre-Freudian psychotherapy movement of 1905–1906, as well as extensions of progressivism in American intellectual life, were possible if the elements of psychogenesis could be discovered. The question of the etiology of dementia praecox had returned.[40]

In 1903 Adolf Meyer published a paper on the "analysis of the neurotic constitution." In it he proposed, based on his personal experience and readings of French authorities such as Pierre Janet, that it might be proper for psychiatry to return to the ancient Greek notion of temperamental, constitutional, or personality "types." Why? "The purpose of characterology is to give a forecast of what a person would do in a considerable variety of emergencies. As alienists, we shall especially have to try and find out whether persons show any combinations of reactions which could make them in our eyes candidates for mental derangement, or which would modify the form of mental derangement which they might happen to get."[41]

In this early statement Meyer is already proposing that "combinations of reactions" characterize a personality type. Different "constitutional types," to use his term, since he always maintained a rhetorical toehold for a theoretical role for physiology or heredity, can be said to characterize already well-received diagnostic categories. Instead of signs and symptoms there are now "combinations of reactions." He identified five types of "nervousness" that were commonly recognized as neuroses (the psychasthenic, neurasthenic, hypochondriacal, hysterical, and epileptic types). Then, in a departure from standard psychiatric divisions, he included a sixth class of types that were considered psychotic disorders, not neuroses: the manic-depressive type, the paranoid type, and the "deterioration type." It is this last type that Meyer claimed to be the personality found in persons who develop dementia praecox.

So what does a child who is a "deterioration type" look like? A child who had a "perfectly exemplary childhood" but was "exemplary under an inadequate ideal" and exhibited "goodness and meekness" rather than "strength and determination." Later, in adolescence, these children developed vivid religious ideas,

> a certain disconnection of thought, unaccountable whims make their appearance, and deficient control in areas of ethics and judgment; at home irritability shows itself. . . . Sensitiveness to allusions of pleasure, health, etc., drive the patient into seclusion; Headaches, freaky appetite, general malaise, hypochondriacal complaints about the heart, etc., unsteadiness of occupation and efficiency, daydreaming and utterly immature philosophizing, and above all, loss of directive energy and initiative without obvious cause. . . . All these traits may not be transient . . . but the beginning of a deterioration, more and more marked by indifference in the emotional life and ambitions, and a peculiar fragmentary type of attention, with all the transitions to the apathetic state of terminal dementia.[42]

In another paper published that year, titled "The Arrest of Development in Adolescence," Meyer picked up this theme: "The adolescent deterioration can very largely be traced to disharmonies of thought, of habits, and of interests which bring about a stunting in one direction or another." After specifically mentioning Kraepelin, Meyer noted, "Unfortunately physicians are rarely in a position really to study the candidates of deterioration during the relatively healthy days."[43]

By January 1905 Meyer would feel confident enough about his growing theory to provide a more detailed exposition of his theory of the cause of dementia praecox. It was due to "habit deterioration." Citing William James as one of his inspirations (James wrote extensively on habit), Meyers presented his new—and vague—theory of dementia praecox: "Instead of merely appealing to cortex changes of obscure correlation, or to equally obscure autointoxications, or to arrest of development, I refer to the disharmony of habits, disharmony of those regulations which shape a well-balanced economy: the intestinal and circulatory functions, the sexual life, and above all the trend of interests depending in its integrity and efficiency on a certain equilibrium." He then indicated that his goal was to "make distinctions of various types of habit disorganization."[44] He and his followers would continue to refer to this paper for the next fifty years with, in the opinion of non-Meyerians, undue and unearned reverence. The material is simply difficult to understand in a concrete way.

By August 1906 he began referring to these "types of habit disorganization" as "reaction types." This was a term that would stick. The human personality, including its constitution, would be reframed as a republic of "reactions," organized into a holistic functional system with the body. In dementia praecox the early premorbid personality in adolescence and perhaps even in childhood is marred by a "deterioration of the habits and undermining of instincts and their somatic components."[45] Meyer warned parents, teachers, and fellow physicians through illustrative case histories about the peculiar, reclusive, daydreaming nature of children who later went on to develop dementia praecox. In 1908 he defined the disease as "most practically expressed as the inevitable and natural development from a deterioration of habits, partly due to developmental defects of the mental endowment, but in part, at least, to the clashing of instincts and to progressively faulty modes of meeting difficulties, and the disability of a proper balance of anabolism and catabolism which they entail."[46] Nowhere in any of Meyer's later writings on the subject is he any clearer than this. And this is precisely the problem.

For decades to come dementia praecox would simply be a "reaction type." Meyer and Kirby compiled a privately printed collection of case histories illustrating these reaction types for their trainees, and Kirby did his best to promote Meyer's new etiology of dementia praecox in print.[47] The few descriptions quoted in the paragraphs above are essentially all that Meyer ever really offered. Needless to say, for those contemporaries of Meyer who were not his disciples, and for historians, these were insufficient.

To one contemporary, the neurologist Michael Osnato, all of this was "exasperatingly vague."[48] To others the problem was not only Meyer's writing style, but something deliberately evasive and elusive about the man himself, almost as if Meyer cloaked himself behind these jargon-laden ruminations on purpose, like an early twentieth-century postmodernist. Meyer "would never make entirely clear what he did believe and resorted to a lot of confusing words, phrases and concepts, which many people accepted chiefly because they had a profound respect for him without any idea whatsoever as to what he meant," complained the psychiatrist Karl Menninger.[49] As these few passages on the psychogenesis of dementia praecox illustrate, Meyer had a difficult time convincing anyone other than his disciples of his originality. According to the historian Edward Shorter, Meyer was "a second-rate thinker and a verbose writer," and "he was never able, in his own mind, to disentangle schools that were absolutely incompatible, and ended up embracing whatever new came along." When, by 1915, the American psychiatric profession had crystallized into only a few local but powerful avenues of influence (Baltimore and Washington, D.C., Boston, New York, Philadelphia), Meyer—and his personality— still dominated the profession: "Paradoxically, the man who came closest to the very center of the highly centralized institutional structure of American nervous and mental disease was a man at once both brilliant and obtuse, thoughtful and undisciplined," wrote the historical sociologist Andrew Delano Abbott. "By virtue of his position, Meyer conferred his flaws on the field."[50]

For Meyer and his disciples, who called psychogenesis a "functional" or "dynamic" approach, the primary enemy was the autointoxication theories of dementia praecox. Throughout his writings on this disease Meyer invariably ridicules or dismisses them as "that simplifying formula which merely exalts the art of purging" and as merely "hypothetical."[51] By 1909 he and his school had become openly critical of the sterility and narrowness of laboratory approaches in medicine and psychiatry. Medical school training that focused only on "a narrow range of laboratory problems" left the student "without help and training to meet some essentials in life."[52] Attitudes such as these served only to pull American psychiatry in a direction that continued to separate it from general medicine. Charles Macfie Campbell (1876–1943), who worked under Meyer at this time, echoed the suspicion of laboratory claims to knowledge shared by many traditional American physicians and alienists:

> To those who work continually with the categories of the physiological and chemical laboratories there seems to be a complete want of contact between the complex disorders of habits and adaptations of individuals . . . and the physical symptoms which have attracted so much attention. These investigators do not realize that this want of contact is their own product; they have divorced the physical symptoms from the setting in which they occur, and have studied them as if that setting were irrelevant. . . . Meyer has formulated a conception of the disorder which takes into consideration many facts which have been neglected by those who have been dominated by auto-intoxication hypotheses.[53]

Divorcing physical symptoms from the setting in which they occur was the hallmark of the specification of diseases in modern medicine. Laboratory-generated knowledge played a key role in this process. It was a defining feature of the rationalization of medicine that had occurred since the mid-1800s. In contrast, retaining an exclusive focus on the singular rise of symptoms in individual cases was an ancient practice of traditional physicians. It was also the preferred medical cognition of the Meyerians and Freudians. The patient, the unique situation, and the patient's style of reaction to the unique situation were all that mattered. Unique circumstances were not generalizable, hence diagnostic labels and conclusions drawn from laboratory research, even psychological research, yielded partial insights at best. By devaluating autointoxication research in psychiatry—indeed by engendering a suspicion of the relevance of laboratory research in general—Meyer, Macfie Campbell, and others of a similar mind endeavored to halt, and perhaps reverse, the process of making Kraepelinian terms like "dementia praecox" into specific, natural, biological "diseases."

At Manhattan State Hospital there was a campaign to reduce the number of dementia praecox cases even if the diagnosis itself could not be banished. Alienists in the front lines of asylum practice found it too useful, and Kraepelinian classification categories based on prognosis served larger bureaucratic needs. But in the elite circle around Meyer the hospital had become a bastion of Meyerian and, to a smaller degree, Freudian philosophy. There is no history of tension between the two approaches: they blended into a seamless, syncretic cognitive chimera in Meyer's mind as well as in those of his acolytes. The annual report for the year ending on 30 September 1909 included a special section explaining the "psychogenic and sexual factors in dementia praecox," a clear expression of the concerns of Meyer and the psychoanalysts. And the institution was pleased to report the following news: "The diagnosis of dementia praecox has grown steadily less frequent since the high mark of 1904, when the term was first introduced into the 'diagnostic tables.' . . . From these percentages it is evident that our conception of what we are justified in calling dementia praecox has undergone a radical change during the past few years."[54]

It had indeed. But other than being psychogenic, what was it? It would be left to Meyer's old friend and colleague August Hoch to try to clarify things.

As indefinite and mystifying as Meyer's ideas were, his explicit argument that the causes of dementia praecox were to be found in maladaptive "responses" or "habit disorganizations" that could potentially be changed through "habit training" was enough to embolden August Hoch and Smith Ely Jelliffe to charge down the same path for the first time in 1907. However, their approaches, as we shall see, were quite different.

After tensions with Edward Cowles had increased to unacceptable levels, August Hoch finally left the McLean Hospital in 1905 and took a position with the relatively new Bloomingdale Hospital in White Plains, New York. The institution had moved into a new building in upstate New York in 1892 from the Morningside Heights area of Manhattan. Indeed the original Bloomingdale Asylum stood on the site where Columbia University's Low Library now stands. While at Bloomingdale Hoch's interests changed markedly. He was no longer a confirmed Kraepelinian.[55] Instead he became interested in psychoanalysis, particularly with the work of Jung at the Burghölzli mental hospital in Zurich. He was fascinated by the possibilities of using the word association test as part of psychoanalytic treatment. The experimental procedure seemed to confirm Freud's ideas about the power of unconscious conflicts in mental life, and the test did so by identifying "complexes," clusters of thoughts, feelings, and images organized around a central theme or motif. His research interests also changed. Following Meyer, Hoch now became interested in exploring the premorbid personality of persons who would later develop psychosis.

Hoch first presented his new views at a meeting of the New York Psychiatrical Society on 6 March 1907. He argued that there was evidence from the case histories of "paranoic states" that "psychogenesis could clearly be traced when the facts of the case were really accessible." He admitted that his own ideas were influenced by Meyer, Freud, Bleuler, and Jung. The cause of a paranoid psychosis was the result of unconscious conflicts—"undercurrents" or "complexes"—created by past experiences that "are not handled properly" and are dealt with by "miscarried attempts at readjustment." He acknowledged that there may be other causes than this as well, such as "influences which increase the strength of the undercurrents, or influences which, in other ways than those indicated, lessen the resistance, such as the action of alcohol, menopause and the like." It was reported in the published summary of Hoch's

talk that during the discussion session that followed, "as to the psychogenic origin of certain types of delusions, Dr. Jelliffe was in accord with
Dr. Hoch," and he suggested turning to novels by Henry James and others for a literary description of how this might happen.[56]

In an article published in June 1907 Hoch proposed that "the study
of mental causes and of the personality" would prove to have bearing
"on the questions of prophylaxis and treatment." The "essential feature" of his view was that "there are certain diseases in which conflicts,
and the reactions of the personality to these, stand in the foreground of
the clinical picture and that in those anatomical or chemical changes,
or indications of them, have thus far not furnished much help for the
understanding of the disease."[57] By January 1908 he was so sure of the
correctness of his position that he could give a lecture with the title
"The Psychogenesis in Dementia Praecox," a radical departure from
the received wisdom about Kraepelin's disease in that era.[58] Hoch, who
for most of his career had put countless hours into autopsying cadavers
and studying the effects of chemical substances on mental performance
and fatigue, had resigned himself to the ultimate futility of those activities. He was now going to devote himself exclusively to the mental
side of things.

Hoch would be most remembered in the decades that followed for
the idea he developed in 1908: that many cases of dementia praecox
developed out of a "shut-in personality." "The insanity grows, as it
were, out of the personality," he maintained.[59] He described the "shut-
in personality" in this manner:

> We find, in dementia praecox, persons who do not have a natural ten-
> dency to be open, and to get into contact with the environment, who are
> reticent, seclusive, who cannot adapt themselves to situations, who are
> hard to influence, often sensitive and stubborn, but the latter more in a
> passive than an active way. They show little interest in what goes on, of-
> ten do not participate in the pleasures, cares and pursuits of those about
> them; although often sensitive they do not let others know what their
> conflicts are; they do not unburden their minds, are shy, and have a ten-
> dency to live in a world of fancies. This is the shut-in personality.[60]

He claimed to have based his notion on a review of seventy-two
case histories he had done with his colleague at Bloomingdale, George
S. Amsden (with whom he would develop a questionnaire to study the

nature of personality). In 35 percent of his cases the relationship of a prior shut-in personality to later dementia praecox was "markedly pronounced," while in another 16 percent it was "indicated," which Hoch inflated to the conclusion that there was "some evidence" of a connection in 51 percent of his cases.[61] The shut-in personality soon became one of those assumed "facts" that have marked the long history of fads in psychiatry. "It is no longer to be questioned that in the genesis of dementia praecox the so-called shut-in type of personality is essentially the type that breaks down with this disorder," said one neurologist in 1915.[62]

In one sense what Meyer and Hoch were attempting to do was medicalize introversion. Being shy, withdrawn, fanciful, and internally directed in childhood soon became a red flag for proponents of the mental hygiene movement. Indeed Hoch presented his warnings about "the early manifestations of mental disorders" at the very first major mental hygiene conference and exhibition, held in New York in November 1912. His warnings about the prepsychotic personality would be echoed by other authors concerned with mental hygiene in later years, for example: "'The shut-in,' or praecox type, is familiar to us all. . . . An important factor in the early recognition of this type of individual is the school physician. Every child should be interviewed personally by the physician at least twice during the school year; a thorough family and personal history should be obtained and any hereditary taint ascertained, and if the child is of a highly nervous temperament, or shows any of the characteristic features of the praecox type, special care should be exercised in his mental training."[63] By 1916 C. B. Farrar would be so convinced of the notion that dementia praecox grows out of a defective personality that he proposed five types of his own (backward, precocious, neurotic, asocial, and juvenile).[64] Hoch's shut-in personality was as protean a concept as dementia praecox.

Hoch's historical research was a far cry from the level of sophistication of his experimental work with Kraepelin in Heidelberg in 1894 and 1897. But as with so many other leading American alienists and neurologists in the first decade of the twentieth century, there was not only a frustration with the slow pace of laboratory science but also an impulse, a collective spirit to create a distinctly *American* contribution to psychiatry.

In 1910 Meyer left the New York Psychiatric Institute (he had changed the name from the Pathology Institute in 1908) and went to Baltimore to become a professor of psychiatry at Johns Hopkins Medical School and to participate in the planning and development of the proposed Henry C. Phipps Psychiatric Clinic. Hoch took Meyer's place as director of the Institute, instilling the strong psychoanalytic influence in that institution that exists even to this day. Both men were now perceived, and rightly so, as wielding considerable power in American psychiatry. Despite their flaws, their ideas had to be taken seriously. When one reads the psychiatric literature of that era one is struck by the lack of criticism of these ideas. Other than the critical asides in the publications of the Harvard neuropathologist E. E. Southard and the articles the neurologist Michael Osnato published in 1918–1919, the only other detailed critiques of Meyer's and Hoch's work on dementia praecox came from two McLean Hospital alienists, E. Stanley Abbot and Earl D. Bond.

Edward Stanley Abbot (1863–?) had been a colleague of Hoch's at McLean Hospital since 1895. After graduating from Harvard Medical School in 1893 he spent two years conducting histological research at Harvard. Abbot came from a well-known New England family. His father, Francis Ellingwood Abbot, was a teacher and Unitarian minister who had written several books of Transcendentalist philosophy before committing suicide in October 1903. In a presentation made at the New York Psychiatrical Society in May 1911, E. Stanley Abbot argued that Meyer's functional view of dementia praecox "runs counter to the prevailing conceptions," specifically the evidence for organic changes and the possible role of toxins. "He thus stands practically alone," Abbot said, "and reverses the general tendency of medical science to take morbid conditions out of the functional class and put them in the organic. It seems like a step backward, and his evidence should be very strong in order to be convincing." Abbot, for one, was certainly not convinced. Particularly problematic was Meyer's claim that "the patient had such and such traits, and afterward had a typical dementia praecox." He accused Meyer of publishing only case histories that supported his theory and not those that were "inconsistent with the theory." Additionally:

> More than half his own most fully cited cases are inadequately reported (though they may have been well-observed).
>
> His own cases fail to demonstrate:
>
> 1. That the antecedents *invariably* show inefficient habits of adjustment; and

2. That the reaction-types shown in the developed psychosis are the necessary developments of the make-up; and they do demonstrate

3. That, when present, the traits do not necessarily determine the reaction-types of the developed psychosis. . . .

Hence his evidence is not strong enough to carry the conviction that we should give up the organic conception in favor of the functional. . . .

We must remember that causes are multiple, and so we need to search diligently, not only in the directions Meyer has indicated, but in these others, including all possible organic changes, as well. . . . He has only pushed the pendulum too far to the other side, and claimed too much for mere habit deteriorations, conflicting instincts, and false adjustments.[65]

In an attempt to replicate the findings of Meyer and particularly of Hoch, Abbot joined forces with Earl Danforth Bond (1878–1968), and together they conducted their own study to see if there was evidence in the histories of their dementia praecox patients for something that resembled the shut-in personality. In the study, published jointly, they took fifty "undoubted cases" each of dementia praecox and manic-depressive patients and analyzed them. They found that "normal traits" seemed to predominate in manic-depressive patients, and "normal personalities" were found more frequently in this group. With regard to "the special 'shut-in personality'" they found evidence in "too small a proportion (20 percent) to substantiate fully the claims made by some writers for its prevalence as an etiological factor in dementia praecox."[66] However, in a larger study conducted by Bond of one hundred admissions "taken in order" at McLean Hospital and then another hundred collected the same way at the Danvers State Hospital (Bond's new place of employment as its pathologist), Bond found that "seclusive personalities are noted . . . in 50 percent of dementia praecox cases," but only twenty-four of the two hundred cases were diagnosed with dementia praecox.[67] The majority (seventy-five cases), particularly at McLean, were diagnosed with manic-depressive insanity. Abbot and Bond may have emboldened other alienists to finally speak their mind as well. H. D. Singer, the director of the Illinois State Psychiatric Institute, claimed that the psychogenic views of Meyer, Freud, and Jung about dementia praecox were "in a realm of pure hypothesis and speculation."[68]

The eruption in 1911—finally—of *public* critical debate about Meyer and Hoch's theory of the psychogenesis of dementia praecox was a sign that psychiatry in America was maturing as a profession. Certainly Abbot's attempted replication of Hoch's work was unprecedented. The charisma of the two Europeans who had injected German medicine into American psychiatry was beginning to wane. Whereas neurologists had tended to be the earliest and sharpest critics of Kraepelin and his disease concept (and Meyer, as a neurologist, should be included in this group), alienists as a rule tended to passively accept the various new ideas emerging from the psychiatric elites in Germany and the United States. The wide acceptance of autointoxication theory around 1905 is just one example; one could also point to the earlier and largely uncontroversial acceptance of the theories of hereditary degeneration or the notion that "mental disease is brain disease" as two others of European origin. The notion of the psychogenesis of mental disorders was in itself a protest against these three earlier biological paradigms. But it was far easier for American alienists to dismiss the ideas of foreign savants than directly—and publicly—challenge the most powerful man in their profession.

Perhaps as another indication that things were beginning to change in America, there is evidence that starting around 1906 some alienists were beginning to refer to themselves as "psychiatrists," as had been the case in Germany for decades.[69] Although the terms "alienist" and "psychiatrist" were used interchangeably in American psychiatry until the 1920s, the year 1917 may have marked a tipping point of sorts. In that year E. E. Southard published an article in which he suggested that the term "alienist" be applied only to those physicians who render opinions in the courts, and "psychiatrist" be the preferred term for clinical practitioners. In addition—another indication of the changing cognitive categories in American psychiatry—Southard argued that the "field" of alienists is "insanity" and "the insane," whereas psychiatrists are concerned with "psychiatry" and "the mentally diseased."[70] By 1922 the American Medico-Psychological Association would become the American Psychiatric Association, and the *American Journal of Insanity* would change its name to the *American Journal of Psychiatry.*

But psychogenic theories of dementia praecox did not disappear. Indeed they thrived in the everyday clinical world of psychotherapy that ran parallel to those of laboratory research and somatic forms of treatment throughout the next sixty to seventy years. Psychoanalysis would be the vector for such ideas.

For at least the first three decades of the twentieth century psychoanalysis had no impact on the practice of the vast majority of psychiatrists in the United States. They worked in asylums and state hospitals with large numbers of chronically insane individuals, often cut off from the intellectual streams of much of professional medicine and psychiatry. Among American neurologists in the northeastern United States, on the other hand, who had long since cornered the market in the private practice treatment of the neuroses (neurasthenia, psychasthenia, hysteria, and epilepsy), there was enough interest in Freud that, by 1922, there may have been as many as five hundred unofficial analysts in New York City.[71] This state of affairs would change by the late 1920s, when asylum psychiatrists too would begin their migration to the more lucrative fields of office practice.

Other than the concerns of a handful of notable members of the psychiatric elite who published articles and books and who were mostly involved in the New York and Washington, D.C., psychoanalytic scenes, this history of psychoanalysis in the United States has very little to do with the story of the rise of dementia praecox. However, psychoanalysis did play a supporting role in the fall of dementia praecox and the rise of its successor, schizophrenia. Although at first a few American alienists tried their hand at applying Freudian techniques in improvised psychoanalytic sessions with asylum inpatients, these few experimental experiences amounted to very little.

Where psychoanalysis could be said to be therapeutic in asylum practice was in its effect on the alienists themselves. Alienists like August Hoch, George Kirby, A. A. Brill, and C. Macfie Campbell used psychoanalytic concepts to help interpret the otherwise bizarre and meaningless delusions, hallucinations, and behaviors of their psychotic patients. At the Manhattan State Hospital in 1910 Kraepelin's "school of formal differentiation" was opposed by a "school of subjective analysis" in which the examination of a dementia praecox patient did not stop at diagnosis but continued with "an analysis of the meaning of the patient's reactions in the context of the patient's inner life."[72] Such interpretations became the new special language of professional consultation and case conference posturing. Intellectually this was stimulating and made for interesting conversations with like-minded colleagues. The alienists had yet another scintillating prism through which to view their insane patients—as well as their colleagues. Gossip took on a Freudian spin. In reality, when the evidence is examined psychoanalytic concepts were simply a seductive new way for doctors to maintain an active interest in hopelessly insane patients who normally would have been ignored.

It was C. G. Jung, not Sigmund Freud, whose psychoanalytic ideas were most influential on American asylum practice in the first two decades of the twentieth century. Jung had achieved a certain level of respect for his experimental researches in psychiatry using the word association test on asylum patients as well as normal subjects.[73] By 1907 his additional interest in Freud and psychoanalysis was already well known to Americans, and he had been published in translation in American medical journals.[74] When his monograph on the psychology of dementia praecox appeared in 1907, synthesizing psychoanalytic ideas and French dissociationist thought with his own experimental researches using the word association test, it sealed his reputation among the American psychiatric elite who could read German.[75] The resonance with asylum alienists was understandable: Jung had worked in an asylum since December 1900 with dementia praecox patients, whereas Freud, who was still largely unknown in 1907, had little experience with such a highly disturbed population and did not write about them. Jung's chimerical theory of the etiology of dementia praecox, which combined psychogenesis with autointoxication (a psychological "complex" might cause the production of a "toxin" that then caused dementia praecox), also had an appeal. So when his book on dementia praecox was translated into English and published in 1909—the first psychoanalytic book to be published in America—it became required reading among professionally curious asylum and state hospital alienists. Interest was further piqued after Jung and Freud lectured at Clark University in the fall of 1909.

Alienists wondered: Was there something to psychoanalysis? Certainly Freud's theory that mental disorders were psychogenic seemed to be congruent with the functional approach of Adolf Meyer. And Jung's emphasis on the dissociation (splitting) of consciousness into complexes seemed to have surface similarities with Meyer's cryptic references to disharmonies of functions or instincts in dementia praecox. Even

Meyer occasionally used Jungian and Freudian terms to illustrate the points of his "functional" or "dynamic" psychiatry.

In the year 1907 the New York neurologist Smith Ely Jelliffe (1866–1945) began to pay closer attention to psychoanalysis after a trip to Zurich to meet Jung and his colleagues.[76] Jelliffe had already been convinced by Hoch and Meyer that some delusions had a psychogenic basis. He discussed the idea with his good friend William Alanson White (1870–1937), the superintendent of the government Hospital for the Insane in Washington, and after a number of years of careful consideration White began to believe in its value as well. These two men, whom Adolf Meyer nicknamed "neuropsychiatric twin brothers,"[77] held nearly identical views about dementia praecox. Even though they are often prominently mentioned in the history of psychoanalysis in America, like most Americans they were "eclectic" and not orthodox Freudians or Jungians.[78] Neither believed, as Jung seemed to argue, that an emotional trauma, or series of them, could create complexes that would alter the biochemistry of an individual to the point that it actually *caused* dementia praecox. Both Jelliffe and White believed that most cases of severe dementia praecox were fundamentally caused by a biological process of some sort, but of course could be made worse through disappointments and traumatic experiences. They did believe that the expressions and behaviors of a person with dementia praecox could be interpreted "symbolically," but they knew better than to claim an arrest of the disease process or a cure.

The personalities of these two close friends could not be more different. Jelliffe was widely read, urbane, colorful, and incautious. White preferred technical literature and was somewhat provincial, gray-scale, and reserved. Jelliffe was a successful consulting neurologist in private practice; White was an alienist who had become the superintendent of one of the largest mental hospitals in the United States. Jelliffe expressed his enthusiasm for psychoanalysis early on, whereas White would always be more carefully balanced in his writings on the subject.[79] Of the two, Jelliffe seemed to have the greater theoretical and therapeutic interest in dementia praecox and published numerous articles on the subject, whereas White tended to express his measured opinions about the disorder in the chapter on the disease in the multiple editions of his textbook, *Outlines of Psychiatry,* beginning in 1907.[80] White followed Jelliffe's lead, and thus it is Jelliffe's views on dementia praecox that require comment.

Jelliffe made multiple trips to Europe to train with distinguished psychiatrists, including periods with Kraepelin in 1906 and 1907. "Thanks to a few ducats extracted from the first Thaw trial I was able to go to Kraepelin in the spring of 1906 and spend six months with him," he quipped.[81] White accompanied him in 1907 to visit Kraepelin in Munich and Jung in Zurich. Through both personal experience and his study of the literature Jelliffe was exceptionally well-acquainted with Kraepelin's views.

In 1907 Jelliffe, like Hoch the same year, raised the issue of the premorbid personality of a person who would later develop dementia praecox. His article on the "pre–dementia praecox" personality was widely cited in the psychiatric literature in the decades that followed. "The whole problem of types of personality has had a new light thrown upon [dementia praecox]," he enthused.[82] He saw the potential fruitfulness of the historical method advocated by Meyer and Hoch. In his article Jelliffe began by anchoring the development of dementia praecox in the research on adolescence and child development of that era as well as that of clinical psychiatry. Disconnections between thought and emotion, and mood and reaction seemed to be key indicators of problems in adolescents. "If I might express it crudely, in dementia praecox we find a state of emotional impoverishment due to the breaking down, perhaps as Freud terms it, a process of conversion, of a rich plexus of associations of many years' growth—the changes in the affective life should be interpreted from the standpoint of a disintegration or analysis of what had heretofore been a developing and fairly fixed personality."[83] The influence of Jung's 1907 monograph on Jelliffe's description of dementia praecox is evident in these passages.

But underlying this disintegration, according to Jelliffe, were the undeniable influences of heredity. Yet "what kind of hereditary influences are most to be feared, or, rather, are certain taints in an ancestry more likely to lead to dementia praecox rather than to other forms of mental disease? We are not yet in a position to state this with definiteness." Based on his own cases of dementia praecox, Jelliffe speculated that what to look for in the family tree of persons with this disease are "dementia praecox itself, alcohol, and abnormal personality or crankiness."[84] As for prevention (prophylaxis), he called for the special training of children and adolescents who exhibit such premorbid personalities and for the legal prohibition of marriage for such individuals—a positive eugenical solution.[85]

In a much more polished presentation of the same views, complete with a more extensive literature review to back up his claims, Jelliffe made the same arguments in a 1911 paper on the hereditary and constitutional features of pre–dementia praecox. Here he sharpened his differences with European psychoanalytic views of psychogenesis: "I am unprepared to accept the Freudian hypothesis that the complex—or group of complexes—of themselves are sufficient to develop the disease in all its phases." Instead he agreed with Bleuler's position that "the complex does not cause the disease, but may determine its symptomatology. In this respect he [Bleuler] rejects the ultra-Freudian views of which it would appear A. Meyer is to advocate."[86] But in 1911 Jelliffe agreed with Meyer enough—"in part," he cautioned—to allow this paper to be published along with those of Meyer and Hoch in the first American book ever published on dementia praecox: *Dementia Praecox: A Monograph*.[87]

Thus by 1911 dementia praecox in America was being promoted by prominent members of the psychiatric elite as a fundamentally psychogenic condition that sprouted from a "pre–dementia praecox" personality defined by "habit disorganization," or an essential cluster of maladaptive psychobiological "reactions" to biological, social, and emotional or psychological events. The few disconnected and confusing biological findings about dementia praecox in the examining room or at autopsy or in the laboratory would be acknowledged, but dismissed as secondary to, or as a result of, psychogenic forces (which increasingly included unconscious inner "conflicts"). This combination of a personality type with a "reaction" or a disease concept would define the conception of dementia praecox favored by the American psychiatric elite for decades to come.

The scientific method employed to arrive at this conclusion was historical research—the case history. This was science in the German sense of *Wissenschaft*. No one in the United States attempted to replicate Kraepelin's longitudinal psychiatric research methods to determine if his conclusions about the course and outcome (prognosis) of mental diseases were valid. It *could* have been done, especially with the considerable resources available to Adolf Meyer at the New York Psychiatric Institute, but was not. As he did at Worcester, Meyer chose instead to devote his energies to administrative reforms and clinical training in the state hospitals of New York, completing these goals by 1907. Rather than initiate conventional scientific research programs, he left the Institute two years later. At the Phipps Psychiatric Clinic at Johns Hopkins he began to collect follow-up data on his discharged patients but did not allow analysis or publication of these data until the 1930s.[88] Nor did E. E. Southard, whether at Danvers State Hospital (1906–1912) or the Boston Psychiatric Hospital (after 1912), use the large Danvers "index of symptoms" database to fashion a new classification scheme (though he intended to, he claimed).[89] Nor did he employ the considerable resources at his command as pathologist for the system of state hospitals in the Commonwealth of Massachusetts between 1909 and 1920, even though longitudinal studies could have been conducted there to verify Kraepelin's claims about the courses and outcome of his insanities. American research methods in psychiatry remained largely historical and anecdotal, and only occasionally quantitative or statistical, until the 1920s.

Also by 1911 even the battles over classification and nomenclature had temporarily subsided. "The disappointment of parental hope and prognostic gloom reside in the term Dementia Praecox," wrote the prominent southern American psychiatrist J. K. Hall in 1910.[90] But perhaps for not much longer. Tens of thousands of persons were now routinely given diagnoses of dementia praecox in asylums and state hospitals from individual alienists whose diagnostic styles were probably highly idiosyncratic; many persons thus labeled seemed to actually improve or completely recover from their illness. If Kraepelin was right, how could this be? Alienists were more apt to question Kraepelin's views on prognosis rather than the self-perceived mastery of their own diagnostic skills. If some insane patients with this diagnosis recovered, then there was hope. The American focus after 1903 on etiology rather than on course or outcome, and on the early recognition of the signs of a premorbid personality type, was designed to serve a greater goal: prevention.

What were the consequences of this uniquely American viewpoint? In effect, Meyer, Hoch, Jelliffe, and others who would later adopt this position greatly expanded the population parameters of Kraepelin's disease. Indeed in many respects by 1911 dementia praecox in America was no longer Kraepelin's disease. The linkage of a pre–dementia praecox personality type with the inevitable development of the later disease meant that there were a great number of young people in the American population who were in trouble. Perhaps the number of "shut-in personalities" and other prepsychotic individuals was greater than the number of individuals who had actually developed the condition and were now in asylums and state hospitals. This was a terrifying thought, a paranoid fantasy that fueled the sloganeering of the mental hygiene movement and its national organization, the National Committee for Mental Hygiene, which Meyer, Clifford Beers, and others helped bring into being in 1909. The mental hygiene movement gave American psychiatry a relevance to the world outside the asylum walls it had never had before. The progressive spirit to prevent and cure mental diseases would extend to efforts to help those with dementia praecox, but largely by focusing on the dangers or warning signs of the pre–dementia praecox personality. Little could be done for those already languishing in state hospitals.[91]

The American conception of dementia praecox (the combined notions of psychogenesis, including unconscious conflicts; the splitting or disconnection of thoughts, emotions, and behavior; and the linkage of the premorbid with the morbid) and the many apparent recoveries from it would provide numerous analogical bridges to an alternative vision of dementia praecox proposed by Eugen Bleuler—schizophrenia—in the years to come. Although 1911 was the year in which Bleuler published his famous volume outlining his new conception of dementia praecox it would take some years before those members of the American psychiatric elite who could read German could disseminate these ideas. But then again, many of these elements of the American conception were already known from A. A. Brill's 1909 translation of Jung's 1907 monograph on the psychology of dementia praecox, which Jung wrote while working under Bleuler in Zurich. And of course Americans such as Frederick Peterson, Brill, Jelliffe, William A. White, and George Kirby had spent time there as well. Knowledge about Jung's dementia praecox and Bleuler's schizophrenia had been transferred across the Atlantic through various channels. But what distinguished the American conception of dementia praecox from that of Jung and Bleuler was the disproportionate emphasis on premorbid "reaction" or "personality" types; the curious lack of interest in detailing variations in the ongoing signs, symptoms, courses, and outcomes of the disease after its onset; and the devaluation (indeed often outright dismissal) of biological, especially autotoxic, causative factors.

Ironically, just as this extreme psychogenic view of dementia praecox gained prominence in the American psychiatric elite, by 1915 the

pendulum would start to swing back toward biology. Even more ironically, it would be introduced by three of the physicians most associated
with the psychoanalytic interpretation and treatment of dementia praecox in 1910–1915: Smith Ely Jelliffe, William Alanson White, and
Edward Kempf (1885–1971).[92] This time around, the seat of the unconscious mind and the roots of the human personality (and its psychopathology) would be viewed as springing from the autonomic or "vegetative" nervous system that had been conditioned to react in certain
ways by the environment and by personal experiences.

In 1915 Jelliffe and White introduced the first edition of their land-
mark book, *Diseases of the Nervous System: A Textbook of Neurology and
Psychiatry.* Jelliffe was responsible for the introduction and all of the neurology in the book, and White wrote the psychiatry sections. It was the
first book of its kind to emphasize the influence of psychosocial factors
(including unconscious conflicts) on the brain and nervous system, particularly the "vegetative" nervous system, which, Jelliffe and White
wrote, "is the historically oldest part of the nervous system." It was during this time that there was much discussion about the experiments on
animals by the Harvard physiologist Walter Bradford Cannon, reported
in his classic 1915 book, *Bodily Changes in Pain, Hunger, Fear and Rage,* in
which he directly demonstrated the role of the autonomic nervous system in producing changes in the endocrine system (the production of
adrenalin by the ductless adrenal glands) in response to stressful conditions, thus discovering some of the underlying physiological mechanisms
of primal emotional reactions. The new experimental knowledge about
the autonomic nervous system that was just coming into awareness about
this time intrigued many psychiatrists: Could this ancient, involuntary,
indeed, *unconscious,* structural and functional part of the nervous system,
with a demonstrated role in the production of emotional responses, be
the foundation of the human personality and its unconscious mind?
What were the implications for psychopathology?

"At the highest level [of the nervous system] stand the mental
mechanisms in which action receives a symbolic representation," Jelliffe wrote in the introduction. "Here the nervous system is also the
medium through which that form of physiological or pathological activity called conduct is brought about. These mechanisms, while operating

consciously, largely through the sensori-motor channels of adjustment, are also intimately related to the vegetative levels where through the emotions they act unconsciously."[93] Jelliffe and White do not hesitate to recommend psychoanalysis as the treatment for mental diseases, including for those with dementia praecox.

The view put forth in this textbook, which united neurology and psychiatry through the operation of the autonomic nervous system (and especially its influence on the endocrine system) and later advocated psychoanalysis as the recommended method for interpreting the "symbolic representations" of symptoms as well as the treatment for them, eventually became known more generally by the term "neuropsychiatry." Neuropsychiatry and its later, Freudian vocabulary would become the paradigm for the understanding and treatment of "shell-shocked" veterans who had developed trauma-induced "war neuroses" or even cases of reversible dementia praecox during combat in the First World War and particularly the Second. The influenza pandemic of 1918–1919 also produced postinfluenza cases of dementia praecox that seemed to reverse five years later. The reversibility of these psychotic conditions with time and treatment lent support to the notion in the 1920s that psychotherapeutic interventions were possible for some individuals with dementia praecox.[94]

Psychologically damaging experiences and maladaptive adjustments to them no longer needed to be linked to the brain, where neuropathological findings had been disappointing, but instead were linked to the conditioning of the autonomic nervous system. The brain was now dethroned in favor of the autonomic nervous system as the most important physical basis of mental disease. This is precisely the argument Jelliffe made in a 1917 article titled "The Vegetative Nervous System and Dementia Praecox." He lists (in alphabetical order) distinct, observable, physical signs that are correlated with dementia praecox: changes in the blood, blood vessels, blood pressure, and pulse; endocrinopathic changes; eye symptoms (including abnormal pupil responses); problems with the gastrointestinal tract; kidney disturbances; and skin abnormalities. All of these were signs of the vegetative nervous system in action, not the higher cognitive functions of the cerebral cortex.[95] Dementia praecox had morphed into the neuropsychiatric disease par excellence. "It would seem to stand midway between the so-called organic and psychogenic psychoses," White wrote in the

1919 seventh edition of his textbook, *Outlines of Psychiatry.*[96] The pendulum had swung again: dementia praecox was a liminal concept, neither fish nor fowl.

Although he left no lasting influence on psychiatry, Edward Kempf is remembered for his energetic attempts to base psychoanalytic theory on a firm neurophysiological footing. Kempf was born in Jasper, Indiana. His father and grandfather had also been physicians. He earned his medical degree at Western Reserve University in Cleveland in 1910 and found a position almost immediately as an assistant physician at the Cleveland State Hospital. In 1911 he moved to the Central Hospital for the Insane at Indianapolis, where he stayed until he was fired near the end of 1912. Kempf was an intelligent, creative man with a difficult temperament. He was fired from his position in Indianapolis for attempting to develop a psychoanalytic treatment program for the insane. He would later claim that he was the first person in the United States to attempt to use psychoanalytic techniques with dementia praecox patients, but Hoch had already done so at Bloomington Hospital, and of course there was already a Freudian colony developing at Manhattan State Hospital. After being fired in Indianapolis he was hired by Adolf Meyer in 1913 to join his staff at the newly opened Henry C. Phipps Psychiatric Clinic of the Johns Hopkins Hospital. He lasted a year there, leaving on his own this time due to intellectual conflicts with his colleagues. William Alanson White hired him away from Johns Hopkins in 1914, a stroke of luck for Kempf. White wanted him to set up an experimental therapy program for the patients at the Government Hospital of the Insane in Washington (which had just been renamed St. Elizabeths Hospital). "In Saint Elizabeths I had complete freedom to think out any problems in psychopathology and psychotherapy and select any male and female cases out of over 3,000 for analysis," he would later remember.[97]

In addition to his clinical research on the applicability of his rather active and directive form of psychoanalysis on psychotic patients, Kempf devoted a considerable amount of time to his biological interests. For one, he set up a primate laboratory at St. Elizabeths to study the sexual behaviors of monkeys in order to follow an evolutionary thread in Freudian theories about humans. He had been inspired to do this after reading an article published in 1914 by G. V. Hamilton, an alienist in Santa Barbara, California, who had set up just such a primate

lab on the grounds of the estate of a wealthy private patient with dementia praecox whom he lived with, Stanley McCormick, for whom
he provided around-the-clock care. Kempf's observations of his monkeys, in his opinion, seemed to place Freudian insights on a Heckelian
evolutionary basis (ontogeny recapitulates phylogeny), which Freud,
Jung, and most psychoanalysts and biologists held to in that era.[98]

Before retiring from St. Elizabeths in 1920 to go into the more
lucrative field of private practice and consulting, Kempf produced two
books that attempted to provide a biological foundation not only for all
of human psychology, but also for psychopathology. The first, *The Autonomic Functions and the Personality,* appeared in 1918.[99] The title says it
all. The biological ground of the human personality, and especially the
actions of the unconscious mind, were rooted in the vegetative nervous
system. The second book, *Psychopathology,* which appeared in 1920, is a
massive whirlwind filled with numerous plates of archaeological artifacts and photos of patients. By including historical and clinical material, Kempf attempts to predicate all of psychopathology on his autonomic theory of the personality, Freudian psychoanalytic concepts,
and comparative historical evidence regarding human sexuality going
back thousands of years. There is a madness in this book that reminds
the reader of one that had appeared in English translation only a few
years before, in 1916, Jung's *The Psychology of the Unconscious.*[100] Although the reviews by Meyer and others were laudatory, it is doubtful
if anyone really understood this volume when it appeared. In both books
Jung and Kempf attempt to place sexuality (the expression of the libido)
on a mythic, evolutionary, and historical foundation. In both books they
argue that the deterioration of ego defense mechanisms led to an eruption of sexualized mythic material of the kind found in primitive peo-
ples, those in the cultures of Hellenistic pagan antiquity, and among
contemporary American Negroes and children. This failure of the de-
fenses causes, or characterizes, the behaviors, delusions, and hallucinations of persons suffering with dementia praecox. *Psychopathology* was
also Kempf's attempt to create a new psychiatric nomenclature. For example, he rarely mentions dementia praecox by name, instead describing
a "chronic pernicious dissociation of the personality," in which in its
"hebephrenic adaptations" one finds the "predominance of excretory
erotic interests." He used case material from St. Elizabeths to illustrate
his points, including a "case of insidious development of anal eroticism

and the tendency to true epileptic orgasms." The volume makes for compelling reading—if one is in the right mood.

Between 1910 and 1913 Adolf Meyer was a professor of psychiatry at Johns Hopkins, preparing for the day when the Phipps Psychiatric Clinic would finally open for business. It would be like Kraepelin's clinic, but smaller—no more than eighty-eight beds, and connected with a major university medical school for teaching purposes. When it did finally open in April 1913, after three days of opening ceremonies that included speakers such as Eugen Bleuler, the creator of schizophrenia, the symbolism was clear: finally, after decades of struggle, psychiatry was publicly recognized as a legitimate branch of general medicine. William Welch, the driving force behind Johns Hopkins and the rise of scientific medicine in the United States, was there to personally anoint Meyer.

But Welch was probably not fully aware of the implications of the fact that the anointed leader of this new medical science of psychiatry was the consummate "mind twist man" who did not believe in specifiable mental disease concepts.

For the many fewer "brain spot men" and autointoxicationists in pathology suites and laboratories, Meyer's ascendency would be seen as only a temporary defeat. Biological psychiatry soldiered on in the shadowlands, far from the bright shining city on the hill at Johns Hopkins. There were many who were going to discover the biological mechanisms behind dementia praecox and develop not only effective rational treatments, but also cures.

For some, the solutions were surgical.

7

BAYARD TAYLOR HOLMES AND
RADICALLY RATIONAL TREATMENTS

In the midst of all the debates over etiology, prognosis, classification, and nomenclature, there was one important fact about dementia praecox that was woefully ignored: treatment. Emil Kraepelin advised no special form of treatment for dementia praecox other than the standard procedures used for all inpatients, regardless of diagnosis: prolonged baths in heated tubs during periods of excitability, some sort of structured activity to keep them active and distracted from their condition, entertainment diversions, a healthy diet, and, only if absolutely needed, sedative drugs or physical restraints. In the United States these were the standard forms of asylum treatment as well—except that American alienists tended to rely heavily on sedative drugs as a form of chemical restraint to keep order in overcrowded institutions. American homeopathic institutions did not rely so heavily on sedative drugs and instead used their materia medica, claiming great success with these treatments. No one really knew what to do to treat insanity.

With the rise of the American psychogenic concept of dementia praecox there was much talk about prophylaxis and other ideals consistent with the growing mental hygiene movement. Adolf Meyer and

August Hoch talked of "habit training" with those young persons suffering from "habit disorganization," but never provided details of what those procedures would be nor published any clinical or research studies concerning such procedures. Hoch, C. Macfie Campbell, Smith Ely Jelliffe, William Alanson White, and Edward Kempf all recommended psychoanalytic techniques in psychotherapeutic encounters with dementia praecox patients who were suffering from milder forms of the illness or were "pre–dementia praecox," but their few publications on this matter largely remained theoretical rather than practical. For the Americans convinced of the psychogenesis of dementia praecox there were only vague suggestions for interventions that would rationally follow the presumed etiology of the disorder. In reality such patients were as heavily drugged as those suffering from any other form of insanity.

But there were those who held to a biological etiology of dementia praecox and had very definite suggestions for treatments that might not only relieve patients of their symptoms, but actually cure them. In an era of medical history when the marvels of bacteriology and endocrinology seemed to demonstrate that each disease had a single cause, and that the treatment or cure of the disease meant eliminating this cause, it was tempting for alienists, neurologists, and other physicians to experiment with radical forms of treatment that were derived rationally from the presumed cause of dementia praecox. In the United States these rational treatments were based on autointoxication theories. Focal bacterial infections or metabolic imbalances (dyskrasias) were the presumed causes of dementia praecox, and surgery and organotherapy (injection with "inner secretions" or "gland extracts" or hormones) were its presumed cures.

Many persons with mental diseases died from these procedures. Looking back, it is far too tempting to be seduced into outrage over the horrors suffered by so many vulnerable persons in the care of their physicians. Such outrage is justified, but, as the historian Gerald Grob observed, "Tragedy is a recurring theme in human affairs, and defines perhaps the very parameters of our existence." Therefore a certain amount of sympathy is appropriate "for our predecessors who grappled—so often unsuccessfully, as we still do ourselves—with their own distinct problems."[1] Dementia praecox was a devastating form of insanity that robbed its victims of their humanity and condemned many of them to the overcrowded back wards of asylums and state hospitals. No one knew what to do about it. But some physicians felt they had to at least *try.*

On 6 February 1905 Ralph Loring Holmes, a seventeen-year-old American boy visiting Jena, Germany, unexpectedly "became sick."[2] When he returned to the United States the boy's father, although a noted Chicago physician, surgeon, and professor of medicine, felt completely helpless when confronted with his beloved son's baffling condition. Following the advice of two physician colleagues, the father placed Ralph in a private institution, "where he was locked up, fed and restrained by pounds, actually pounds of sedatives."[3] The diagnosis was dementia praecox. The boy would never recover from this illness, and it is listed on his death certificate as the official cause of his death at Lakeside Hospital in Chicago on 23 May 1916.[4] Many death certificates of that era blamed dementia praecox for extinguishing the flame of life in mostly young, mostly male, and mostly forgotten insane persons such as this one.

The psychotic illness of Ralph Loring Holmes enters the history of American medicine and psychiatry through its influence on the life of the boy's father, Bayard Taylor Holmes (1852–1924).[5] Holmes was personally devastated by his son's illness. His anguish was exacerbated by feelings of impotence, for although his professional life was devoted to improving medical education in Chicago, like most physicians he had a complete lack of expertise in psychiatry. Holmes, however, had a combative nature, and he decided to tackle his ignorance and his son's illness head-on. Weary of relying on the advice of colleagues and some of the most respected alienists in America while watching his son deteriorate further, Holmes partly retired from his surgical practice and his position as professor of surgical pathology and bacteriology at the College of Physicians and Surgeons in Chicago to care for his son himself. He also vowed to use his scientific expertise to find both a cause and a cure for dementia praecox. He soon became a prominent advocate for reforms in the institutional care of the mentally ill, compiled a bibliographic collection of more than eight thousand international scientific articles, dissertations, and books relevant to laboratory studies of dementia praecox, and from 1918 to 1922 was the editor of what is believed to be the first medical journal named after a mental disease: *Dementia Praecox Studies.*

Using equipment and bench space loaned by medical colleagues, in January 1915 Holmes began his own laboratory studies of dementia praecox. Within a few months, to his satisfaction, he hit upon a viable organic theory of the cause of the disease. In the spring of the following year, 1916, he developed and experimented with a rational treatment based on this theory, testing it further on additional patients with dementia praecox between April 1917 and February 1918 at an experimental inpatient unit known as the Psychiatric Research Laboratory of the Psychopathic Hospital, Cook County Hospital, in Chicago.

The organic etiology of dementia praecox that Holmes believed he had discovered was grounded firmly in medical theories that were popular during the First World War: autointoxication or focal infections located somewhere in the body that reached the brain and produced severe mental and physical disorders. His bibliography of publications in support of the autointoxication or focal infection theory of dementia praecox is perhaps the most comprehensive summary of this obscure literature in the history of psychiatry.[6]

The rational treatment that Holmes derived from his specific theory—abdominal surgery and daily colonic irrigations—claimed the life of the first dementia praecox patient in history to receive it as an experimental procedure. Ralph Loring Holmes died at the hands of his own father, a medical misadventure known at the time by family friends and some prominent medical colleagues, such as Adolf Meyer.

In his fascinating book *Madhouse: A Tragic Tale of Megalomania and Modern Medicine,* the historian Andrew Scull details the story of Henry A. Cotton (1876–1933) of the Trenton State Hospital in New Jersey and his reliance upon radical surgical procedures to alleviate or "cure" persons afflicted with severe mental diseases (such as dementia praecox) that he believed were caused by focal infections arising from the mouth (rotting teeth), the colon, the stomach, the thyroid, the cervix, and other areas of the body.[7] The story is a horrific one. Many died from complications following these surgeries. However, although Scull's tale is instructive about the reception and application of focal infection theory in America, it is incomplete. For example, although Cotton worked under Kraepelin in Munich for two years and certainly must have known of Kraepelin's speculation that dementia praecox was probably caused by an autointoxication, this influence on Cotton's later thinking is not explored. But more important for our purposes here, nowhere in Scull's volume is there a mention of Bayard Taylor Holmes or the fact that it was Holmes, not Cotton, who was the first to try abdominal surgery as a treatment of dementia praecox.

There is no evidence that these two men met or corresponded. However, Holmes knew of Cotton's work by the early 1920s and was supportive of it, although he criticized the emphasis on the removal of teeth, organs, or tissues rather than the daily colonic irrigations that his method offered.[8] Cotton never mentions Holmes in his publications, but probably knew of him through his many publications or from their mutual colleague, Meyer. Like Holmes, Cotton produced two sons, performing abdominal surgery on the second, Adolf Meyer Cotton, in a preventive measure to halt the development of any mental disturbance later in life.[9] He had already extracted the permanent teeth of both sons and later, his wife. Unlike Cotton, Holmes had a deeply personal stake in finding the cause and cure of dementia praecox. Unfortunately he suffered the sacrifice of his own son to achieve it. But any parent of a child with a devastating chronic mental illness would understand his complex motivations, for what is done out of love is beyond good and evil.

What follows therefore is essentially a contextualizing preface to Scull's gothic tale: the biographical and scientific case history of a forgotten man in the history of psychiatry. An examination of the life and work of Bayard Taylor Holmes provides us with a narrative perspective through which to view the application of early twentieth-century laboratory medicine to the devastating problem of dementia praecox. In order to comprehend the rationale for his etiological theory of dementia praecox, and his treatments for it, I will explore the various stages of his research program in great detail. Such a narrative, I believe, also gives us insight into the creative space opened in psychiatry by theories of autointoxication and focal infection, a rich field of possibilities for medical experimentation that, in the era before antibiotics, perhaps could have logically ended only with surgical tragedies such as those brought about by Holmes and Cotton. It is useful to remember, as the physician and historian Joel Braslow argued, that "during their heydays . . . most of the therapeutic practices . . . generally conformed to standards that constituted legitimate evidence for efficacy."[10]

The story of Bayard Taylor Holmes also documents the influential role played by Adolf Meyer in the tacit promotion of focal infection theory in American psychiatry through his personal contacts with

Holmes and Cotton and his uncritical acknowledgment of their rational treatments. This is remarkable considering Meyer's antipathy toward autointoxication theories. But Cotton had worked under Meyer at the Worcester Insane Hospital and was as devoted a disciple as George Kirby had been. By the time Cotton began his program of surgical solutions in Trenton, Meyer had undergone a decline in power and influence in American psychiatry, and his attachment to, and tolerance of, Cotton may be understandable when this is taken into account. Meyer is anchored at the center of the Holmes story just as he is in the Cotton story, with not only Holmes but two of the researchers working under him, Julius Retinger and Horry M. Jones, reaching out to Meyer for support at various stages of their research on the causes and treatments of dementia praecox.

Why have Holmes and his *Dementia Praecox Studies* been forgotten?

There is a revelatory silence in the literature of the history of psychiatry about Bayard Taylor Holmes, his journal, his laboratory studies of the etiologic and pathologic processes of dementia praecox, and the experimental treatment unit in Chicago. All of the major histories of psychiatry completely ignore him. And Holmes was hard to ignore: he published no fewer than sixty-two articles on dementia praecox between 1911 and 1922. But indeed even in his own time neither his publications nor those of his research team in Chicago were cited by prominent figures in psychiatry and neurology. Why?

First and foremost his professional credentials as a surgeon and bacteriologist and his utter lack of formal training in psychiatry may have been reason enough for the prominent alienists of his day to disregard Holmes and his work. Hence, with the passage of time, the historical trail grew cold. "I know very well that I have no education or University training, such as your colleagues have, and that it is ridiculous for me to tell you what I think of your letter," he wrote to his old acquaintance Adolf Meyer on 19 February 1912.[11] The men met at some point during the two years (1893–1895) that Meyer was in Illinois. "Somehow I have always maintained a warm feeling for you as one of my early acquaintances," Meyer wrote to Holmes. "When I heard your son was ill, I really thought often of what might be done for him."[12]

But perhaps more distasteful to alienists than a surgeon dabbling in psychiatry, Holmes had made it quite clear in numerous opinion pieces in medical journals such as *The Lancet-Clinic* from 1910 until his death in 1924 that he detested the psychiatric profession for its lack of interest in laboratory science and for making false claims to the unsuspecting public about scientific knowledge of causes and effective treatments. The frustrating experience of trying to find competent help for his son led him to charge that the psychiatrists of his time were not true physicians, but merely "keepers":

> I am shy at using psychiatrist for a man who devotes himself to the professional custody of the crazy and yet denies that they suffer of disease or that there is any need of pathological study of their condition or any hope of cure. . . . I prefer to term them keepers of the insane rather than physicians. It seems to me that a group that denies to dementia praecox a place among diseases and disparages it by relegating it to the "reactions" can not claim to be psychiatrists in the medical sense.[13]

This did not win him the respect of psychiatrists, and they responded by refusing to cite his published work and by leaving him out of the histories of their profession that they would subsequently write. Additionally Holmes was exceptionally out of step with the changing political tide in professional psychiatry by being a vocal skeptic of Freud and psychoanalysis. "It is a distinctly mystical theory," he wrote in 1914, "insusceptible of either proof or refutation."[14] Edward Kempf had an unpleasant encounter with Holmes over the issue of psychoanalysis, and, as was the sectarian belief in Freudian circles, criticism of Freud could come only from the unresolved complexes of the critic:

> The viciousness of the attacks upon psychoanalysis is so utterly ill-founded and unjustifiable that it automatically directs attention to the source of the prejudices in the personalities of these critics. One man, a surgeon of national reputation, has written severe attacks upon the psychoanalytic method without a justifying study of the literature. At a medical society meeting in which he presented an interesting theory on the pathology of dementia praecox, he said, when informed that I desired to discuss the physiology of the emotions in relation to the pathology of dementia praecox, that he did not care anything about the emotions, and, further, that since he was an older man, it was only courtesy

that I should withhold my discussion. So, to please his personal prejudice, science and fairness had to be aborted. Later, I learned that his
prejudice was, at the least, related to repressions which were intimately
associated with a psychopathic tragedy in his family.[15]

Holmes also rejected the Meyerian notion that dementia praecox,
like all other mental diseases, was merely a jumble of psychogenic "reactions." Like some others, he believed that Meyer deliberately used a
deceptive style of idiosyncratic psychiatric jargon to divert attention
away from the fact that little was known about dementia praecox and
nothing could be done about it. "You are probably the most respected
man in psychiatry in the United States and what you say ought to mean
a lot to me," Holmes wrote to Meyer in 1912. "As a matter of fact, I
cannot understand hardly anything in your letter and I believe that
some of it, in spite of its interrogatory form, is designed to deceive."[16]

Holmes was also a critic of eugenics, which he referred to as a
"pseudoscience."[17] This too set him apart from contemporary trends in
science and from prominent figures in psychiatry and neurology associated with the Eugenics Record Office, such as Adolf Meyer and E. E.
Southard, though he maintained superficial professional contacts with
both of these men.

Taken together, the absence of Holmes in the literature of his day
can be understood by the incongruity of his views with those of the
American psychiatric elite. He was at right angles to almost every aspect
of the conventional wisdom about dementia praecox and the claims to
therapeutic knowledge offered by prominent alienists. Indeed Holmes
had found himself on a collision course with the status quo throughout
his life, for his trajectory was an unusual one.

Bayard Taylor Holmes found his way to medicine rather late in life. He
was thirty when he entered the Homeopathic Medical College in Chicago in the fall of 1882. Having spent the previous ten years teaching
science in the schools of Kendall, De Kalb, and La Salle Counties in Illinois, he began an aggressive self-education program that went far beyond
his formal training. He received his M.D. from the Homeopathic Medical College in 1884, interned for eighteen months at Cook County Hospital in Chicago, then entered the College of Physicians and Surgeons in

the fall of 1885 for further medical training by "regular physicians." He received his second M.D. from this institution in the spring of 1888, just before his thirty-sixth birthday.

Holmes began his training just as the bacteriological breakthroughs of Louis Pasteur and Robert Koch offered the possibility of challenging new career paths for scientifically ambitious medical students. Although he was already no stranger to microscopic work and was of course aware of the work of Pasteur and Koch, a single chance event steered him in the direction of bacteriology. While on his way to a series of histological lectures at Rush Medical College in the summer of 1883, he happened to see a notice for a lecture on tuberculosis accompanied by an autopsy to be given by W. T. Belfield at the County Hospital Morgue. Having just returned from Europe, Belfield summarized the latest developments in bacteriology. The lecture ended with Belfield inviting the medical students in the audience to his side to observe as he squeezed fluid from the lungs of a cadaver, smeared a specimen from it on a glass microscope slide, then gave these curious students their first look at what some were calling *Bacillus tuberculosis.*

Profoundly moved by the experience, Holmes initiated a course of activity that eventually led to a position in 1885 as an assistant to Christian Fenger (1840–1902), a noted pathologist who had introduced Lister's antiseptic operative methods to the staff of Cook County Hospital in 1878 and who was then professor of surgery at the College of Physicians and Surgeons in Chicago.[18] Holmes made an impression on Fenger the year before being offered this prestigious post, when he was the first to show Fenger microbes growing in nutrient material. Fenger had had no experience with the techniques of cultivating bacteria, and he responded to the sight with "childlike delight."[19] Holmes's bacteriological work and his association with Fenger opened doors for him in Chicago. In 1889 he became attending surgeon at Cook County Hospital; in 1891 he was appointed professor of surgical pathology and bacteriology at the College of Physicians and Surgeons. Holmes personally oversaw the design and construction of a six-story laboratory building at the College, and his advocacy of laboratory science in medicine influenced medical training not only at the College but also at other medical schools in the United States. In the opinion of Holmes, a professor of medicine held little credibility unless he could hold his own at the laboratory bench. "A man can easier preach without being converted," he argued, "than he can preach without being inspired, and the laboratory will show up a false teacher in the shortest time."[20]

Together with Fenger, Holmes wrote "Antisepsis in Abdominal Operations: Synopsis of a Series of Bacteriological Studies," which was published in the *Journal of the American Medical Association* in October 1887.[21] This was Holmes's second publication, and it is remarkable for introducing two professional preoccupations that became very personal ones. Indeed during the years of the First World War they would frame the fateful trajectory of his work on dementia praecox: infections as causes of disease and abdominal surgery as a cure of disease.

Bayard Taylor Holmes married Agnes Anna George on 14 August 1878. Their first child, Bayard Jr., was born in 1879. He would follow in the tradition of his father and become a physician in Chicago. Their only other child, Ralph Loring Holmes, was born in Chicago in 1887. He was a highly intelligent young man who could read both German and Latin and spoke German fluently.[22] Ralph too was expected to become a physician. However, it was during the middle of his first year of medical school that he was unexpectedly disabled by his illness. Unfortunately he then quickly became, as his father put it in 1918, one of "the 130,000 pitiable wrecks" suffering from dementia praecox who were periodic inmates in approximately "four hundred hospitals for the insane" in the United States.[23]

The psychotic breakdown of his beloved younger child awakened Holmes to the extreme prejudice against the mentally ill not only in society as a whole, but also among his colleagues, close friends, and even his own family. Despite his disregard for Meyer's professional opinions, Holmes was grateful for a letter he wrote in response to Holmes's increasingly polemical editorials and articles about the deficiencies in the care of persons with dementia praecox. In fact Meyer's letter was the first response he received from anyone in the field of psychiatry. In his response to Meyer on 19 February 1912, worth repeating at length here, Holmes wrote:

> I am grateful to you for the first letter which my editorials or reprints have brought forth. At the end of your letter you refer to the calamity to my son Ralph. A few days after the boy was taken away to

Jacksonville, I had a beautiful and helpful letter from Doctor Bernard Sippey [a Chicago physician], who had undergone a similar experience. Yours is absolutely the second letter from any person, except Ralph's attendants, in which his existence or misfortune has been mentioned. My own scattered family in their numerous and intimate letters to me have never once during these six terrible years mentioned his name or recognized by holiday token or birthday present his past or present existence. Not one of my medical friends in Chicago and elsewhere, many of whom in their family bereavements or professional misfortunes, have called upon me for sympathy and sometimes for succor, rendered at my own great risk, not one of them have volunteered me by letter or by word of mouth in all these terrible years, one single inquiry for my boy or one suggestion of sympathy or token of support. The dozens of internes and assistants and the hundreds, even thousands of students, and I may say, the public itself which has been entertained so freely at my house, not one of them has ever once written me one word of sympathy or recognition of the catastrophe which ruined my son and has taken away my own zest of life.

In my first helplessness I called on two colleagues, who advised in a cold and fateful manner, and withdrew. I followed implicitly their advice, yet they have never asked me how this advice eventuated. Ralph was put in a private institution, where he was locked up, fed and restrained by pounds, actually pounds of sedatives, as his history shows.

At this time I wrote a letter to the two acquaintances whom I considered most likely to offer helpful advice. They were both men most distinguished in their particular spheres. It would be hard for you to imagine with what anxiety I watched for days and weeks for some answer to those two letters which might reprieve my imprisoned hopes, but until today none ever arrived. Professor Jacques Loeb, of California, likely thought my request impertinent, and in your letter today you say that you sent me literature at the time.

It seems hardly likely to me that had I had a daughter and she had blazonly gone into public prostitution, would my colleagues have been as silent.[24]

During the first year of his son's illness Holmes threw himself into his work and relied on his "most distinguished colleagues in the United States" for advice rather than doing any reading on dementia praecox himself. "They gave one cheerless and discouraging reply, if they did not hedge or neglect to answer. They agreed to a man that the disease was of unknown pathology, unknown etiology and of an invariably unfavorable prognosis. Hopeless custody was the substitute for treatment." But when Ralph returned home after spending eight months in a private sanitarium, Holmes decided to use his expertise to find the cause of his son's devastating illness and to save him by finding a cure. He began visiting psychiatric institutions and was horrified when he finally saw the inmates on the "back wards": "When at last I discovered the result of the disease, the realization of the victims' pathetic condition threw me into a new frenzy. Terrible as my affliction was already my agony had not yet begun. So this was to be my son's end!"[25]

Holmes gradually retired from teaching but continued his medical practice and began a review of the medical literature on dementia praecox. His first impression of the scientific status of psychiatry appalled him. He wrote to Meyer, "It will be impossible for you to imagine my astonishment and confusion on reading text books, journals and monographs to find that in this branch of medical literature, the same method, the same argument and the same obscurity prevailed as in the literature of religion and occultism."[26]

By 1920 Holmes had complied more than eight thousand references relevant to the pathological, biochemical, histological, and bacteriological laboratory findings on dementia praecox. He kept these references in a card catalog which he donated to the John Crerar Library at the University of Chicago. This database would prove to be of decisive importance when he returned to the laboratory to do the critical work himself. He never lost his certainty that clues to the etiology, prophylaxis, therapy, and eventually cure of dementia praecox were somehow buried in this gigantic and seemingly disconnected body of evidence. To Holmes continual consultation of the medical literature was as necessary for a practicing physician as clinical experience and basic laboratory skills.[27] The problem that plagued him for years, however, was how to discern which of the thousands of published laboratory findings on dementia praecox led to the truth about this disease. One new lead after another was followed and then abandoned in favor of the latest new laboratory technique or organic finding. As Holmes frantically tried to master this immense literature and begin his own laboratory studies, the years rolled by and Ralph continued to deteriorate.

Holmes turned his revulsion for the psychiatric treatment of his son into a public crusade. He was temperamentally well-suited for this. As a man of rather benign rural origins, he had been appalled at social conditions in Chicago when he moved there to attend medical school. He was especially angered by the living and working conditions of immigrants and the poor. He involved himself in the education of illiterate workers, the inspection of safety conditions in factories, and child welfare. He founded an organization called the National Christian Citizenship League, which recruited volunteers to engage in various social welfare projects among the destitute of Chicago. His social conscience led him into politics, and in 1895 he was the unsuccessful Chicago mayoral candidate for both the People's Party and the Socialists of Eugene Debs, coming in third behind mayor-elect George Bell Swift. "He is a man of moods," reported a Chicago newspaper in the days following Holmes's nomination. "The doctor's personal peculiarities are intense. He is a fighter when aroused, and frequently it takes very little to arouse him. He has been known mercilessly to flay with tongue or pen those with whom he differed or whom he thought deserved a flaying as a matter of principle."[28]

Three years after Ralph became ill, Holmes published his first clinical article with a psychiatric theme when he wrote a warning about the use of chloroform with dementia praecox patients.[29] However, it would be several years before he published further clinical contributions in psychiatry. Instead he used the pages of the Cincinnati-based medical journal *The Lancet-Clinic* as his bully pulpit and wrote one short essay after another that deplored the conditions in state hospitals, demanded more state funding for laboratory research on dementia praecox, and denigrated just about every prominent school of thought in psychiatry. The first eight of these essays appeared in 1910, but Holmes, mimicking William Osler, used the pseudonym E. Y. Davis, M.D. for them.[30] He continued writing editorials for this journal until 1916. These essays were collected and published under his actual name in two volumes: *The Friends of the Insane, the Soul of Medical Education, and Other Essays* and *The Insanity of Youth and Other Essays*.[31] Beginning in 1914 he sent out reprints of his articles as circulars under the heading *Dementia Praecox Studies*. Holmes became peripherally involved in the mental hygiene movement, but it would not be until the year after his son's death that he founded his own organization.

Holmes lobbied for the creation of such an organization during the annual meeting in Chicago of the Alienists and Neurologists Associa-

tion, held from 10 to 12 July 1917.[32] However, although several prominent conference participants signed the initial petition, only Holmes's
Illinois colleagues committed themselves to the proposed organization.
On 13 July 1917 Holmes was joined by two Illinois physicians, Hermann
Campbell Stevens of Chicago and George Mitchell of Peoria, as elected
officers of the Society for the Study of Dementia Praecox. The purpose
of the society was "to stimulate further research and to co-ordinate work
already in progress in different parts of the world."[33] The main method
for achieving these goals was the publication of a quarterly scientific
journal that would be distributed internationally, *Dementia Praecox Studies: A Journal of Psychiatry of Adolescence.*

In the opening pages of the 1 January 1918 inaugural issue of *Dementia Praecox Studies* the editors unabashedly expressed their "faith" in
the hypothesis that "disease of the mind is the result of organic disease
of the body." "In spite of the magnitude of this problem there is a great
scarcity of books and monographs dealing with the physical, chemical
and biologic conditions of the unfortunate victims of this disease"; thus
they "urge[d] the publication of a journal devoted exclusively to the
study from the organic point of view, of one part of the field of mental
disease, viz., dementia praecox."[34]

Dementia Praecox Studies continued to be published through five
volumes, ending in 1922, when Holmes's health began to fail. During
those five years it published a wide range of articles on dementia praecox,
many of them republished or translated from international journals. Unfortunately for Holmes and his colleagues, in an era dominated by an
American conception of dementia praecox that was largely psychogenic,
the journal had little impact on accelerating research. But fortunately
for historians it chronicles the path of Holmes's own research in the cause
of dementia praecox, the rise and fall of one dementia praecox research
laboratory and the failed plans for two others, and the results of the experimental treatment that he devised and believed until the day he died
was more effective than anything psychiatry had to offer.

Like many physicians of his era who were trained in the new science of
bacteriology, Holmes believed that each disease had a single cause and a
single cure. Rationally discover the cause of the disease in the chemical,
bacteriological, hemolytic, or physiological laboratory, and a rational

treatment or even a cure would soon follow. Dementia praecox would yield its secrets just as tuberculosis, syphilis, yellow fever, typhus, and cholera had done in Holmes's lifetime. He was convinced from his earliest bibliographic researches that dementia praecox was a physical disease with an organic, mechanistic etiology. Psychogenic causes for dementia praecox were not rational ones, in his opinion, and therefore he completely discounted them. Holmes could not discount the role of heredity in the insanities, but he felt that these distal influences were secondary to more powerful, ongoing proximal causes in dementia praecox that could be found in living bodies and effectively treated. The theory of the hereditary cause of dementia praecox should, he felt, therefore be taken with a grain of salt. He often illustrated his position by arguing that heredity also had been considered the greatest etiologic factor in pulmonary tuberculosis and syphilis until the discovery of their respective pathogenic bacteria led to the abandonment of that theory.

By the winter of 1909 Holmes's literature review of laboratory studies of dementia praecox had led him to conclude that "most of the investigations came to zero for their aggregate result."[35] However, he felt that there were eight firm findings in the literature: (1) the identifying symptoms of the disease were well described and could lead to a reliable diagnosis after a single observation of the patient; (2) the prognosis for recovery was uniformly poor; (3) spontaneous recoveries were rare; (4) many dementia praecox sufferers improved, and some completely recovered, following an acute infectious disease accompanied by a high fever; (5) brain weight was heavier than normal in dementia praecox; (6) chronic cases of dementia praecox often manifested left-sided internal hydrocephalus; (7) no fundamental histopathology of dementia praecox had been discovered, and its existence was often denied; (8) in several highly suggestive cases, rapid polycythemia (an increase in the number of red cells in the blood) resulted in an alleviation of symptoms in dementia praecox, especially if the red cell count increased by 2 million within an hour.

This last finding particularly intrigued Holmes. He had been following with fascination the transformation of the clinical laboratory since 1900 brought about by the serological and immunological contributions of Karl Landsteiner (1868–1943) and others, such as August Wasserman (1866–1925) and Emil Abderhalden (1877–1950), who followed in his wake. When, in 1909, the German researchers Much and

Holtzman published their study of differences in reactivity to cobra venom of the blood of dementia praecox patients when compared to normals, Holmes was encouraged. Blood changes measured in dementia praecox victims were, in Holmes's mind, convincing evidence—especially to himself—that persons such as his son Ralph were "really sick" due to a recognized organic disease rather than a psychogenic mind twist or hereditary taint (which would locate the cause of his son's illness directly in Holmes himself).

Blood held the secret to solving the mystery of dementia praecox. Therefore, in congruence with his training as a bacteriologist, between the years 1909 and 1916 Holmes largely followed a *serological* program in his search for a cause of dementia praecox.[36] From this point on he was intrigued by spontaneous rapid changes in the relative numbers of red and white cells in the blood, a phenomenon termed a "blood crisis," particularly if they were linked to specific diseases and not found in normals. Holmes found the work of two dementia praecox researchers particularly relevant in this regard. The first, Halvar Lundvall of Lund, Sweden, had reported in Swedish publications as early as 1907 some initial success in improving the symptoms of dementia praecox patients by injecting them with sodium nucleate (salts of yeast acids used in the treatments of anemia, rheumatism, and gout).[37] Sodium nucleate had long been known to increase the number of white blood cells (leukocytosis) and had been used with success in the treatment of septicemia and paresis, and the fact that it seemed to work in dementia praecox suggested that its symptoms too might be due to an infectious process, perhaps even a bacterial one.[38] The second, Gunnar Kahlmeter, found that very abrupt changes in the relative numbers of white blood corpuscles, red blood corpuscles, and the percentages of the neutrophile leukocytes, lymphocytes, and eosinophile cells could be directly correlated to disturbed mental states.[39] "The blood crisis of Lundvall and Kahlmeter is prognostic of change in the mental symptoms and this crisis is sudden, almost explosive," wrote Holmes.[40] Holmes was also fascinated by the studies of Willi Schmidt in which the typically low blood pressure of dementia praecox patients (or so it was assumed at the time) could not be raised by an intramuscular injection of 0.5cc of 1/1,000 adrenaline solution.[41] Holmes suggested that adrenalin injections could be a possible diagnostic test for dementia praecox since they produced this paradoxical response.[42]

In January 1915 Holmes returned to the laboratory to do his own serological work on an intermittent basis with a colleague, Peter Gad Kitterman (1877–?). Holmes and Kitterman had coauthored a short, amateurish monograph on ancient Egyptian medicine.[43] At first they had no lab of their own, nor any money for their own equipment, so from 1 January to 1 April 1915 they used a laboratory room at the Ricketts Laboratory in Chicago belonging to Dr. H. Gideon Wells, director of the Otho S. A. Sprague Institute and a researcher at the University of Chicago. This work was conducted during off hours whenever they could steal the time from their busy lives. Holmes knew it was to be the beginning of a long research program: "My first thesis was to demonstrate the first evidences of disease in dementia praecox patients and the absence of the same evidence in other patients."[44]

The decisive factor in the return of Holmes to the laboratory was his discovery in late 1913 of the techniques of the Abderhalden defensive ferment reaction and the fact that it had been used with some success by researchers in Germany and Italy. He was particularly convinced by the claims of the Stuttgart researcher August Fauser (1856–1938) that Abderhalden's test could differentially diagnose dementia praecox from other disorders and from healthy controls. "Here then, it seems that we have found an almost certain, if not absolutely certain, method of diagnosing dementia praecox," Holmes enthused in a short medical report published on 12 February 1914.[45]

The dialyzing method of Abderhalden purported to recognize in the blood specific defensive ferments (enzymes) connected with specific protein molecules that formed the basis of specific organs or glands. If cells of an organ or gland (such as the brain, liver, heart, lungs, appendix, thyroid, or gonads) are injured, molecular detritus ends up in the blood; this arouses a reaction, that is, production of the defensive ferments that catabolize or break down these molecules into ones small enough to be eliminated by the body. The specificity of the "positive reaction" of the ferment in the Abderhalden dialysis method was thought to be directly linked to damage to specific parts of organs, including very specific areas of the brain. For example, a colleague of Holmes consistently found positive reactions in "the lower part of the motor area in the cortex corresponding to the trunk, shoulders, arms and in a lesser degree that representing the head."[46] Therefore just by drawing the blood of a patient and analyzing it, it was assumed one could see into the living body without opening it surgically and be able to discern focal areas of disease.

At the Ricketts Laboratory, Holmes reported, he "examined the blood of seventy lodging house tramps by the defensive ferment reactions of Abderhalden" and found that "the blood of the average tramp does not contain ferments that would lead to the diagnosis of dementia praecox" because "these bloods did not give reactions to the cerebral cortex or to [a] testicle," as had been found and reported in the European studies. From 1 April to 1 August 1915 Holmes continued his studies in a lab at Lakeside Hospital in Chicago, but added a new experiment: taking blood from a dementia praecox patient (probably his son Ralph) and injecting it into a goat and a rabbit to see if the "passive transmission of the defensive ferments" could be accomplished. It was. However, because Holmes did not have any blood from a "recovered patient," the defensive ferment against the cause of dementia praecox could not be injected into an animal for the purposes of producing a serum against the disease to later be used in humans if the animal also began producing these same defensive ferments.[47]

By his own admission, his application of this complex technique was rather crude, but this problem was soon rectified. On 1 August 1915 Holmes and his team were joined by a skilled biochemist, Julius Retinger, Ph.D. (1885–?), who had received his degree from Leipzig in 1913 for a thesis on a method of preparing ninhydrin, an essential component of one of the various procedures for the Abderhalden reaction test. Holmes was given the money to pay for Retinger's services by a grateful former patient. But it was a small amount, and Retinger too could work only part time on finding the cause of dementia praecox. Retinger's hiring coincided with Holmes's move to the laboratory of the Psychopathic Hospital of Cook County Hospital at the invitation of Adam Szwajkart, M.D., its director. The Psychopathic Hospital, which had opened in 1914 and occupied the corner of the Cook County Hospital grounds at Wood and Polk Streets, averaged about eighty psychiatric admissions a week who remained only a few days before being released or transferred to various Illinois state hospitals.[48] Thus Holmes and his new colleague now had daily access to a rich supply of dementia praecox subjects for their studies.

During the last five months of 1915 Retinger devised an "improvement" on the Abderhalden method. After examining thirty dementia praecox patients he concluded, "It can now be seen that the organs mostly involved in dementia praecox are the cerebral cortex, pons, optic thalamus, genital organs, and the small intestine."[49] With reliably replicated results such as these, the Abderhalden reaction test seemed to be a breakthrough in psychiatric research.

The problem with the test, as many researchers soon discovered, was that it was not a quantitative test, but a subjective one. The reaction was real only if tissue from a particular organ gave off a bluish or purplish color during the process. Some researchers always saw the color, a few more sometimes saw the color, but many others never did—and the doubters eventually began to speak out against Abderhalden. By 1920 Abderhalden's defensive ferments had fallen into general disrepute in the United States, although it continued to be used in Germany for several more decades. Until the end of his life Holmes would never lose his faith in the method. But by the end of 1915 the Abderhalden test had already outlived its usefulness as a source of new knowledge, for as Holmes believed, based on Retinger's research, it had repeatedly confirmed which internal organs were implicated in the etiology or pathophysiology of dementia praecox. But it had not led to the development of a serum that would cure dementia praecox, as had been hoped.[50] Other methods were needed to detect the true *vis morbi* of dementia praecox, the cause of the "blood crisis" and other unusual physiological phenomena.

In a few short months Holmes believed he had found the cause of dementia praecox.

In January 1915, the month that Holmes began his laboratory studies and completed his preface to *The Insanity of Youth and Other Essays,* he was confident that he had identified a cluster of five organic signs that, taken together, were pathognomonic of dementia praecox: (1) adrenal mydriasis (pupil dilation produced experimentally by two or three drops of adrenalin solution); (2) cyanosis, particularly in the hands; (3) the blood crisis of Lundvall; (4) the positive reactions of the defensive ferment test of Abderhalden for the sex glands, thyroid, and cerebral cortex; and (5) the positive response to artificial hyperleukocytosis induced by injections of sodium nucleate.[51] What was missing was an adequate pathologic "disturber," as Holmes often put it, that would link all these physical phenomena to an underlying cause.

It was Holmes's careful reading of the medical literature that provided him with the clues. While searching the literature for parallels to the paradoxical lowering of the already chronically low blood pressure in dementia praecox patients with adrenaline injections, he found an animal study in which this phenomenon could be produced, but only if the injection of adrenalin followed a prior dosing with ergotoxine (tyramine). Because ergot was then commonly used to induce uterine contractions, Holmes found this same paradox occurred in obstetrical cases. Women who had been given ergot or peturiterin and then injected with an adrenalin solution (5 cc. 1/1,000) had their blood pressure lowered. Thus in the winter and spring of 1915 Holmes began an intense study of the chemistry of ergot and the history of epidemic ergotism. It was this latter literature that led him to consider a connection between the toxic amines of ergot and the symptoms of dementia praecox—an analogical transfer familiar in studies of the history of science in which a previously solved medical problem (in this case, ergotism) serves as a source for solving a new target problem (the illness of his son and others diagnosed with dementia praecox).

Of the ten or more toxic amines in ergot described in the biochemical literature of that time, Holmes seized upon histamine (beta-iminazolylethylamine) and indolethylamine as possible pathogens capable of producing the symptoms of dementia praecox. But it was histamine in particular that attracted his attention. In June 1915 he published a paper in which he detailed the striking similarities of the physiological effects of histamine on the body to the symptoms of dementia praecox.[52] Histamine lowered the blood pressure and produced various effects on the conditions and number of the red and white corpuscles in the blood similar but perhaps not identical to the blood crisis of Lundvall. Because cyanosis and adrenal mydriasis also occurred in persons who had ingested ergot, four of the five core pathognomonic signs of dementia praecox could be explained by the actions of the toxic amines found in ergot, particularly histamine. The fifth sign, the results of the Abderhalden test, could not be used to detect toxic amines in the blood. Other research methods needed to be found.

Serological analysis allowed for the detection of evidence of an excess of indolethylamine in the blood, but not for histamine. Urine tests were inconclusive. Holmes and Retinger, who had been hired specifically to pursue the ergot-like toxic amine hypothesis of Holmes, found literature documenting the presence of catabolized products of indolethylamine in the urine, but again histamine could not be detected. Because their theory of the cause of dementia praecox depended heavily on the assumption of "hyper-histaminemia," they were running out of options. Finally, after work conducted during the latter half of 1915 and early 1916, Holmes and Retinger wrote, "The examination of the feces alone was left to us. If there had been excessive production of histamine in the intestine from any cause, bacterial or non-bacterial, 'endogenous' or 'exogenous,' some moiety of this excess might be found entangled in the stool." And so it was. Retinger found no histamine in normal controls and in "one perfectly sane patient" who had spent three years in an asylum with catatonic dementia praecox. However, the six dementia praecox patients at the Psychopathic Hospital had excessive amounts of histamine, as did one patient with the "gastric crisis of tabes."[53] When this last patient was injected with adrenalin the gastric pain stopped immediately and the blood pressure dropped—the same paradoxical effect found in people who had ingested ergot and in dementia praecox patients. This patient provided another clue: they found a tender spot on the right side of the patient's abdomen. Was this the locus of an infectious process that sent poisons to the brain?

Evidence found in the medical literature supported their hypothetical locus of infection. They also learned that other researchers had found that *B. aminophilus intestinalis,* a bacterium discovered in the cecum, reduced histadine to histamine. All the pieces fit.

Holmes was now on familiar territory. He was a specialist not only in bacterial infections but also in the organs of the abdomen. His ten-year quest to find a cause and a cure for dementia praecox that had begun in 1906 brought him right back to his major areas of expertise as a physician and a scientist. His autodidactic mastery of the gigantic and confusing medical and psychiatric literature, his years of consultations with alienists, neurologists, and other medical colleagues, his data resulting from the adoption of new laboratory methods—all of these disparate sources of evidence now made sense when he assimilated them to his preexisting cognitive schema. Perhaps this trajectory was inevitable. Indeed as early as 1908 Holmes had speculated, "It is my opinion that there are many cases of insanity which are due to exogenous toxemia that should be sought for in the infection of some of the natural cavities of the body . . . possibly of bacterial origin."[54]

Similar odysseys by laboratory researchers looking for the causes and cures of dementia praecox had all ended in shipwrecks. The vast majority of those scientists moved on to other, more fruitful voyages at the bench. But not Holmes. Because of the constant reminder of his son's illness, Holmes was simply not going to give up; he was going to *comprehend* dementia praecox. And with this knowledge he was going to save his son.

With these new clues to the puzzle Holmes worked fast. Getting the cooperation of Cook County Hospital for technical support, during the late months of 1915 he and his colleagues began to use the relatively new technique of the fluoroscope to observe barium meals being passed through the digestive system. It was quickly determined that in dementia praecox patients it took 60 to 120 hours to pass a barium meal, but only 4 to 6 hours for normal controls. The barium meal tended to be stuck in the cecum and proximal colon for this abnormally long time in dementia praecox patients. A spasm of the sphincter of the colon, the "ring of Cannon," was blocking the passage of the meal. Holmes and Retinger offered their conclusion in the article that Holmes believed to the end of his life was his greatest single scientific contribution to the world, "The Relation of Cecal Stasis to Dementia Praecox," published in the 12 August 1916 issue of *The Lancet-Clinic*: *"The time necessary for the development of the toxic amines is furnished by the stay of the residue in the cecum."*[55]

Holmes had found the mechanisms of dementia praecox: ergot-like toxic amines produced in the cecum that poisoned many organs of the body, including the brain. The poisoning of the brain resulted in a mental disorder with psychotic symptoms. All the sufficient links in the mechanistic causal chain were present. In Chicago some very important physicians, politicians, and benefactors learned of Holmes's success and were offering to help him fulfill the next logical step: the establishment of a laboratory and experimental unit where new treatments and even a cure for dementia praecox could be realized.

The etiologic theory of dementia praecox proposed by Holmes was highly congruent with theories of self-infection, autointoxication, and focal infection in medicine and psychiatry that were peaking in popularity during the First World War. Perhaps the most significant validation for his theory came from a prominent Chicago physician Holmes knew personally, Frank Billings (1854–1932). Billings, the dean of the faculty at Rush Medical College and a past president of the American Medical Association (1902–1904), generated publicity for his own focal infection theory of disease after giving a series of lectures on the topic at Stanford University Medical School in September 1915.[56] His theory proposed that the primary focus of infection in the body was the mouth, where rotting teeth, inflamed tonsils, and bad oral hygiene produced toxic bacteria that were inhaled into the lungs or swallowed or otherwise entered the blood stream and caused systemic diseases such as rheumatoid arthritis, endocarditis, and nephritis. As a founder of the Otho S. A. Sprague Memorial Institute in 1909 and president of its Board of Trustees, Billings was instrumental in funding and at times directing laboratory research on focal infections as they related to systemic disease.[57]

Holmes and Retinger's new publications in primarily local and regional medical journals and Holmes's promotion of the new autointoxication theory of dementia praecox at various Chicago medical and charitable societies attracted the interest of Billings, who wanted to extend his focal infection theory to psychiatry. It also attracted state and local officials excited by the prospect of finding new treatments for the insanities that would empty institutional beds. In October 1915 Holmes began negotiations with H. Gideon Wells, the director of the Sprague Institute, and the alienist George Zeller of the Board of Administration of the State of Illinois, to establish a "cooperative research laboratory" at the Chicago State Hospital at Dunning. The mission would be to conduct research into Holmes's focal infection theory of dementia praecox and to develop possible cures for this disease. The Board of Administration approved the idea in a resolution dated 15 October 1915, and, with the endorsement of Wells, Billings and his Board of Trustees of the Sprague Institute voted to fund the project in a meeting on 17 December. Holmes and Retinger accordingly began slanting their articles to signal their approval of Billings and his ideas.

The contract of the Cooperative Research Laboratory at Chicago State Hospital was modified, extended, and then signed on 3 April 1916.[58] The Board of Administration ordered the emptying of patients from an isolated building known as Ward W, and blueprints were drawn up to divide the building into five laboratories, including an experimental treatment unit. But this never happened. The Sprague Institute suddenly balked at further cooperation with Holmes. The building remained vacant for eight months and then, due to the crowded conditions at the Chicago State Hospital, was filled with patients.

Holmes was furious, writing to a colleague, "The contract failed . . . because of the neglect of the director of the Sprague Institute, Dr. H. Gideon Wells, or of the trustees of the institute behind him."[59] "The Sprague Institute abandoned the undertaking without notice or apology," he continued to fume years later.[60]

Why did Wells, Billings, and the Sprague Institute distance themselves from Holmes and his work on dementia praecox after April 1916? Perhaps it had something to do with the sudden shift in focus from basic research to radical treatment that followed the signing of the contract for the proposed laboratory by the newly emboldened, and temperamentally incautious, Bayard Taylor Holmes.

April 1916 was the high-water mark of Holmes's career. He had articulated an autointoxication or focal infection theory of dementia praecox that was congruent with current medical thinking and had conducted primary research that, he believed, provided compelling evidence supporting it. He had received the blessing of the powerful Sprague Institute and was promised financial backing for a complex of laboratories to be devoted solely to work on his discoveries, a dream of his since 1911.[61] And it was in this month that Holmes submitted for publication the paper he regarded as his most significant contribution to science, "The Relation of Cecal Stasis to Dementia Praecox."

Holmes also underwent a personal transformation in his thinking at this time. The careful laboratory researcher had become impatient, and the physician and healer in Holmes now overtook the cautious scientist. As he himself later noted when reflecting back on his career, "[This article] was offered for publication in April 1916. The facts it contains seemed to me irrefutable at the time and I determined to act upon the rational indications without delay."[62] And so he did.

As the months of stalling by the Sprague Institute dragged on, Holmes refused to wait for the opening of the Cooperative Laboratory to conduct more foundational research before trying out experimental treatments: "It has been forced upon me as a conviction that in a condition so desperate, treatment should be begun even before absolute scientific demonstration of a theory could be reached."[63]

Cecostomy or appendicostomy, followed by daily irrigations of the cecum, would be the new rational treatment of dementia praecox. If the irrigations were performed daily to prevent fecal stasis in the cecum, the toxemia symptoms of dementia praecox should diminish or disappear entirely. For Holmes this treatment was rational in two senses: first, it followed logically from his theory of the cause of dementia praecox; second, it was consistent with contemporary medical practice. Surgical removal of teeth, tonsils, and sections of organs or other bodily tissue had long been the only effective treatment available to believers in the focal infection theory of Billings. Others, such as the surgeon William Arbuthnot Lane (1856–1943), believed that removing the entire colon was an appropriate measure for treating constipation and preventing autointoxications that might arise from fecal stasis.[64] In Britain autointoxication due to intestinal stasis is still known as Sir Abuthnot Lane's Disease.

As the late medical historian Roy Porter pointed out, focal sepsis was a "fashionable interwar diagnosis" that led to numerous medical misadventures.[65] It was literally cutting-edge medical science in 1916. If dementia praecox was a true physical disease caused by a focal infection in the cecum, it made perfect sense to Holmes, a specialist in abdominal surgery who had written a textbook on the subject in 1904, that surgical intervention was a rational response. Like many surgeons, Holmes had an almost fetishistic fascination with one specific bodily structure, in his case the appendix, which he considered "the most mournfully interesting and unique structure in the body."[66]

In May 1916 Holmes applied his rational treatment for dementia praecox to his son Ralph. It made sense for a man of Holmes's ideals and sense of honor to risk his own son first before daring to operate on another family's child. The result, as we know, was tragic.

Holmes never admitted in any of his publications that he had killed his own son, but in recounting the history of his contribution to medical science he lied about his first experimental subject: "The first patient that I performed appendicostomy upon was a boy of 20 who had been sick only two years."[67] This boy was actually the second. Holmes conducted the operation on "A. H." on 25 July 1916 at Lakeside Hospital in Chicago, some three months after resolving to put his rational—but still experimental—treatment to a test.

A very small incision was made as if for an appendectomy, and the appendix brought into the wound. No gross pathology was observed in this region. The appendix was rather large but not inflamed. About two-thirds of the mesentery of the appendix was ligated and cut away. The cecum was stitched to the peritoneum and fascia of the abdominal wall on both sides of the wound. The short incision was then closed around the appendix in layers with fine lasting catgut. The skin was closed and last of all the protruding portion of the appendix was cut off a quarter of an inch from the skin, one half at a time, and fastened open with silk stitches holding the mucosa and serosa together and fastening both to the skin.[68]

Penetrating the resulting stoma (opening) with a glass-tipped rubber hose, Holmes performed an irrigation of the cecum using water mixed with magnesium sulfate. Later he taught the patient and his father how to do the daily irrigations.

During the following six months his father irrigated the colon through the appendix with water, in which a small amount of magnesium sulfate was dissolved. The patient sat on the stool in the bath room. The ten-quart pail was hung about five feet above the stool and connected by an ordinary rubber tube with a dull glass point to the appendix. When the irrigation was begun the father read aloud to his son, thus passing the time profitably.

According to Holmes, the patient was less delusional and much improved after the operation even five years later, though there remained a "pronounced mental defect."[69]

Holmes eventually came to believe that his treatment would work best, perhaps even curing dementia praecox, if it was performed either before or directly after the first psychotic break. Patients who had been sick for many months or years, such as his son, would probably not be helped very much by the procedure. Like Henry A. Cotton, Holmes believed that early surgical intervention could prevent the chronic course of the illness.[70]

Holmes operated on a second dementia praecox patient, a twenty-one-year-old male, on 3 October 1916 at Lakeside Hospital. The young man had become ill in March 1915 and was removed from Elgin State Hospital in Illinois for the experimental surgery. Upon recovery he was returned to the hospital. No improvement in his condition occurred until five months of daily irrigations had taken place. After being released in March 1917 the patient continued the irrigations himself at home and had a full recovery.[71] Holmes enthusiastically used this patient as living proof of the correctness of his new treatment, mentioning his case in many of his later writings and encouraging him to give testimonials of his cure at professional meetings of Holmes's medical colleagues. Holmes would routinely publish the names, addresses, and intimate details about the lives of the patients who received this experimental treatment so that others could verify his new treatment and possible cure of dementia praecox.

Shortly after operating on this young man, Holmes rushed into print a description of his new rational treatment for dementia praecox in late October 1916, claiming prematurely that he had operated on two patients and that they were both "apparently improved."[72] Obviously he neglected to mention the fate of his own son. Holmes began to convince his colleagues of the soundness of the new experimental treatment. Two more dementia praecox patients were operated on for Holmes at Cook County Hospital by Wyllis Andrews, M.D. In all, by 31 December 1916, Holmes reported that five patients received this experimental treatment: "Two of the operated patients are now at the Elgin State Hospital where the irrigations are being continued. Three of them are at home. The first patient was operated on in July, the last one in December. All of them have improved in weight, and the blood pressure has approached normal. The mental condition is said to be better."[73]

With the demise of the dream of the Cooperative Research Laboratory, and with his own work with Retinger abruptly halted on 1 April 1916, when private funds ran out and all their lab equipment was taken from the Psychopathic Hospital space and returned to Cook County Hospital, all Holmes could do was operate and convince others to do so. But this situation was soon to change.

Holmes lobbied hard for a new laboratory and convinced the Board of Commissioners of Cook County, Joseph Miller, M.D., the medical director of Cook County Hospital, John Nuzam, M.D., the head of the clinical laboratories at Cook County Hospital, and Adam Szwajkart, M.D., the director of the Psychopathic Hospital to approve his proposal. On 18 April 1917 the top floor of the Psychopathic Hospital was formally designated the Psychopathic Research Laboratory of the Psychopathic Hospital, Cook County Hospital. The space contained a full hydrotherapy suite with four continuous tubs, but the facility had never been used. Holmes and his colleagues covered the tubs with tall laboratory tables where they could work while standing. One large room was filled with ten beds for experimental subjects with dementia praecox. Other large rooms became laboratories for bacteriology and physiology, and a smaller one became a "blood laboratory." An "animal house" was constructed on the roof.[74]

Before the Psychopathic Research Laboratory closed in February 1918, having been open for only ten months (the entry of the United States into the war in Europe in 1917 led to the reallocation of funds by Cook County and disruptions in medical and nursing staff), Holmes served as its director and Retinger as its biochemist. The remainder of the clinical staff were Horry Matthew Jones, bacteriologist, who had received his Ph.D. in bacteriology from Northwestern University in 1916; Walter Ford, M.D., psychiatrist; H. C. Stevens, Ph.D., M.D., psychologist; James Henderson, blood morphologist; Paul Headland, clinical assistant; and Leola Sexton, A. B., in charge of the patients' entertainment and reeducation. During its brief existence the laboratory admitted thirty patients to its experimental research inpatient unit, but ten remained only a few days before being discharged or sent elsewhere because they were not suffering from dementia praecox or permission for experimental treatments could not be gained from parents or guardians. Of the twenty genuine dementia praecox patients treated, ten were discharged as "recovered" or "greatly improved," three were committed to state hospitals at the request of the researchers, and seven were still residing in the laboratory when it closed.

Three experimental treatments were tested. The first consisted of administering calcium lactate with meals to bolster calcium levels in the body. Holmes had read clinical reports that indicated a lack of calcium led to muscle spasms, including those in the intestinal sphincter known as the "ring of Cannon," which Holmes had come to believe was causing the cecal stasis in dementia praecox patients. No improvement was ever found with this treatment. A more promising remedy was intravenous injections of saline, which led to improvements in the symptoms of two of eighteen dementia praecox patients on whom it was administered. But the third and most effective treatment was appendicostomy and daily irrigation of the cecum and colon. Eight patients underwent this surgery and procedure, and all were among the ten discharged as "recovered" or "greatly improved."[75]

But right from the start all was not well in the lab. During the official opening-night reception the neurologist Sidney Kuh (1866–1934), a powerful physician at Cook County Hospital, made remarks critical of Holmes and his research program, and this emboldened others who were rubbed the wrong way by Holmes's fiery temperament. Prominent among these was Julius Retinger, who had begun to resent Holmes. Two months into the operation of the laboratory Holmes wrote Retinger an emotional letter on 4 June 1917, confiding at first, "You know that I love you like a son and admire you and your splendid intellect." But Holmes then issued a sharp rebuke for the "very many deficiencies" in Retinger's work "due to neglect." He ended with a threat: "You must be more attentive to your own work, less conspicuous elsewhere, or I shall be obliged to terminate our business relations and I shall do it on June 30."[76] The chill in relations between the two men progressed to the point that Holmes fired Retinger in December 1917. "My laboratory has had a sort of revolution and Retinger is discharged," Holmes wrote to one of his most generous financial backers, George Fuller. "The trouble began in what Dr. Kuh said the night of the opening Apr. 18, Dr. Retinger took his cue from that and began intriguing for my displacement and his own elevation."[77]

Retinger also did not get along with the newly hired bacteriologist, Horry M. Jones. On 5 September 1917 Holmes wrote to Adam Szwajkart, the director of the Psychopathic Hospital, "During the past three months there has been a constant condition of petty quarreling between Dr Retinger and Dr Jones and it has been necessary for me to take them aside and discuss matters with which the laboratory has absolutely nothing to do." Holmes then asked Szwajkart to fire Jones and keep Retinger.[78] But there may have been another reason Holmes wrote this letter: Jones had participated in the same research as Holmes and Retinger, but had arrived at entirely different interpretations of the data. Furthermore Jones had been vocal in raising serious methodological questions about the scientific soundness of their work. He was fired in September 1917 and replaced by Enrico Ecker. Stunned, Jones wrote to Adolf Meyer for guidance. The letter is worth quoting in its entirety:

Dear Doctor Meyer:— I have just been summarily dismissed from the Cook County Hospital Psychopathic Laboratory by Dr Bayard Holmes for my inability to agree with him and his chemist regarding their theory on the etiology of Dementia Praecox. However, during the investigation, I have collected a mass of data and observations, which I am anxious to publish, although directly opposed to every phase of their theory. For example, some Xraygraphs to which I have access, entirely disprove Dr Holmes statements in regard to the cecal-stasis caused by the constriction of the ring of Cannon. This statement although not fundamental to their theory has been made so often, and if true, ought easily to be proved by them with actual Xraygraphs, instead of Dr. Holmes' freehand drawings.

Early in the investigation I made a comparison of the bacterial flora of the stools of normal controls and of Dementia praecox patients. Among the organisms isolated for study was found one which I later proved was able to produce histamine from histadine and which proved to have all the ear-marks of a B. aminophilus intestinalis of Berthelot and Bertrand, an organism which Dr. Holmes now refers too so freely as being a constant inhabitant of the intestinal tracts of Dementia Praecox patients. This organism, which, as my daily records will show, was isolated from the stool of the Chemist himself, was then mixed in definite proportions with feces and plated on a specially prepared or selective medium and found to be easily recovered and recognized directly on the plates. (In all the specimens examined, thirty-eight counting the controls, no other organism was found which in pure culture produced detectable quantities of histamine from histadine.) This selective medium was then used for direct plating of the stool of the patients, and in no case was it possible to recover a single colony of this organism on plates showing as high as five hundred colonies per plate with ten plates to each sample of stool. In other words, I tried hard to find the organism. The chemist, however says he finds histamine in the stools of the patients but I am able to say positively that since I have been here he has not examined one single specimen from normal controls to see if it may not also be found in persons other than Dementia Praecox patients, in spite of the fact that I detected in a normal stool and demonstrated in his presence a substance giving the Pauly reaction and the oxytocic reaction of tyramine, a substance produced by the same peculiar action of the histamine producing organism.

At present I am looking for a position where I shall not be forced to pervert my laboratory findings to fit some preconceived theory, but I am writing to you primarily to learn your opinion of the worth of this theory in the light of your knowledge of the disease, and also for your advice as to how I can get the data I have accumulated into print.

Very sincerely,

(signed) H. M. Jones[79]

Meyer's response, if any, has not surfaced. Jones quickly composed a scientific paper that has stood the test of time as the only serious attempt at scientific criticism of the research of Bayard Holmes.[80] The editors of the *Journal of Infectious Diseases* received the paper from Jones on 5 October 1917, less than a month after he was fired. By early 1919 he had found a position in the Department of Pathology and Bacteriology at the University of Illinois College of Medicine in Chicago. It is clear from the information contained in this letter that Holmes's own dictum, "The laboratory will show up a false teacher in the shortest time," had come back to haunt him.

Ignoring the serious scientific objections to his theory of dementia praecox, Holmes continued to dispense his cure. In the autumn of 1917 he received a request for a consultation from Leonard C. Mead, M.D., the superintendent of the Yankton State Hospital in South Dakota, who wrote concerning the misfortunes of the Lauer family, who had a son and two daughters in his hospital, all with dementia praecox. Holmes offered to go to Yankton and help in any way he could.

In the latter half of November 1917 Holmes made presentations to the medical staff of the Yankton State Hospital on his theory of dementia praecox and on the therapeutic successes achieved by abdominal surgery and the postoperative regimen of regular irrigations of the cecum. Impressed by this apparent medical breakthrough, Mead and his medical staff agreed to cooperate in a grand experimental test. Seven dementia praecox patients underwent the appendicostomy: the three afflicted members of the Lauer family and four other inpatients. In a two-year follow-up assessment of the treatment, the results were mixed. Of the members of the Lauer family, one (the son) died from peritonitis following the operation, one made no improvement whatsoever, and the third, who had just been admitted for the first time, completely recovered and by September 1919 took only an "occasional irrigation." Of the four unrelated patients, one female recovered after eight months and was working and doing well; one male recovered after nine months and also was working and doing well; another female showed no improvement, and a final female improved after eighteen months but was still not well and had to be taken care of at home.[81]

By the time of the closing of the Psychopathic Research Laboratory in February 1918, Holmes or other surgeons who had been instructed by him had performed appendicostomies on at least twenty-two dementia praecox patients.[82] Neither Holmes nor his colleagues performed any more surgical procedures on dementia praecox patients after this date.

Just a few months later, in July 1918, at the Trenton State Hospital in New Jersey, Henry A. Cotton conducted the first of 645 major surgical procedures (laparotomies, colectomies, hysterectomies, thyroidectomies, and so on) over the next fourteen years, one-third consisting of dementia praecox patients, one-third of manic-depressive patients, and one-third of patients with milder psychiatric illnesses.[83] By Cotton's own reckoning, 25 to 30 percent of these procedures resulted in the death of the patient.[84] Like Holmes, his rationale for targeting specific areas of focal infection in the body was based on his early use of the Abderhalden defensive ferments reaction test, which, also like Holmes, he abandoned after being convinced of its findings.[85] Of the twenty-two dementia praecox patients operated on by Holmes or his colleagues, only two died from complications following surgery, confirming Holmes's claim that his surgical treatment for mental illness was superior to that of Cotton's, which "crippled" his patients: "A small number of cases have been treated by this method [appendicostomy] under favorable conditions, but too many have been 'operated on' and then left without carrying on the months long irrigation of the colon and years long re-education of the crippled patient."[86]

"I shall be at Fairhope, Ala., for the next few months," Holmes wrote to the editor of *Medical Life,* Victor Robinson, on New Year's Day 1923. "I have been quite sick and must lay up."[87] He revealed that he had been suffering from a "toxic myocarditis" for quite some time. In fact an infection of his left hand had developed into an inflammation of his heart and had rendered him a semi-invalid by August 1922. Holmes knew the game was up. He gathered his personal papers relating to his scientific and political careers and donated them to the John Crerar Library at the University of Chicago. He also wrote a farewell address for those interested in his research program on dementia praecox that was published posthumously. "And so it has come to this," he told Robinson. "I can personally do no more. Spiritually and physically I am disheartened. . . . I am down and out, but not melancholy."[88]

While Henry A. Cotton of Trenton State Hospital had become a medical celebrity in the popular press in America, due to his own self-promotion, for his surgical treatment of the focal infections that caused the insanities, Holmes followed the traditional ethical path of physicians of his era and resisted such a strategy. Despite his keen knowledge of the power of the press, which he had used to his advantage in his political campaign for mayor of Chicago and his public health crusades, Holmes did not seek out journalists to sell his cure. But sticking to the tried and true path of aiming his publications at medical colleagues ultimately failed him. As his life neared its end, he suffered intensely from the fact that his own major medical contributions, his hypothesized cause for dementia praecox and its rational treatment, had been resoundingly ignored by the scientific community. The fact that Cotton never referenced him in any of his publications, nor gave him credit for the priority in developing surgical treatments for dementia praecox, must have particularly galled him.

Holmes would further weaken and eventually die at his Alabama home on 1 April 1924. He was buried in the cemetery in Fairhope. On the front page of the 11 April 1924 issue of the *Fairhope Courier* the article "Dr Bayard Holmes Passes to Rest" is prominent above the fold. The piece contains a description of a memorial service held at his home. "No man ever gave more than he gave—no one ever loved more than he loved his son—no one served better than he served," said Mrs. John O'Connor, a friend and neighbor from Chicago. "His ambition had been centered in this son, so he retired from his practice to minister to him in the home they had built together—a great man—who had made the great sacrifice in the eyes of the world."[89] A letter to Victor Robinson from a Fairhope neighbor also identified the agony of the father with the fate of his son: "I knew Dr Bayard Holmes in Fairhope, Ala., know his beautiful home, and know him by sight only. There was something sad about it all, and it must have been the 'mental' illness of his son that made of him a 'recluse' in Fairhope."[90]

But perhaps it was not the mental illness of his son, but the gnawing memory of how it had ended that eventually drove Holmes to retreat into his Alabama sanctuary. Ralph had died one month after his father's decision "to act upon the rational indications" of his theory of dementia praecox "without delay." One week after Ralph's death, Adolf Meyer composed a letter of condolence to Holmes. "A sad fate fulfilled—unlike many others, having been a factor in the great call for more knowledge," he wrote.[91] We can only wonder if, at the end of his life, when reflecting on Ralph, Holmes may have wished for a more patient temperament and moderation in his quest for more medical knowledge. Martyred by his father, the son cannot tell us if the "great sacrifice" was worth it.

Holmes and Cotton were not the only American physicians to consider surgical solutions to dementia praecox. Charles Eucharist de Medici Sajous (1852–1929), a Philadelphia physician and a pioneer in American endocrinology, also believed in the rationality of this form of treatment. "The cause of [dementia praecox], whether tonsillar, dental, intestinal, etc., of the thyroid erethism [causing hyperthyroidism], must be removed. Bayard Holmes and also myself have cured severe cases by flushing the colon through the abdominal opening."[92] As Sajous indicated, the thyroid gland was also a focus of interest as the possible source of etiology. Certainly Emil Kraepelin had considered this hypothesis in 1896 in the fifth edition of his textbook, when he grouped dementia praecox with myxedematous insanity and cretinism, two conditions caused by thyroid dysfunction, as mental diseases caused by metabolic autointoxication. In the United States some physicians attempted to alleviate or cure dementia praecox through rational treatments such as the alteration of thyroid activity through organotherapy or, if that didn't work, surgery on the thyroid gland.

Just such an infamous experiment took place in the Baltimore Insane Hospital at Bay View in 1897. In that year Henry J. Berkeley (1860–?), a clinical professor of psychiatry at Johns Hopkins Hospital, selected eight insane patients who "had either passed, or were about to pass, the limits of time in which recovery could be confidently expected," in order to test the poisoning effects of administrations of thyroid gland extract. He had done such experiments on guinea pigs, mice, and dogs and wanted to see the effect on humans. There was no indication in his published report that he was doing so to improve the mental state of the patients—a fact that would later cause an uproar when antivivisectionists learned of the experiments. Berkeley started the patients off on "5 grains" of preparations of thyroid gland per day for three days, then "10 grains" per day, and then, if the reaction was not too severe, "15 grains per day" (one apothecary grain is equivalent to 64 mg today). All of the patients lost weight and had circulatory symptoms such as tachycardia and skin changes that made their forehead feel gelatinous. But the behavioral changes were the most dramatic: "Irritability and a greater or less degree of mental or motor excitement were remarked in all cases. . . . Two patients became frenzied, and of these, one died before the experiment had subsided." Berkeley then published his findings in the *Bulletin of the Johns Hopkins Hospital* in July 1897.[93]

Antivivisectionists protested the use of vulnerable human subjects who were not capable of understanding the dangers of the experiment. The scandal played a part in the eventual adoption of ethical rules for human experimentation by the American Medical Association, but that would be years in the future. When a U.S. Senate committee debated legislation in 1900 that would regulate vivisection in the District of Columbia, one senator raised the issue of the infamous Berkeley experiment. William Osler, who was in attendance, leaped out of his seat and exclaimed, "Mr. Chairman, those experiments were *not* made in Johns Hopkins Hospital!"[94] As the historian Susan Lederer noted, Osler defended Johns Hopkins against Berkeley's experiments, "condemned improper experimentation on patients," and "insisted that the medical profession absolutely opposed non-therapeutic experiments in patients."[95]

But in psychiatry, which was still largely regarded as a sect separate from the community of physicians, such experiments continued. Berkeley himself continued to use the insane patient population at Bay View for such experiments, but was careful in the future to assert they were rational experimental treatments for specific insanities, such as dementia praecox. In 1907 he teamed up with Newdigate M. Owensby (1882–1952), an alienist at Bay View, to put Kraepelin's metabolic autointoxication theory to a test.[96] Thyroid extract seemed to make dementia praecox patients worse. They developed tremors, hyperidrosis, muscular spasms or rigidity, increased reflexes, leukocytosis, and weight loss. Perhaps, they thought, this meant that dementia praecox was not caused by too little thyroid activity, but too much. So they decided to start a new phase of experimentation involving the surgical removal of portions of the thyroid gland.

In June 1907 they received permission to operate on two insane patients who were in advanced states of catatonia.[97] The first was a nineteen-year-old girl with religious delusions. She had become so unmanageable and destructive in her behavior that she was admitted to the hospital in March 1907. In the asylum she became mute, apathetic, and untidy in hygiene and grooming and developed a "mask-like expression." The second patient was a twenty-one-year-old man who presented with the same catatonic symptoms, but who exhibited more muscle rigidity and tremors. In each case the surgeon, R. H. Follis, removed four-fifths of the right lobe of the thyroid gland. Within forty-eight hours after the procedure both patients seemed to improve and were eventually discharged.

In November 1907 two more catatonic Bay View patients underwent the operation and also improved to the point that they could be discharged. Had a cure for dementia praecox been found? The news media at the time certainly thought so. In fact perhaps the first newspaper article in the United States to discuss dementia praecox in a medical context concerned these surgical procedures on the thyroid gland. In the 20 December 1907 issue of the *New York Times* the following item appeared:

CURES DEMENTIA PRAECOX
Surgeon Discovers Operation to Relieve Disease of Mind

Baltimore, Md., Dec 19.—A cure for one of the most pitiable forms of insanity, hitherto considered by experts as 80 per cent incurable, has been found, it is hoped, in the use of the surgeon's knife by Dr. Newdigate M. Owensby, physician in chief at Bayview Insane Asylum. This form of insanity is known to the profession as dementia praecox.

It attacks persons generally between the ages of 15 and 30 years. It destroys the qualities of resistance, thought, and speech, rendering the victim little more than an idiot.

The disease resembles in certain symptoms the more familiar forms of cretinism and myxoedema, and it was this similarity that first led Dr. Owensby to conceive of an operation. The two latter diseases originate, it is thought, by a lack of secretion in the thyroid gland, located near the windpipe. A fairly effective cure was found in the administration of extract of thyroid glands taken from sheep.

Following this line of treatment in dementia praecox, Dr. Owensby found that instead of reducing the symptoms the treatment seemed to accentuate them. He concluded that instead of the disease arising from a lack of secretion, there was a likelihood of oversecretion, due to diseased blood vessels in the gland. This suggested using the knife to cut away the diseased portion, giving opportunity for new blood vessels to form.

Dr. Owensby last July performed the operation on the worst case in the asylum. The case was kept under close observation for two months, without the slightest indication of a return of the symptoms. In October the case was dismissed. The man has secured employment and is doing intelligent work.

Of four other cases operated upon, three showed the same return of intelligence.

Berkeley and Owensby later performed this operation on a twenty-five-year-old man with the catatonic form of dementia praecox who had been mute, refusing food, and sitting in the same bodily position for four months. The surgery was a success. But when the two physicians tried their procedure on three dementia praecox patients at the Second Hospital for the Insane of Maryland, there was no effect. These patients were more chronic and had apparently passed the point of recovery.

After these paradigmatic experiments the conventional wisdom was that surgery could, in some instances, cure dementia praecox, especially in its catatonic form. Hyperthyroidism was now considered by some to be the cause of Kraepelin's disease. Sajous would later report with authority in his textbook, "In dementia praecox we have . . . hyperthyroidia as the underlying cause," for which he recommended the surgical procedures of Berkeley and Owensby as the solution.[98]

Emil Kraepelin followed these reports of American experimental treatments for dementia praecox "with expectancy," but noted in 1913 that the "partial *excision of the thyroid gland*" had yielded mixed results. There is no evidence that Kraepelin himself ever attempted such surgical treatments. However, for a time he did experiment with organo-therapy, probably in the 1890s in Dorpat or Heidelberg: "Many years ago I endeavored for a long time to acquire influence on dementia praecox by the introduction of preparations of every possible organ, of the thyroid, of the testes, of the ovaries and so on, unfortunately without any effect."[99]

Throughout the first three decades of the twentieth century there would be other occasional reports here and there of experimental surgical procedures that were performed on dementia praecox patients

(such as a study published in 1924 on the effects of vasectomies performed on one hundred patients at the Manhattan State Hospital), but
all would ultimately fail as therapeutic alternatives.[100]

Dementia praecox was stronger than any gland extract or scalpel.
No medical treatment was ever found that could alter its tragic
trajectory.

8

THE RISE OF SCHIZOPHRENIA IN AMERICA,
1912–1927

August Hoch remembered the day he introduced schizophrenia to American alienists and neurologists.

Hoch, then the director of the New York Psychiatric Institute, had been following with interest and admiration the work of his fellow Swiss psychiatrists at the Burghölzli mental hospital in Zurich. Just a few years earlier he himself had been there to train with Jung and Bleuler, the energetic, empathetic, and kindly man who was the chief of that institution. When Bleuler published a thick volume in 1911 containing his own new ideas about dementia praecox, Hoch studied it carefully and wrote an insightful review of it.[1] Hoch remembered that he had "balked" at Bleuler's proposed new name for dementia praecox, schizophrenia, which he found "a rather uncouth term." But he was fascinated by Bleuler's new perspectives on the disease and found himself in agreement with many of them. Hoch then presented a summary of his review at a meeting of the New York Psychiatrical Society in 1912. "All of them made a lot of fun at the term," he recalled. "But it is remarkable what one can get used to."[2]

Such was the ignoble birth of schizophrenia in America.

Although many in Hoch's audience may have been unfamiliar with the term, there were other Americans who had been personally introduced to schizophrenia by its creator. Like Hoch, Smith Ely Jelliffe and William Alanson White had also worked with Bleuler and Jung in Zurich in 1907. A. A. Brill was there in 1907 and 1908, the critical years during which the "Zurich school" was developing the concept. After Brill returned to the United States he assumed positions as a clinical assistant at Columbia University's Vanderbilt Clinic (an outpatient neurological clinic) and at Bellevue Hospital in New York City. In July 1909 he published the case history of a man he had treated in Zurich with "schizophrenia (dementia praecox)"—apparently the first use of Bleuler's term in an American medical journal. Brill treated the man for one month, discharging him to his father on 31 January 1908 with a "schizophrenia" diagnosis. The condition was neither "a dementia nor a praecox," so Brill stated, rather strongly, "My former chief, Prof. Bleuler, to whom I am indebted for this case, repudiates this meaningless term, dementia praecox, and uses Schizophrenia." Other Americans who had not made the pilgrimage to Zurich certainly knew of schizophrenia. In 1910 I. W. Eggleston, an assistant physician at the New York State Hospital at Binghamton, used the term schizophrenia "as a synonym of dementia praecox," adding, "This would appear to be far better adapted to the condition than dementia praecox."[3]

But the reaction of Hoch's distinguished audience during a public forum recognized for being the place to introduce new ideas into American neurology and psychiatry indicated that schizophrenia was an unknown entity. Given Hoch's position as the director of the Psychiatric Institute on Ward's Island, his enthusiastic endorsement of Bleuler's clinical vision of schizophrenia, if not its name, meant Bleuler's disease would now be taken very seriously in American psychiatry.

Bleuler's disease was not Kraepelin's disease; dementia praecox and schizophrenia were not true synonyms. Hoch realized this right away, and soon a select few others in the American psychiatric elite would too. Most American alienists and neurologists would not.

One of the most confusing aspects of American psychiatry in the first half of the twentieth century was this interchangeable use of the terms "dementia praecox" and "schizophrenia" in clinical publications, in everyday diagnosis, and even in research. The source of this problem can be laid directly at the doorstep of Bleuler himself. His introduction of the hyphenated bridge "Dementia praecox—Schizophreniegruppe ('Dementia praecox—Schizophrenia group')" in the title of the 1908 article in which he introduced schizophrenia, as well as the either/or option in the title of his 1911 monograph, *Dementia praecox oder Gruppe der Schizophrenien (Dementia Praecox or the Group of Schizophrenias)* directly led to this misconception.[4] Although some American physicians (such as Hoch, Meyer, Jelliffe, and Southard) recognized that the option of a differential diagnosis choice *between* dementia praecox and schizophrenia was possible in the case of certain patients, a minority within an educated elite engaged in an intellectual discourse far from the day-to-day world of their hundreds of psychiatrist colleagues in North America.

What, then, was schizophrenia? And how was Bleuler's disease different from Kraepelin's disease? Let us first remember Kraepelin's conception of the disorder in 1899. Dementia praecox was a disease with an onset after puberty characterized by a progressive deterioration process that would result in an irreversible "mental weakness" or "defect." The progression could be fast or slow, and the terminal phase might vary as to the amount of permanent cognitive deterioration. The symptoms during the onset of the illness, as well as during its middle stages, were not predictive of the course or the outcome (prognosis). Only one symptom— *Zerfahrenheit,* a word used by Kraepelin that is perhaps best translated as "distraction" or "incoherence"—seemed to be a constant. Two persons with the same dementia praecox diagnosis could differ markedly in clinical picture when it came to the combination of symptoms they presented (delusions, hallucinations, motor abnormalities, language abnormalities, mood alterations, and so on). No symptom or cluster of symptoms was necessarily pathognomonic (disease-identifying) of schizophrenia, and thus none of the characteristic symptoms was any more important than any other in this regard. The disease progressed with occasional flare-ups (delusions, hallucinations, behavioral abnormalities) that would be regarded as signs that further progressive deterioration was taking place. The mental weakness or defect persisted between such episodes (unlike manic-depressive insanity, where such permanent defect was far less common but not unheard of). Complete recoveries were so rare that Kraepelin doubted their existence. Dementia praecox was thus diagnosed by its prognosis—which was uniformly grave.

Exactly how the very different concept of schizophrenia emerged from within the walls of a mental hospital in Zurich is a story that remains largely untold. The basic contours of the narrative, however, are clear. From 1886 to 1898 Bleuler was the medical director of the backwater asylum in Rheinau, Switzerland, then replaced August Forel as the head of the Cantonal Psychiatric University Hospital and Clinic of Zurich (the official name of the institution that was more commonly referred to as the Burghölzli Mental Hospital). One of his new responsibilities was teaching, and content from his lectures found its way into his publications on schizophrenia. Bleuler certainly drew his primary insights from his many years of intense devotion to his patients, a character trait admired even by his subordinates, from whom he expected exceptional personal discipline (abstinence from alcohol being one example) and long hours of work. He was renowned for his ability to establish an "affective rapport" with even the most alienated of psychotic patients, and therapeutic results in individual cases were certainly far more important to Bleuler than to Kraepelin. The same could be said for his sometimes volatile second in command, Carl Gustav Jung, who had a keen interest in therapeutic change. After his arrival in December 1900 Jung also played a key role in fashioning the schizophrenia concept, providing experimental support for the core metaphoric assumptions of Bleuler's fully articulated revisioning of dementia praecox. Both men were influenced by French dissociationist psychology as well as the psychoanalytic ideas of Freud, and the Burghölzli was the first academic and clinical institution where psychoanalysis was applied. These ideas also shaped the schizophrenia concept. Both men played an early role in the psychoanalytic movement, but both had distanced themselves from it by 1914.

Their personal relationship was increasingly conflicted by the time Jung left in 1909, but over the years they remained cordial, even attending spiritualistic séances together in the 1920s. Whether their shared fascination with spiritualism and parapsychological phenomena played a role in their construction of the schizophrenia concept is an interesting question. Certainly both men became increasingly candid about their own metaphysical speculations in the decades after their association, with Bleuler publishing a book on "the natural history of the soul" in 1921. Jung—and his disciples—went even further afield, by 1916 positing a transpersonal "collective unconscious" and transforming psychotherapy into a spiritualistic ritual of initiation and rebirth that was based on Jung's deep reading of the classical scholarship on the Hellenistic mystery cults of pagan antiquity.[5]

Eugen Bleuler formally introduced schizophrenia to the world at a meeting of the German Psychiatric Association in Berlin on 24 April 1908. But it was earlier, certainly by 1907, that he and Jung had begun the process of turning Kraepelin's disease inside out. The two key features of Kraepelin's concept—prognosis and the central assumptions about the progressive dementia—were directly challenged by a study that Bleuler, Jung, and other members of the staff of the Burghölzli conducted around 1907 using the records of 647 "schizophrenics" admitted to their institution over a period of eight years. The outcome of the cases was the focus. The pattern of outcomes contradicted Kraepelin's pessimistic conclusions from his own studies. Various patterns of course and outcome, including cases of many of those who were able to return to employment in the community, were documented. Dementia praecox therefore was not necessarily the terminal cancer of psychiatry. However, as Bleuler noted, he never encountered a case, even with the best of outcomes, that did not have some sort of residual cognitive weakness or defect. No one was ever "cured" of schizophrenia. Bleuler wrote, "When the disease process flares up, it is more correct, in my view, to talk in terms of deteriorating attacks, rather than its recurrence. Of course the term recurrence is more comforting to a patient and his relatives than the notion of progressively deteriorating attacks."[6]

The second major revision of Kraepelin's disease concept concerned the central, defining characteristic of lasting "dementia." For Bleuler, the deteriorating process was not caused by the disease process itself, but was a *secondary* result of other, more primary symptoms. Bleuler considered dementia one of the "secondary symptoms" of the disease, "which arise as reactions of the ailing psyche to environmental influences and to its own strivings."[7] Needless to say, language like this in Bleuler's seminal article and then later, in his 1911 volume, eventually caught the attention of the Americans. The Meyerian American psychogenic conception of dementia praecox developed between 1906 and 1911 interpreted the symptoms of the disease as a republic of "reactions" to environmental stressors and internal conflicts that often had their roots in early childhood.

In contrast to Kraepelin, Bleuler argued that there were some symptoms of dementia praecox that were caused directly by the disease process—which was ultimately biological—and those that were not. *Primary symptoms* included some signs associated by Kraepelin, and

Americans such as Jelliffe, with the vegetative or autonomic nervous system, such as "fibrillary twitching, muscular excitability and pupillary disequilibrium." Psychologically the primary symptom was "a change in associations. . . . The thread of ideas very easily becomes lost in unfamiliar and incorrect pathways. Associations are then guided by random influences, particularly by emotions, and this amounts to a partial or total loss of logical function." There is also "a kind of stupor and a slowing down of all mental processes which cannot be explained as arising from secondary sources." Additionally "confusional states may be attributed to the primary cerebral disorder."[8] Although Bleuler differentiated dementia from stupor and confusion, in practice most alienists might not. By dementia Bleuler had in mind a sort of intellectual impairment such as is found in senile dementia, such as memory problems and a decline in overall intelligence. *Secondary symptoms* were dementia, hallucinations, delusions, flat affect, and catatonic symptoms. They were not caused directly by the disease process. The biological disease process causing the primary symptoms could come to a standstill at any point in the illness, Bleuler added, but the secondary symptoms, which are often dramatic, may remain indefinitely. Irreversible damage had been done.

Bleuler thus argued that dementia praecox or schizophrenia could be diagnosed on the basis of these primary symptoms alone. This rationalized a "cross-sectional" approach to diagnosis based on a list of symptoms. In practice, outside of Kraepelin's clinics, this was probably how dementia praecox had always been diagnosed by alienists: they looked for signs of something that resembled their own personal view of what constituted dementia or deterioration, perhaps noted a few delusions or hallucinations or bizarre behaviors, and that was enough.

Whereas for Kraepelin, the central mechanism of his disease was progressive deterioration *(Verblödung),* for Bleuler (by 1911) there were two mechanisms: the dissociative psychological process of "splitting" *(Spaltung)* and "indifference" *(Gleichgültigkeit).* What were split from each other were different mental functions (called "faculties" in nineteenth-century psychiatry and philosophy), such as thought, feeling, and volition. Even the core metaphors of the two disease concepts were vastly different in nature.[9]

Schizophrenia was never Kraepelin's dementia praecox, which is why Bleuler's opening paragraph in his 1908 article is so confusing:

In using the term dementia praecox I would like it to mean what the creator of the concept meant it to mean. To treat the subject from any other point of view would serve no purpose, but I would like to emphasize that Kraepelin's dementia praecox is not necessarily either a form of dementia nor a disorder of early onset. For this reason, and because there is no adjective or noun that can be derived from the term dementia praecox, I am taking the liberty of using the word *schizophrenia* to denote Kraepelin's concept. I believe that the tearing apart or splitting of psychic functions is a prominent symptom of the whole group and I will give my reasons for this elsewhere.[10]

In 1911 Bleuler presented a more comprehensive view of "the schizophrenias." The symptoms of schizophrenia were organized according to a bottom-to-top vertical splitting process that began with disturbances in three fundamental functions that cascaded into a fractured tree of disabling symptoms.

The "fundamental symptoms" of schizophrenia were divided into "simple" and "compound." The simple functions of thought, feeling, and volition that were disturbed were *associations* (how thoughts are bound together), *affectivity* (feelings as well as subtle feeling tones), and *ambivalence* ("the tendency of the schizophrenic psyche to endow the most diverse psychisms with both a positive and a negative indicator at one and the same time").[11] Only these three simple fundamental symptoms were posited by Bleuler to be directly caused by the underlying biological disease process (which he thought was most likely due to the effect of "toxins" on the brain).

The "compound" fundamental symptoms (which were the psychological effects formed out of combinations of the three simple fundamental symptoms) were *autism* (a word Bleuler coined in 1910), disturbances in *attention,* disturbances in the *will* (volition), a disturbance in the sense of self or the *person* (a split ego), *schizophrenic dementia* (disorders of intelligence and memory), and disturbances in *activity and behavior.* These compound fundamental symptoms were not caused directly by the underlying biological disease process.

The "accessory symptoms"—*hallucinations, delusions, illusions,* and so on—were also not caused directly by the primary disease process, nor related to the fundamental symptoms, and were *purely* psychogenic. These were reactions to inner conflicts (complexes) and to external, environmental events. But these accessory symptoms were regarded as perhaps the most troublesome because they were usually responsible for having the schizophrenic finally brought to a hospital or clinic for treatment.

Kraepelin made no such hierarchy of symptoms nor regarded any as exclusively psychogenic. All were ultimately derivative of an underlying disease process, the biological origins of which would be discovered one day. Because hallucinations and delusions could be produced in states of intoxication, he viewed them as evidence in support of a metabolic autointoxication process and not as derivatives of the concerns or life experiences of the patient with dementia praecox.

Throughout his book Bleuler referred to Freudian mechanisms of symbolization in attempts to offer meaning to the various *secondary* or *accessory* symptoms of schizophrenia that he discussed. Such kinds of symptoms were symbols to be decoded and interpreted within the context of a schizophrenic's past history. Jung had been the first to present essentially the same approach to dementia praecox in his 1907 monograph, reflecting the collective mind-set of the staff at the Burghölzli working under Bleuler in that year. Kraepelin never made such speculations and did not believe that the symptoms of dementia praecox could be construed as having any special or deeper level of meaning to them. Psychoanalytically oriented American alienists and neurologists such as Brill, Hoch, C. Macfie Campbell, George Kirby, Jelliffe, and White—all of whom had admired Jung's monograph and had long advocated the psychogenic nature of some symptoms of dementia praecox and the facility with which they could be interpreted "symbolically" by psychoanalytic concepts—would eventually recognize and welcome Bleuler's psychoanalytic vision of dementia praecox. This would be true even long after he had distanced himself from psychoanalysis. In the 1911 monograph schizophrenia was a disease concept that seemed to reflect more Freud—and French dissociationists such as Pierre Janet—than Kraepelin. Furthermore psychological processes that were split could, theoretically, be reunited; hence the door was opened for psychotherapeutic intervention.

Here, then, was the compelling attraction of Bleuler's schizophrenia: nested within the concept was the promise of therapy. With treatment schizophrenic patients might be returned to life and their proper place in the social order. Kraepelin's dementia praecox offered no therapeutic hope—an excuse, indeed a justification, for therapeutic nihilism. Rejoining society was not an option. Asylums would always be necessary to separate such individuals from the larger social world in which they could never be productive participants. Kraepelin's disease would prove politically uncongenial to government officials seeking to reduce the financial burden of state institutions, and philosophically repugnant to American nervous and mental disease specialists increasingly fascinated with the possibilities of psychotherapy. Furthermore, for the practicing alienist or neurologist who often had to make a diagnosis under stressful and time-limited conditions, Bleuler said such a determination could be made based on the cross-sectional image of the structure of thought. For Kraepelin a proper diagnosis was—in theory and in research at least, if not in daily practice in his own clinic— predicated on the longitudinal observation of the clinical course of the illness.

There was another feature of Bleuler's disease that would prove to be congenial to the American conception of dementia praecox in 1911. This was Bleuler's linkage of the premorbid with the morbid. He made this link by broadening schizophrenia to include two groups rarely found in asylums and hospitals: "simple schizophrenics" and "latent schizophrenics."

Bleuler followed Kraepelin in recognizing that dementia praecox had three basic but fluid forms: the catatonic, the paranoid, and the hebephrenic. Bleuler stretched the paranoid form to include forms of paranoid psychosis that Kraepelin believed were separate from dementia praecox, thus greatly expanding the boundaries of this form. As for the hebephrenic form, the milder forms were split off and put in their own category. Bleuler followed the suggestion made in 1903 by Otto Diem that there was a fourth identifiable form of dementia praecox, the "simple" form.[12] Diem had also worked under Bleuler in Zurich, so Diem's article probably bears the imprint of the general ideas being formed by the Zurich school. In his 1911 book Bleuler renamed this form "schizophrenia simplex," simple schizophrenia.

According to Bleuler, in simple schizophrenics the fundamental symptoms are present, but the accessory symptoms (delusions, hallucinations, and so on) are absent.

This group is rarely found in hospitals, but outside it is as common as any of the other forms. In private practice, we often see it, indeed as frequently in the relatives who bring the patients as in the patients themselves. On the lower levels of society, the simple schizophrenics vegetate as day laborers, peddlers, even as servants. They are also vaga-bonds and hoboes as are other types of schizophrenics of mild grade. On the higher levels of society, the most common type is the wife (in a very unhappy role, we can say) who is unbearable, constantly scolding, nagging, always making demands but never recognizing duties.[13]

Bleuler observed that when simple schizophrenics did end up in a hospital it was because of an exacerbation of their symptoms, "a criminal charge," or "a pathological drinking bout." "Such mild cases are often considered to be 'nervous' or 'degenerated' individuals."[14] Bleuler's words would be remembered in the clinics, courts, and culture in the United States for the next seventy years. School guidance counselors, social workers, judges, probation officers, private practitioners, and state hospital staff would all be familiar with the simple schizophrenic.

The same would eventually hold true for another of Bleuler's cre-ations, the "latent schizophrenic." "I am convinced that this is the most frequent form," he wrote, without providing statistics, "although, admit-tedly these people hardly ever come for treatment." They are "irritable, odd, moody, withdrawn or exaggeratedly punctual people" who "arouse, among other things, the suspicion of being schizophrenic." Furthermore every form of schizophrenia "may take a latent course."[15] Hoch recog-nized the "shut-in tendencies" (his words) of the latent schizophrenic, and the similarities between his own concepts and those of Bleuler are ad-dressed early in his review of Bleuler's schizophrenia.[16]

Could there now be any introverted or troubled child, adolescent or adult who was *not* a potential latent schizophrenic? Theoretically almost anyone could be under suspicion. Which was precisely the problem with both Bleuler's disease and the American conception of dementia praecox that had solidified by 1911. Dementia praecox in America was already a concept firmly linked to simpler or latent forms: Meyer's "deterioration" reaction-type, Hoch's "shut-in personality," Jelliffe's "pre–dementia praecox" personality, and (later, in 1916) C. B. Farrar's five premorbid personality types (backward, precocious, neurotic, asocial, and juvenile). Kraepelin's disease was not. Kraepelin's dementia praecox had already fallen before Bleuler's schizophrenia had even arrived on the scene.

But it would be another fifteen years or so before schizophrenia would begin to widely assert itself in the vocabulary of American neurologists and psychiatrists. Unlike Kraepelin's dementia praecox, Bleuler's disease would follow a more indolent course. Thanks to Adolf Meyer, who was singularly responsible for bringing dementia praecox to America and, early in his career, introducing it into American asylums as a diagnostic category, American alienists and neurologists had become used to the term. Also, because Bleuler used the terms interchangeably, it was easier and less confusing to stick with Kraepelin's term. Another factor that prevented a quicker adoption of the term was the fact that Bleuler's descriptions of schizophrenia were not immediately translated into English; indeed his 1911 volume, *Dementia Praecox oder Gruppe der Schizophrenien,* was not translated until 1950.

So there was no Bleulerian revolution in classification and nomenclature that immediately followed Hoch's introduction of schizophrenia to the elite of American neurologists and psychiatrists in New York City. Schizophrenia would first have to endure a latency period in the shadow of dementia praecox before becoming manifest. In the meantime dementia praecox was a protean concept that would shove its roots deeper into the American psyche.

Heredity had always been considered a factor in mental disease, and dementia praecox was no exception. In 1910 there were still many who believed that the insanities were the result of a multigenerational process of hereditary degeneration, though degeneration theory in medicine would fall out of favor after World War I. Many agreed with sentiments such as those expressed by the British physician Frederick W. Mott, who conducted pathological and hereditary studies on the patients of the London County Asylum. Mott noted that "the general tendency is for insanity not to proceed beyond three generations. . . . Not infrequently the stock dies out by the inborn tendency to insanity manifesting itself in the form of congenital imbecility or insanity of adolescence—dementia praecox." This was actually a good thing, according to Mott. "Thus rotten twigs are continually breaking off the tree of life, and I will now illustrate these facts by some examples of pedigrees."[17] His pedigree chart of "two sisters and a brother now in an asylum suffering from dementia praecox" may be the earliest in the English-language medical literature for this disease.[18]

These iconic images of dementia praecox pedigree charts would become familiar in the United States through the publications of the

Eugenics Record Office, based in Cold Spring Harbor, New York, after its foundation in 1910. The eugenics movement advocated both positive (legal prohibition of the marriage of insane persons) and negative (involuntary sterilization) measures to eliminate "the unfit" from society. The eugenics movement synergistically fused with the mental hygiene movement, which started at about the same time. Both Adolf Meyer and E. E. Southard were associated with the progressive efforts of the Eugenics Records Office as well as the National Committee for Mental Hygiene (founded in 1909).

In the decade between 1910 and 1920 dementia praecox became a particular concern of American courts dealing with the problems of crime and juvenile delinquency. The disease would be linked to notions of hereditary criminality in the "eugenical jurisprudence" of that era.[19] In Chicago the eugenics movement found an ally in Harry Olson (1867–1935), the first chief justice of the Municipal Court of Chicago, which had been established in 1906. In 1909 Olson established the Psychopathic Institute, the first American court-affiliated psychiatric clinic, which was attached to the country's first juvenile court. Its first director was William Healy. The purpose of the laboratory was to conduct psychiatric evaluations, including the administration of psychological tests of intelligence, in order to advise judges on the disposition of cases (jail or a mental hospital were the two usual options). As one legal historian argued, "The idea [of the Psychopathic Laboratory] marks a turning point from the traditional policy of society of treating the delinquents as a single large class . . . without consideration of the various individual characteristics which distinguished them."[20]

A second psychopathic laboratory was established specifically for the Municipal Court of Chicago in 1914 to handle cases from the specialized courts (the Boys' Court, the Morals Court, and Domestic Relations) for offenders seventeen and older. Olson was the driving force behind the establishment of both of these laboratories. For the proposed psychopathological laboratory of the Municipal Court he wanted an alienist with European training. He found what he was looking for in William J. Hickson (1874–1935), who became the first director in 1914. Hickson had spent two and a half years studying in Germany in the laboratories of Kraepelin and Theodore Ziehen and spent a year on the staff of the Burghölzli under Bleuler. In addition to these impressive credentials, he shared Olson's eugenical philosophy.

Not surprisingly given his experiences with the two leading experts on dementia praecox, Hickson was particularly interested in the relationship of this disease to criminal behavior. In October 1915 he characterized many of the criminal cases that were referred to him for examination in the Psychopathic Laboratory as suffering from "predementia or latent dementia praecox."[21] In his view many individuals who had been previously classified as mental defectives or "feeble-minded" were in fact misdiagnosed cases of latent dementia praecox, or "propfhebephrenia." Of the 929 cases that judges had referred to the Psychopathic Laboratory for evaluation by Hickson during his first year, 15.6 percent had dementia praecox as defined in this broader sense.[22] But by the end of the decade Hickson was finding dementia praecox in 84 percent of all criminals. He said, "We see the determining role of dementia praecox as the great causative factor of crime."[23]

Many of these individuals were sent to colonies for the feeble-minded, but these institutions quickly became overcrowded. There had to be other long-term solutions to the dementia praecox problem. Olson advocated involuntary sterilization.[24]

Thus the use of the expanded boundaries of the dementia praecox diagnosis as defined by both the American and Bleulerian concepts of the disease was having a profound effect on the lives of Americans in the criminal and civil court systems in 1920. Some certainly were being sterilized. In places that adopted the broader diagnostic parameters of dementia praecox the numbers of cases also began to rise.

The Manhattan State Hospital on Ward's Island is a case in point. The absence of Adolf Meyer and the presence of August Hoch may have had an effect on the number of cases diagnosed with dementia praecox upon first admission. As we have seen, in 1912 Hoch had made the connection between his "shut-in personality" type and Bleuler's latent schizophrenia and simple schizophrenia. He now directed the physicians under his command to look for signs of the shut-in personality in their new admissions. And of course they found what they were told to look for: "The life histories of cases of dementia praecox show very definitely a marked predominance of certain types of personality which have been described as the 'shut-in' makeup. These constitutional traits appear to have a pretty definite relation to a defect in the sphere of sexual adaptation. Approximately 60 percent of the cases of dementia praecox show clearly a shut-in type of personality."[25]

Although the trend between 1904 and 1912 was an overall reduction in the use of the diagnosis at Manhattan State Hospital, during the
1912–13 fiscal year this pattern shifted, and the percentage of dementia
praecox cases started to rise again. For the year ending 30 September
1914 21 percent of all new admissions were dementia praecox patients—
the largest diagnostic group. The report for the year ending in September 1915 concluded, "During recent years the number of cases placed
within the dementia praecox group has increased somewhat, due no
doubt to certain modifications of views as to the circumscription of the
group."[26] As for the institution itself, which was designed to hold 3,596
patients, by September 1915 the average daily census was 4,992 patients.
The nightmarish conditions on Ward's Island were only getting worse.

But there was a psychiatric institution in Baltimore in 1915 that did
not have a single case of dementia praecox. Adolf Meyer was its chief.

Before the Henry Phipps Psychiatric Clinic of the Johns Hopkins Hospital was ready to open, Meyer had begun the process of selecting his
staff. He chose Charles Macfie Campbell, his former colleague at the
New York Psychiatric Institute, to be his associate physician and second
in command. Macfie Campbell would be the head of outpatient services
and would direct the Clinic in Meyer's absence. Next in rank was David
K. Henderson, another Scot, who had also worked under Meyer in New
York between 1908 and 1911. Henderson would be the chief resident
physician. The two assistant resident physicians were Ralph Truitt and
Edward Kempf, who was fresh from being fired from an Indiana state
hospital for attempting to treat patients with psychoanalysis. Five interns,
most from the Johns Hopkins Medical School, were also part of the staff.
According to Henderson, who left behind a vivid memoir of the early
days of the Phipps Clinic, when he arrived in Baltimore to begin work
the building, and his accommodations in it, were not yet finished, so he
stayed with Meyer and his wife for some time. As for the building itself,
it was regarded as perhaps a bit too lavish in the opinion of some members of the staff of the older hospital, a building one jealous employee
considered to be "more consistent with a 'general paralytic's dream' than
with stern reality."[27]

The red brick building had two wings and an enclosed garden.
There were four floors and rooms of various sizes (including private

rooms for wealthier clients), but no room held more than eight beds. The institution itself was designed to house eighty-eight patients. In the basement of the building was the hydrotherapy suite (for extended baths, as Kraepelin had used as his primary form of treatment in both Heidelberg and Munich), a gymnasium, and the outpatient and social services departments. On the top floor was a recreation area and a large professional library. The building also had a roof garden. On other floors were laboratories set up for various medical, psychiatric, and psychological uses.[28] After eight years in the midst of the chaos of thousands of patients on Ward's Island, Meyer must have thought he was the luckiest man in the world.

During the three days of opening exercises of the Clinic held between 16 and 18 April 1913 there were welcoming addresses and formal scientific presentations by William Welch and William Osler of Johns Hopkins, F. W. Mott from London, and Stuart Paton (who had been influential in promoting psychiatry as a medical science at the Johns Hopkins Medical School), among others. August Hoch presented a paper on "personality and psychosis" in which he detailed the premorbid personality types that developed into dementia praecox and manic-depressive insanity.[29] Meyer's fellow Swiss acquaintance, Eugen Bleuler, was on hand to deliver a lecture on autism as a mode of thinking in both normals and schizophrenics.[30] Henderson remembered meeting Bleuler for the first time at Meyer's home, describing him as "a vivacious active man who never walked upstairs, he took them running two at a time."[31]

The first patient was admitted to the Clinic on 1 May 1913. The rooms soon filled with patients, and the outpatient and social services departments were quite busy by the end of the year. As he had done in Worcester and New York, Meyer emphasized the extensive documentation of a patient's life. But what he could not do at other institutions—eliminate the Kraepelinian classification system that he himself had introduced into American psychiatry—he did at the Phipps Psychiatric Clinic. In a presentation of the first year's work at the Clinic made to the American Medico-Psychological Association in 1914, Meyer said, "We have pushed as far as possible the etiological factors, and those components of the conditions which are decisive for the outcome and the treatment."[32]

But to identify the causes of "conditions," these conditions had to have names. So Meyer invented a new diagnostic scheme in which all of these conditions were "reactions." Dementia praecox was not one of them. Instead, as he had done for Kraepelin's disease in Worcester in 1896, Meyer's clinic became the first institution in the United States to formally label patients with Bleuler's schizophrenia. In Meyer's nomenclature, schizophrenia became a "schizophrenic reaction." Thus there was someone in Baltimore in 1913 who crossed Meyer's doorstep who may have been the first institutionally identified case of schizophrenia in the United States.

But how were Meyer and his staff defining this term? And did a change in name lead to a change in prognosis?

An unpublished typescript from 1915 of "a few rough notes on the work of the clinic," prepared by Henderson for Meyer, gives us some clues. Henderson records that between the opening of the clinic on 1 May 1913 and 31 January 1915, out of 717 patients admitted, "91 women and 71 men showed a schizophrenic reaction type." Henderson explained the new nomenclature as follows: "The term reaction type seems to have most value when applied to those cases which we have been in the habit of designating manic depressive psychosis and dementia praecox. For the former we have come to substitute the term affective reaction type, and for the latter schizophrenic reaction type." The dire prognosis associated with Kraepelin's term is the only justification given by Henderson for Meyer's decision to rename the condition: "In regard to the use of the term dementia praecox, and practically whenever that diagnosis is made, it is immediately assumed that the prognosis is bad and that the patient will probably live a life of ease for the rest of his or her days in an asylum." And yet, he confessed, "In the main I believe the above suppositions are true."[33]

Henderson's belief about the poor prognosis of dementia praecox or the schizophrenic reaction type was vindicated by the data of follow-up studies conducted at the Clinic between 1936 and 1951. These data—which were found in an unused, locked closet in the Clinic in the mid-1980s—were, in true Meyerian style, extensively collected and organized but not fully analyzed or published. A 1986 analysis of these original records found that, of the 8,172 first admissions between 1913 and 1940 (the years of Meyer's reign at the Clinic), 17 percent (1,357) received diagnoses roughly equivalent to the 1980s diagnosis of schizophrenia. These were "schizophrenic reaction type" (55 percent), "parergasic reaction type" (26 percent), "dementia praecox" (12 percent), "allied to schizophrenia" (4 percent), and "catatonia" (3 percent). ("Parergasia" was a term coined by Meyer in the mid-1920s that he believed should replace schizophrenia in clinical usage. It never caught on.) The original follow-up data, which contained after-care information for 89 percent of these schizophrenia analogue cases, revealed that a full 62 percent of Meyer's patients remained "unimproved" at an average of ten years after discharge. "The sizeable difference in rated discharge status between schizophrenia and affective disorders patients obviously supports Kraepelin's prognostic nosology to which Meyer vigorously objected," concluded the authors of the 1986 analysis of the data. In other words, simply changing the name of this group from dementia praecox to schizophrenic reaction to parergasia did nothing to improve the prognosis of the patients within it. Perhaps it was wise for Meyer and his colleagues to leave these data in a locked closet.[34]

"Already the term schizophrenia seems to have taken a firm root in many camps," observed Southard in July 1915.[35] But Meyer's clinic seems to have been the only *institution* that officially diagnosed schizophrenia (as a reaction) in its patients. Many, such as the powerful Philadelphia neurologist Francis X. Dercum, refused to use the new concept. "The term, schizophrenia, is not distinctive and I trust it will not survive," he declared in August 1916. "Perhaps in the future some term will be invented which will convey the idea of endogenous deterioration in adolescence, but until then we had best adhere to the name, dementia praecox."[36] Of the very few references to schizophrenia to appear in the medical literature between 1910 and 1925, most were from psychoanalytically oriented private practitioners such as the neurologist Smith Ely Jelliffe.[37] Americans were slow to welcome schizophrenia.

With the fall of Kraepelin's disease by 1911 and its replacement in the literary discourses of American psychiatry by a greatly expanded, psychogenic construct that emphasized etiology as a path to get to prophylaxis, the issues of classification and nomenclature began to resurface as concerns. Should American alienists and neurologists still refer to "dementia praecox" when the American and Kraepelinian concepts were now so far apart? There is no doubt Meyer's adoption of "schizophrenic reaction" at the prestigious Phipps Clinic brought this issue to the fore. But there were other problems as well that went beyond dementia praecox.

While psychiatrists could point with pride to the opening of the Phipps Clinic at the revered Johns Hopkins Hospital and its association with the medical school—the best in the country and the center of the new laboratory-based scientific medicine—the situation across the forty-eight United States and its territories in the year 1913 remained an embarrassment. Not only were asylums and state hospitals overcrowded and infected with therapeutic nihilism, but clinical issues relevant to psychiatry as a medical science remained unimportant. This was reflected in the hundreds of annual reports issued from across the vast American continent. Most asylums were located in rural areas, far from the intellectual centers of Boston, New York, or Baltimore and Washington, D.C. Perhaps the most glaring omission from these annual reports, which otherwise included finely detailed expenditure sheets on farm equipment, ducks or "piggeries," or lists of entertainment "diversions" such as magic lantern shows, silent movies, and musical events was the lack of statistical tables that broke down the patient populations into their diagnostic forms of insanity.

As Gerald Grob noted when reviewing such statistics, even from those mental hospitals that did report diagnostic categories, "the task of describing the institutionalized mentally ill population with any degree of accuracy is almost impossible."[38] "The invisible patient," as Grob termed it, became a concern for those members of the American psychiatric elite eager to follow the rationalizing procedures of the social sciences that had been borrowed with useful effect by other professions, including other branches of medicine.[39]

The issue came to a head after a persuasive presentation by James V. May, a physician who was on the board of the New York State Hospital Commission, in June 1913 in Niagara Falls, Canada, at the annual meeting of the American Medico-Psychological Association. The bulk of May's address was to present the detail and clarity of the system of keeping statistics within the large New York state system of hospitals and to illustrate their usefulness. But his main goal was to call for the adoption of similar uniform statistical record keeping in all psychiatric institutions throughout the country. In 1913 the situation was chaotic. With respect to identifying the forms of insanity in each institution, May reported, "Some still follow classifications in vogue twenty or thirty years ago; others have adopted various modifications of Kraepelin's ideas, while the great majority give no information whatsoever regarding the various forms of insanity."[40] In essence, in most asylums and state hospitals in the United States and its territories superintendents and alienists alike regarded diagnosis as irrelevant to asylum management. The patients were "insane," and that is all.

May's plea fell on receptive ears. The Association set up a standing Committee on Statistics. May of course was on the committee, but its chair was Thomas Salmon (1876–1927). Salmon, not an alienist but a bacteriologist and physician, had risen to professional prominence the year before, when he was appointed the first medical director of the National Committee for Mental Hygiene. Whereas Meyer was respected, Salmon was revered. His death was considered a great loss by many in the profession.[41]

Over the next several years the committee met to discuss four issues of concern and to make recommendations for them: (1) the desirability of uniform statistics relative to mental diseases and the operation of institutions for the insane; (2) the classification of mental disorders; (3) forms to be used in reporting statistical data; and (4) the means to be adopted to secure uniform statistical reports.[42]

The committee presented its recommendations at the May 1917 annual meeting of the AMPA, which was held in New York City. For the first time in the history of American psychiatry, a uniform classification of mental disorders was proposed that was to be followed by all institutional psychiatrists. The committee also submitted drafts of eighteen different forms that institutions could use to report various statistical data. The responsibility for collecting and analyzing these forms fell to the National Committee for Mental Hygiene, which was no doubt a major contribution of Salmon's work with the committee. He knew—in fact they all knew—that leaving such an administrative headache to an AMPA committee of busy psychiatrists who met together only a few times a year was not going to work. The final approval for these proposals was left to future meetings.

The proposed classification of mental diseases listed twenty-one broad diagnostic categories and one for "not insane." No clinical descriptions of signs and symptoms were offered, just category headings. Number 15 was "Dementia praecox," and it was further defined by four forms: paranoid type, katatonic type, hebephrenic type, and simple type.[43] Thus already in May 1917 we see the influence of Bleuler's ideas entering the cognitive categories guiding the practice of American psychiatrists. But schizophrenia is not mentioned.

Number 13 was "Manic-depressive psychoses" and had the following forms: manic type, depressive type, stupor, mixed type, and circular type.[44]

"The present condition with respect to the classification of mental disorders is chaotic," said the psychiatrist Owen Copp, who presented the committee report to the conference. "Some states use no well-defined classification. In others the classifications used are similar in many respects but differ enough to prevent accurate comparisons. Some states have adopted a uniform system, while others leave the matter entirely to the individual hospitals. This condition of affairs discredits the science of psychiatry and reflects unfavorably on our Association, which serves as a standardizing and correlating agency for the whole country."[45]

There was one person in the audience who was seething quietly with anger at the report of the Committee on Statistics: Adolf Meyer. The recommendations for a uniform classification of mental disorders used none of his "reactions" as proposed diagnostic categories. Indeed the very fact that his colleagues in the AMPA were going ahead with such a classification was yet another reminder to Meyer was he was no longer the sole arbiter of innovations in American psychiatry. Meyer had resisted all classification proposals and had refused to participate in the committee's activities. He wanted to continue to use his considerable influence to keep American psychiatry pluritheoretical, pragmatic, and eclectic, but by 1917 a new generation of physicians had begun to push back against the derationalization of the profession that Meyer had encouraged.[46] It was a loss of power for him. To some degree he felt betrayed.

And so, when he rose to make his own scheduled presentation later in the conference, Meyer drew an analogy to the committee's actions with the declaration of war on Germany that the United States had been made just the month before, in April 1917. It was "a distressing surprise" that "our own committee on statistical classification should at this late hour have sworn allegiance to the German dogma," he scolded.[47] The meaning was clear: he considered them traitors.

A final draft of the classification of mental diseases was constructed at a meeting of the Committee on Statistics of the AMPA in New York City on 7 February 1918. Also at the meeting were representatives of the National Committee for Mental Hygiene. The Committee on Statistics added brief clinical descriptions to each diagnostic term, based on a document that had been designed for the staff in the state hospital system in New York.[48] It was at this gathering that the fate of schizophrenia was sealed for future generations.

Something had happened between May 1917 and January 1918. Perhaps it was the growing anti-German sentiment now that America was at war, coupled with the knowledge that Emil Kraepelin was being very vocal about his nationalist sentiments. Certainly there was an attempt to placate Adolf Meyer. We may never know the full details of what happened at that meeting.

But when the final draft of the uniform classification of mental diseases was published later in 1918, "schizophrenia" was promoted as an alternate term for "dementia praecox." As part of the parameters for diagnosing dementia praecox, the document also included the notion of a prepsychotic personality type that Meyer, Hoch, Jelliffe, and Farrar had long ago inserted into the American reframing of Kraepelin's disease and that corresponded with Bleuler's "simple schizophrenia" and "latent schizophrenia." Because it is the foundation document of all twentieth-century efforts by the American Psychiatric Association to define dementia praecox and schizophrenia, it is worth quoting at length:

> This group cannot be satisfactorily defined at the present time as there are still too many points at issue as to what constitute the essential clinical features of dementia praecox. A large majority of the cases which should go into this group may, however, be recognized without special difficulty, although there is an important smaller group of doubtful, atypical allied or transitional cases which from the standpoint of symptoms or prognosis occupy an uncertain clinical position.
>
> Cases formerly classed as allied to dementia praecox should be placed here rather than in the undiagnosed group. The term "schizophrenia" is now used by many writers instead of dementia praecox.
>
> The following mentioned features are sufficiently well established to be considered most characteristic of the dementia praecox type of reaction:
>
> A seculsive type of personality or one showing other evidences of abnormality in the development of the instincts and the feelings.
>
> Appearance of defects of interest and discrepancies between thought on the one hand and the behavioral-emotional reactions on the other.
>
> A gradual blunting of the emotions, indifference or silliness with serious defects of judgment and often hypochondriacal complaints, suspicions or ideas of reference.

Development of peculiar trends, often fantastic ideas, with odd, impulsive or negativistic conduct not accounted for by any acute emotional disturbance or impairment of the sensorium.

Appearance of autistic thinking and dream-like ideas, peculiar feelings of being forced, of interference with the mind, of physical or mystical influences, but with the retention of clearness in other fields (orientation, memory, etc.).

According to the prominence of certain symptoms in individual cases the following four clinical forms of dementia praecox may be specified, but it should be borne in mind that these are only relative distinctions and that transitions from one clinical form to another are common.[49]

The manual then briefly describes the paranoid type, the catatonic type, the hebephrenic type, and the simple type ("cases characterized by defects of interest, gradual development of an apathetic state, often with peculiar behavior, but without expression of delusions or hallucinations").

With this document, the first edition of *The Statistical Manual for the Use of Institutions for the Insane,* American psychiatry's first diagnostic manual, we see the official sanctioning of the American conception of dementia praecox that had existed since 1911 and its merger with Bleuler's schizophrenia concept. Other than the name of the disease and its first three forms, there was little that could be traced back to Kraepelin in this description. *Nothing was said about course or prognosis.* This was an official repudiation of Kraepelin's disease concept.

The diagnostic boxes were now in place. Dementia praecox or schizophrenia was *expected* to be found and counted in every institution for the insane in the country. And to this day something called schizophrenia—but certainly not Bleuler's schizophrenia—is diagnosed by psychiatrists because it is *expected.*[50]

But change did not happen overnight. It took three years, until 1921, before all institutions were using the AMPA-approved forms and uniform classification system and including them in their annual reports to the National Committee for Mental Hygiene.[51] At least from a statistical point of view, patients were no longer as invisible as they had been just a few years before. They could be counted according to diagnosis, and therefore, in some sense, they and their afflictions were real.

Dementia praecox was real. So was schizophrenia. And as far as American psychiatry was concerned in 1918, they both referred to the

same thing. But for some, like E. E. Southard, such terminological ambivalence was a symptom of psychiatry's continued scientific immaturity.
Southard knew the terms referred to two very different concepts. But
which one should be chosen over the other?

E. E. Southard was elected to the presidency of the American Medico-
Psychological Association for 1918–1919. In his presidential address,
which he delivered in June 1919, he confessed, "I still contemplate
with astonishment my election to the office of president in your association." He was not a hospital superintendent, he said, and was probably closer to the habits and ways of thinking of a typical assistant physician. Adolf Meyer was probably equally astonished; tensions between
the two had been exacerbated over the classification and nomenclature
changes the previous year. In his presentation Southard, as was the cus-
tom in such addresses, reflected fondly on certain persons and events in
the history of American psychiatry. Then he got to Meyer: "I myself
believe that no greater power to change our minds about the problems of
psychiatry has been at work in the interior of the psychiatric profession
in America than the personality of Adolf Meyer. If he will pardon me
the phrase, I shall designate him as a ferment, an enzyme, a catalyzer. I
don't know that we could abide two of him. But in our present status we
must be glad there was one of him."[52]

As a man obsessed with words and their clear expression (and constantly irritated by Meyer for his deficits in these areas), Southard made
many suggestions for improving classification in psychiatry. These,
however, were among his least influential contributions. His plea for a
"pragmatic psychiatry" based on a deductive process of "diagnosis by
exclusion" through a "pragmatic sequence of consideration" of eleven
groups of mental disorders, including one termed "the Schizophreno-
ses," was never taken seriously in American psychiatry.[53] But after the
AMPA adopted its uniform system of classification in 1918 there was
really no longer any place for proposals such as Southard's. However,
the AMPA's Committee on Statistics still met on an ongoing basis and
had the power to suggest changes in classification and nomenclature.
Southard was not willing to wait for the dust to settle and already had
ideas for changes to be made—especially with regard to dementia praecox and schizophrenia.

In an exchange of letters with Meyer in mid–December 1918,[54] Southard said he was unsure about the propriety of using his position as president of the AMPA to induce "a small controversy at the next meeting of the Association" concerning the issues of classification and nomenclature, but that's what he wanted to do, and he wanted Meyer to participate. In reply Meyer signaled his rejection of such public engagement. Southard attempted to negotiate common ground with Meyer and get him at least to agree to a need for broad classification groups, since Southard said he regarded the "nomenclature question" as "subordinate."

"The statistical committee could give as synonyms such names as it chose to regard as synonyms for the leading names of its list," Southard wrote on 11 December 1918. "Let any psychiatrist, however, use what name he chooses." This was a signature stroke of Southard's cognition: the glossing over of details in the service of constructing broad categories in order to classify items analogously and by surface similarities. Identifying broad categories of seemingly related concepts would then be a starting point for deductive analysis later on. Southard gave Meyer the promise of allowing psychiatrists to use Meyerian terms such as "reaction-types" if they preferred, but within the general outlines of an agreed-upon classification grouping. But in his replies Meyer never gave ground. Rather than initiating yet another nosological debate so soon after *The Statistical Manual* had been distributed, Southard opted instead to fight a battle that he might win: convincing his colleagues to adopt the term "schizophrenia" in place of "dementia praecox."

On 20 February 1919 Southard delivered a lecture to the Boston Society of Psychiatry and Neurology titled "Non-Dementia Non-Praecox." It was his clearest statement on the unsuitability of Kraepelin's term and concept of dementia praecox and his argument for the adoption of Bleuler's schizophrenia as a more palatable replacement. At the time Southard was president of the AMPA, and this fact added weight to his argument for a change in nomenclature. It was easier to argue for a change in a term rather than revisions of entire classes of mental diseases, but Southard was going to try. He prepared the text of his lecture in a typescript form that was intended for publication, but like so many other projects in his life he never completed the task. In less than a year's time he would be dead.

Southard made several key points in his paper.[55] First, the neuropathological evidence was not pathognomonic for an actual "entity" that could be named dementia praecox or schizophrenia. Second, Bleuler's dissociative metaphor for schizophrenia was a better fit for what Southard calls the "psycholytic" nature of the phenomena that would be placed in this broad classification group. Third, Meyer's preferred nomenclature of "reaction-types" or "reaction-complexes" was equally welcome in a classification group that included the alternative terms "dementia praecox" and "schizophrenia." Fourth, a classification project aimed at synthesis (in other words, accepting a classification group large enough to contain the concepts, if not the terms, of Meyer, Kraepelin, and Bleuler) was consistent with Kraepelin's own grand synthesis of hebephrenia, catatonia, and paranoia into dementia praecox, and any idea that Kraepelin "created" a new entity is wrong. Fifth, the term "dementia praecox" itself was "horrible" and gave the wrong impression about prognosis. Sixth, "schizophrenia" was a term from which adjectives could easily be formed (e.g., schizophrenic), whereas such word forms could not be derived from "dementia praecox." And seventh, Kraepelin himself had given up his original 1899 concept of dementia praecox, multiplying the number of forms and relabeling some patients with Bleuler's suggested schizophrenia, in the 1913 volume of the eighth edition of his textbook, *Psychiatrie.*

Southard's last point requires some comment. It was indeed true that in the third volume of the eighth edition of *Psychiatry* Kraepelin himself broadened his dementia praecox concept even further to ten subtypes or forms of the disease. Sections from this edition were translated into English and published in 1918. However, other than Southard, who had published a comprehensive review of the four volumes (1909–1915) of Kraepelin's eighth edition, no one in America seemed to pay particular attention. Americans had already decided for themselves what dementia praecox would be. The nomenclature for the three forms of dementia praecox that Kraepelin identified in 1899—the paranoid, the catatonic, and the hebephrenic—would be all that would survive in the American psychiatry of the twentieth century.[56]

In December 1918, in order to prepare for his lecture and its planned publication, Southard wrote to several psychiatrist colleagues and surveyed them on the comparative suitability of dementia praecox and schizophrenia for the new American nomenclature in *The Statistical Manual.* Only a few responses have survived. George H. Kirby told Southard that he was not happy with either term, nor how they were applied in practice. "My experience in the Army has made me keenly aware of the existence of a widespread, extremely loose and wholly unjustifiable use of the term dementia praecox. . . . I do not think 'schizophrenia' is a good substitute and American psychiatrists have never used the term in nearly so wide and all-embracing a sense as Bleuler who introduced it. . . . I feel that several terms must eventually be devised to provide for the breaking-up of what is now included under dementia praecox."[57]

"We use the term schizophrenia and speak of benign and grave forms and residual states," replied Adolf Meyer. "I hope that the elimination of the term schizophrenia will follow, as too broad an entity."[58] He may have wished to see the term eliminated, but by May 1921 Meyer was using it interchangeably with dementia praecox in public presentations and publications.[59]

August Hoch, who had played a key supporting role in forming the first draft of the new uniform classification system, cogently listed the reasons why "dementia praecox" was an unsuitable term, but was lukewarm to replacing it with "schizophrenia." "I am not at all certain whether I shall definitely abandon the term dementia praecox, since everyone has gotten so used to it, but I quite agree that the term is not good. . . . I guess my personal antagonism against discarding dementia praecox completely and standing up for schizophrenia is in part due to a feeling that after all they both imply all sorts of things which are not proven."[60]

Albert M. Barrett, the director of the Psychopathic Hospital in Ann Arbor who chaired the Committee on Statistics when the final draft was approved in February 1918, was the only respondent to Southard who was unequivocal in his support of adopting schizophrenia and dropping dementia praecox. "For some time past, in this clinic, we have been using the term 'dementia praecox' less frequently," he wrote to Southard. "Without having taken a fixed attitude in the matter we have happened to use the term 'schizophrenia' in a more or less interchangeable way with dementia precox. . . . The term schizophrenia is less committal as to the outcome. It emphasizes more the aspect of the development of the disorder and places etiological factors in the foreground that may be taken advantage of in therapeutic directions. . . . On the whole I believe that the term 'schizophrenia' is preferable to dementia praecox."[61]

Southard's preference for adopting schizophrenia was also based on personal clinical experiences in diagnostic case conferences. He knew that a differential diagnosis could be made *between* dementia praecox and schizophrenia, as they were not identical concepts. He was one of the few psychiatrists in the United States who really understood this. But Bleuler's widening of the dementia praecox concept to include prepsychotic simple schizophrenics and latent schizophrenics made it a more useful diagnosis in everyday clinical practice for the many cases he encountered at the Boston Psychiatric Hospital that could not be characterized using Kraepelin's classification system.

For example, at one staff meeting held in 1917 the goal was to determine the diagnosis of a forty-seven-year-old man with a history of heavy drinking and vagrancy. "What can we say for dementia praecox?" Southard asked. The man presented with a certain "silliness," odd mannerisms, and an unusual emotional tone. But, as Southard pointed out to his colleagues, the man had no hallucinations. As a whole this pointed away from Kraepelin's dementia praecox, but Southard said that psychiatrists could still "build up quite a case for schizophrenia." And yet in this particular case Southard expressed doubt that he could go along with a schizophrenia diagnosis either. Instead the staff psychiatrists decided on the usual alternative: manic-depression.[62]

This was not an unusual pattern of decision making. Since its introduction into American asylums, manic-depressive insanity was the convenient category used for patients who were mentally disturbed in some significant way, perhaps even delusional or disorganized, but who had qualities that made them seem likely to have a better prognosis than "praecox patients." If manic they could be emotionally engaging, perhaps infuriating, or entertaining; if depressed, evocative of sympathy or exasperation. Either way they made the alienist *feel* something.

On the other hand, "praecox patients" were strange, remote, bizarre. "What is characteristic of the condition is something very elusive," said C. Macfie Campbell in 1929. "The physician feels in his interview with the patient that there is something lacking which is essential to the normal bond between two people in ordinary intercourse. The physician cannot feel himself into the life of the patient."[63] How alienists felt in their gut when in the presence of a new patient drove diagnostic decisions. This was especially true because of two important constraints on institutionally based alienists: the lack of a proper or accurate history of the patient and the lack of observational time needed to make a more accurate diagnosis and prognosis. In truth, upon initial presentation many persons could have easily fit into either diagnosis.

Two studies of Massachusetts institutions illustrate this point. In 1909 E. S. Abbot published an analysis of the 14,770 admissions to Massachusetts state hospitals between 1 October 1903 and 1 October 1908. Of these, Kraepelinian diagnoses of dementia praecox (3,096 cases) and manic-depressive insanity (2,111 cases) comprised the two largest groups out of a range of forty-seven different terms, many of which were archaic survivals from the alienism of the nineteenth century. Abbot said that the "probable error of diagnosis" was large. Even so, a sizable number of cases (512) were confounding enough to be "undiagnosticated." "The difficulties of diagnosis lie chiefly between dementia praecox and manic depressive insanity, or between these and involutional psychosis," admitted Abbot.[64] At the Boston Psychopathic Hospital a sampling of records between 1912 and 1921 indicated that the most common diagnosis was dementia praecox (26 percent), followed by manic-depressive insanity (11 percent). Southard and his colleagues may have relied upon the sex of a patient as a factor in making this difficult differential diagnosis. As the historian Elizabeth Lunbeck observed, "Men . . . were twice as likely to receive a diagnosis of dementia praecox, to be classified as incurable and destined to deteriorate. Neither social class nor ethnicity came into play in this determination."[65] But other than sex and a guess at possible prognosis, or those anecdotal reports of an eerie "praecox feeling" of strangeness or emotional remoteness that an alienist might detect, how could these great Kraepelinian diseases be distinguished?

In 1920 even Kraepelin himself admitted defeat. Alas, the master could not always recognize his two creations using his own published diagnostic criteria. He too had great difficulty in distinguishing between manic-depressive insanity and dementia praecox in actual clinical practice: "No experienced physician would deny that cases occur with unwelcome frequency in which, despite the most assiduous observation, it is impossible to reach a diagnosis. The experience that we cannot significantly reduce the number of mis-diagnoses has a crippling effect on one's job satisfaction. . . . However, it is becoming increasingly obvious that we cannot satisfactorily distinguish these two diseases." Kraepelin insisted, however, that the two disease processes were "distinct" despite the areas of overlap.

Kraepelin further complicated the issue, however, by developing an argument that Bleuler's schizophrenic symptoms (loss of drive and destruction of the will, stereotypic behaviors, automatic obedience, negativism, neologisms, and so on) "are in no way confined to dementia praecox" but may also be found in manic-depressive insanity. Confusingly Kraepelin spoke of schizophrenia as a "clinical sign," not a distinct disease, but also spoke of "schizophrenic illnesses," of which dementia praecox was the best example.[66] To some degree he was moving away from his earlier conviction that dementia praecox and manic-depressive insanity were discrete natural disease entities.

Kraepelin used Bleuler's schizophrenia concept to bridge his two great insanities, making the argument that the areas of overlap between dementia praecox and manic-depressive insanity were to be found in their common "schizophrenic symptomatology." "We shall have to get accustomed to the notion that our much used clinical checklist does not permit us to differentiate reliably manic-depressive insanity from schizophrenia in all circumstances; and that there is an overlap between the two, which depends on the fact that the clinical signs have risen from certain antecedent conditions." These "antecedent conditions" might be "heredity" or the "human personality."[67]

Kraepelin did acknowledge "diseases of the personality," particularly in the eighth edition of *Psychiatrie* (1909–1915). And it is true that in 1913 he seemed to indicate a shift in his thinking about the etiology and pathogenesis of dementia praecox that put more weight on the destruction of the "unitary complement of mental functions," the core intellectual coherence of the personality, than on organic hypotheses (whether neuropathological or autotoxic). However, as the historian and psychiatrist Paul Hoff noted, "Kraepelin developed and maintained a skeptical attitude towards subjective, especially biographically determined aspects of mental disorders, which could not be studied experimentally."[68] But by 1920 most American psychiatrists, long lost in a swirl of Meyerian reaction types, Freudian mechanisms, "shut-in" personalities, and autotoxic hypotheses, had essentially stopped reading Kraepelin for almost two decades.[69]

Except for E. E. Southard. As noted earlier, in 1916 Southard published an extensive review of Kraepelin's eighth edition of *Psychiatrie* and continued to read and summarize the periodical literature in German. Although he died before the appearance of Kraepelin's 1920 ar-

ticle on "the manifestations of insanity," Southard was aware of Kraepelin's attempts to introduce the term "schizophrenia" as a clinical sign
(not a separate disease entity) that cut across various disorders. He certainly knew the passage in the third volume of the eighth edition in
which Kraepelin wrote of "that inner *disintegration,* those 'schizophrenic'
disorders, which we meet with in dementia praecox."[70] Indeed it was
probably Southard who was responsible for including schizophrenia as
one of the dozens of signs and symptoms on the loose-leaf checklist that
was included in individual case files at the Danvers State Hospital in
April 1918.[71] Thus for a brief period of time, and perhaps only in Massachusetts, schizophrenia was a sign or symptom and dementia praecox
was a disease.

By the time of the June 1919 annual meeting of the American
Medico-Psychological Association, Southard had decided to drop the
subject of schizophrenia. As was his nature, he was already distracted by
other issues. After Southard no one bothered to raise the issue of conceptual incompatibility again. For the time being at least, dementia praecox
and schizophrenia would be used synonymously. But it is clear from the
historical record that at some point in the 1920s "schizophrenia" became
the preferred term. How and when did that occur?

One way to discern the reception of a new diagnostic term is to trace
its use in the titles of medical publications. This is an imperfect method,
as it reflects the usage of a term in the discourses of the minority of the
members of the psychiatric profession, who recorded their changes of
mental habit in print. Fortunately evidence for this temporal and cognitive discontinuity in the history of American psychiatry can be documented through an analysis of the bibliography of English-language
publications (medical articles, monographs, book chapters, books, dissertations) that used either "dementia praecox" or "schizophrenia" in
their title in *The Index-Catalogue of the Library of the Surgeon-General's
Office.* This useful source is a compilation of medical publications in
the Library of the Surgeon-General's Office, U.S. Army, which was
published in five series in sixty-one volumes between 1880 and 1961.
The U.S. National Library of Medicine of the National Institutes of
Health has digitized this massive resource and made it available for
electronic searches through its online website, *IndexCat.*[72] Although

this bibliography omits some publications (such as Bleuler's seminal 1908 article on dementia praecox and A. A. Brill's 1909 case history, added here) and duplicates others (eliminated here), a decade-by-decade comparison of the use of the two terms results in the following pattern:

	Dementia praecox	Schizophrenia
1900–1910	67	1
1911–1920	268	6
1921–1930	152	73
1931–1940	89	153

Only four English-language titles used the term "dementia praecox" between 1941 and 1950 (one each in 1941, 1943, 1944, and 1948), the last being Leopold Bellak's *Dementia Praecox: The Past Decade's Work and Present Status. A Review and Evaluation,* in 1948.[73] This was a curious choice of title, for by this time "schizophrenia" was the preferred term both in the everyday world of clinical practice and in publications. Rather than reviving Kraepelin's term in clinical practice and research through its use in the title of his book, Bellak instead punctuated the end of an era in the history of psychiatry. Except for the 1950 appearance of the translation of Bleuler's 1911 volume, *Dementia Praecox, Or the Group of Schizophrenias,* after 1948 "dementia praecox" vanishes.

The year 1927 was the first in which "schizophrenia" appeared in more titles than did "dementia praecox." Except for three nonconsecutive years (1930, 1932 and 1936) in which dementia praecox had a slight advantage, it is clear that schizophrenia had become the preferred alternative. The collapse of Kraepelin's term was effectively completed by 1938, with only two such titles appearing in 1939 and 1940 each.

Thus we can pinpoint with relative certainty the late 1920s as the era in which Bleuler's term began to supplant Kraepelin's. But why? As with any historical transition, multiple factors must be considered.

One obvious factor was the widespread adoption by 1921 of *The Statistical Manual for the Use of Institutions for the Insane.* "Schizophrenia" was now an officially recognized term for statistical, clinical, and research purposes.

Another important factor in tilting preference toward Bleuler's term was the 1924 publication of Brill's translation of the fourth edition of Bleuler's textbook on psychiatry.[74] Chapter 9, "Schizophrenias

(Dementia Praecox)" was the first detailed presentation of Bleuler's ideas on schizophrenia to be published in English. The time was ripe for considering an alternative to dementia praecox, a term that almost everyone, including Kraepelin, agreed was problematic.

There were other reasons for the Americans to embrace Bleuler. Kraepelin's boorish vocal expression of his fervent German nationalism in the postwar era, combined with his equally vocal disregard of psychoanalysis, had generated a certain antipathy toward him among his colleagues in the United States. For example, when Kraepelin visited for a few months in 1925, he and Felix Plaut (a colleague from the Munich clinic) attended a dinner hosted by Smith Ely Jelliffe. George Kirby was there and reported the following to Meyer in a letter:

> We had an interesting evening, but the conversation turned more to the war and political issues than to psychiatric topics. We all felt quite disappointed to learn that Professor Kraepelin can see no solution of the Franco-German problem except another war and the ultimate domination of France by Germany. He seems to be not at all interested in any plan whereby mutual confidence and understanding could be established between the two countries.[75]

Thus Bleuler had the right nationality (Swiss), the right temperament (noncombative), and the right ideas (a dissociative model of schizophrenia that held out the promise of therapy and recovery). The translation of Bleuler's textbook generated considerable interest, and many psychiatrists and psychoanalysts were receptive to its new nomenclature.

But it took a well-publicized scientific conference on schizophrenia to bury dementia praecox for good.

A signal event in the adoption of schizophrenia in the United States was the meeting of the Association for Research in Nervous and Mental Disease held in New York City on 28 and 29 December 1925. Almost all of the prominent figures in American neurology and psychiatry were in attendance, reflecting the three dominant power centers of the profession's elite: from New York came Charles Dana, M. Allen Starr, Frederick Peterson, Bernard Sachs, Louis Casamajor, Walter

Timme, Michael Osnato, Charles B. Dunlap, A. A. Brill, Smith Ely Jelliffe, George H. Kirby, Ralph P. Truitt, and Thomas Salmon; from Boston, C. Macfie Campbell, George M. Kline, E. W. Taylor, George A. Waterman, and Morton Prince; from the Baltimore and Washington, D.C. area came Adolf Meyer, William Alanson White, Walter Freeman, Nolan D. C. Lewis, and Harry Stack Sullivan. The second tier of power and influence in the United States was represented by Charles W. Burr, Earl D. Bond, and Edward A. Strecker of Philadelphia, and Karl A. Menninger from Topeka, Kansas. Less influential physicians from Chicago and the psychopathic hospital in Ann Arbor were also in attendance.

Except for Adolf Meyer, every participant used the term "schizophrenia" instead of "dementia praecox" in the title of their presentation. This unprecedented uniformity was almost certainly the result of a consensus decision that had been reached months in advance—a clear signal to the profession, and to the public, that "schizophrenia" would now be the preferred term. Rather than committing to schizophrenia, Meyer, true to his oppositional nature, unsuccessfully promoted his own substitute term for dementia praecox: the "parergastic-paranoid reaction-types."[76]

The publicity generated by this conference led to the first appearance of the word "schizophrenia" in the *New York Times* on 29 December 1925.[77] By virtue of the highly centralized triune power structure of American psychiatry at this time, which could pivot the entire profession if all three local centers were in harmony, schizophrenia had become the newly anointed American madness virtually overnight. Following Kraepelin's death in October 1926 and the decline of "dementia praecox" in titles of medical publications in 1927, schizophrenia rose in importance in American psychiatry.

This same geographical trinity of power, patronage, and knowledge-transfer networks was directly responsible for the relatively rapid and decisive shift to psychoanalytic theory in the American psychiatric elite by the mid-1930s. Freudian ideas were imposed from the top by a handful of politically powerful physicians who dominated key training and research institutions and high-status local professional organizations. Because Meyerian "anything goes" eclecticism remained strong among American psychiatrists well into the 1930s, indeed dominating medical school training in psychiatry in that decade under his new blurry slogan of "psychobiology," many psychiatrists were open to psychoanalytic ideas without becoming confirmed converts. That would change by the late 1940s, when the Freudians made "psycho-analysis" and "psychiatry" synonyms in American culture. Until then, at the peripheries of power, most isolated state hospital physicians across the American continent were largely ignorant of what seemed to be the latest fad hatched in an irrelevant fairyland. But soon enough they too would have to speak Freudian when talking about their schizophrenic patients.

Throwing the allegiance of the profession to Freudian mental mechanisms and away from natural disease entities, or even syndromes, would decisively split psychiatry from neurology by 1934. Neurology embraced the doctrine of disease specificity and its requirement of bio-logical mechanisms, and thus became an uncontroversial branch of medical science. Psychiatry did not. The license to practice as a psy-chiatrist would thereafter depend in part on psychoanalytic fluency. Many of the men who played important roles in this later paradigm shift were in attendance at the 1925 conference on schizophrenia.

The widely divergent content of the conference presentations, and the revelatory fluidity of medical cognition in the more informal dis-cussions that followed, were an expression of American eclecticism at its incoherent finest. The broad spectrum of psychogenic to biogenic speculation was represented, sometimes within the same presentation. Although still muted to a large degree, the discourse of Freudian de-fense mechanisms (especially regression and projection) was already in motion as an interpretive framework for the delusions, hallucinations, neologisms, and withdrawn behaviors of schizophrenics. To cite one example: during the discussion session that followed a presentation of laboratory findings about metabolic and blood sugar abnormalities in schizophrenic patients, Jelliffe argued that because the "psychoses are flight phenomena," "may not the high blood sugar content be under-stood better of the flight phenomenon, and similarly the low metabo-lism? Might they not all be interpreted as aspects of running away from reality?"[78] Such flights of ideas would become increasingly common-place among American psychiatrists during the next half-century.

Along with psychoanalysis came the surrender of the quest for the Holy Grail of disease specificity in the sense understood by the other medical sciences. Freudian defense mechanisms would be all that American psychiatrists required, not biological mechanisms. Meyer and a few other eclectic American psychiatrists had already rejected the relevance of the European medical doctrine of the specification of diseases (the assumption of natural disease entities with typical onsets, signs and symptoms, syndromes, courses, outcomes, and biological mechanisms). This was a doctrine at the core of the medical philosophies of both Emil Kraepelin and Eugen Bleuler, and this fact alone was enough to keep the issue open in the minds of many American psychiatrists in the 1920s, particularly with regard to the "functional psychoses" (dementia praecox, schizophrenia, and manic–depressive insanity) that often seemed so biological in presentation.

But the Freudians would eventually dissolve the controversy over disease specificity to a point where many psychiatrists would not remember a time in their careers when it was ever a serious issue. Perhaps this was to be expected. For, as the sociologist Andrew Delano Abbott noted, "the notion of disease itself vanishes from Freud's writing rather early, suggesting the separation of analysis from medicine that he himself wished. Once he worked out his theories of psychic mechanism, he reconceptualized symptoms as indicative of certain states of disordered personality. At that point he and the nervous and mental disease specialists were no longer observing the same reality."[79]

Psychiatry would soon develop its own parallel universe of unfalsifiable psychoanalytic insights to rival competing claims to expert knowledge from the laboratory. Some psychiatrists who followed Meyer and Freud in the glorification of the uniqueness of the individual human life were openly scornful of statistical and laboratory studies. They expressed an emotional, visceral reaction against quantification and generalization. They resisted the disenchantment of the world wrought by the rationalizing methods of science. Other psychiatrists developed chimerical theories that attempted to translate biochemical and physiological processes into Freudian concepts, and vice versa.

But American eclecticism did not just enable the rise of psychoanalysis. It also kept the door open for biological psychiatry and its promise of disease specificity. Beginning in the 1920s the number of published laboratory studies on mental diseases would proliferate. To some degree this was the result of a broader program of biomedical research funding by American philanthropic foundations associated with the Rockefeller and McCormick families and, to a much lesser degree, the Scottish

Rite Masons. Most of these researchers had little concern for Freud. Many were biochemists and endocrinologists, not psychiatrists. Schizophrenia was their most frequent object of inquiry. Some of these studies concerned the effects of experimental somatic treatments. Such research was critical for the survival of the profession: American psychiatry needed to legitimize the claim that it was a branch of modern scientific medicine and not a queer survival of a nineteenth-century therapeutic sect.

The fatal flaw in all such studies, whether statistical or biomedical, was the absence of a uniform definition for schizophrenia. Results could therefore not be generalized, compared, or interpreted in a meaningful way. Should the patients they selected for research, those they separated from the others as definitely schizophrenic, match the descriptions found in Kraepelin or in Bleuler? Or should the subjects be culled from state hospital wards using the diagnostic criteria of some other expert? Most of these studies did not reveal how they selected their subjects. But all understood that the new term "schizophrenia" did not necessarily carry with it the assumptions of Bleuler.

Always insightful, especially when being irreverent, Smith Ely Jelliffe illustrated this point at the 1925 schizophrenia conference when he addressed his distinguished colleagues:

> In many fields of medicine it must be frankly admitted that our conception of this or that "disease" is a purely fictional one; an artifact, even though of value. . . . What position may we assume with reference to the infinitely less precise nosological fiction which we term schizophrenia? On the one hand, we are loath to ally ourselves with those pessimistic attitudes of Hoche, Bumke and many others who would even overlook the logical value of nosological fictions, and hold up our hands and say the problem is hopeless of solution and, furthermore, of no value. On the other hand, are we ready to accept the wide, marshy extensions of the schizophrenia concept as Bleuler has so masterfully outlined it, or the more incisive etching of Kraepelin with his brilliant gift for "knapp und klar" clinical delineation?

As for himself Jelliffe declared, "We shall accept as part of our point of view the purely logical fiction value . . . of all nosology—not in the pessimistic sense of being of no value . . . but in the pragmatic sense."[80]

American psychiatry would not concern itself with the issue of whether or not schizophrenia was a natural disease entity, as it had with dementia praecox. It would not refight the previous war. It would tolerate ambiguity and paradox. It would embrace logical fictions.

Kraepelin's disease survived in America in name only. In the years that followed it would be attached to Bleuler's term as "dementia praecox (schizophrenia)" or, more frequently, as "schizophrenia (dementia praecox)."[81] But there was one notable exception to this trend. In 1936 Nolan D. C. Lewis published a book-length review of the literature published between 1920 and 1934 on this subject under the title *Research in Dementia Praecox* and used the term "dementia praecox" throughout. Interestingly he largely dismissed the "earlier literature" of the pre-1920 period as unworthy of scientific interest. He observed that in 1935 " 'schizophrenia' and 'dementia praecox' are used interchangeably in many psychiatric hospitals," but "when used interchangeably and indiscriminantly, create additional confusion in a situation which is at best exceedingly complicated."[82] Despite Lewis's warning, confusion continued to reign. Between 1918 and 1952 it was entirely acceptable to publish clinical or research reports using five terms interchangeably: dementia praecox, schizophrenia, schizophrenic reaction, dementia praecox (schizophrenia), and schizophrenia (dementia praecox).

But did the new term advance American psychiatry? Charles Macfie Campbell didn't think so. In 1920 he left his second-in-command position under Adolf Meyer at the Phipps Psychiatric Clinic in Baltimore and had replaced the deceased E. E. Southard as director of the Boston Psychopathic Hospital. Together with his appointment as a professor of psychiatry at Harvard Medical School he had finally secured his place (with Meyer, Kirby, and White) at the highest level of influence in the American psychiatric elite. His opinions now mattered more than ever before.

"I think the paralyzing effect of Kraepelin's psychiatry has been the assumption of a 'Krankheitsvorgang (course of disease),' " he said in 1925. As for dementia praecox, "the use of this term has done serious injustice to many patients and both in physician and nurse it has tended to paralyze therapeutic effort."[83] But replacing dementia praecox with schizophrenia, he said in December 1929, "recalls Hoche's relevant remark that one does not make muddy water clearer by pouring it from one jug to another." In a private letter to a colleague five years later he was more forthcoming: "I do not believe that there is such a thing as schizophrenia, and on the other hand I think it is the most important topic for investigation in our field. To put it another way, I do not think there is a *disease* schizophrenia, but, on the other hand, it is useful at this period to have some group term for an extremely large number of cases of mental disorder of the more serious type."[84]

Not much had changed in the thirty-four years since May 1900, when an alienist from St. Louis said that he found "dementia praecox a very comfortable, if I may say vulgarly, dumping ground."[85] The historian Edward Shorter once wrote that with "dementia praecox, or schizophrenia," psychiatry had been handed "its most powerful term of the twentieth century."[86] Perhaps the source of its power has been its ability to expand and contract the parameters of inexplicable madness, to simultaneously take on all meanings, and no meaning, all at the same time.

As they did with Kraepelin's dementia praecox, Americans seemed to merely borrow Bleuler's term and prognostic assumptions without adopting the theoretical fullness of his concept. Whatever schizophrenia was in American clinical practice after 1925, it most certainly was not Bleuler's schizophrenia. Bleuler himself did not seem to notice or care. By the 1920s he had long distanced himself from psychoanalysis (and, by default, from some increasingly dogmatic Freudian partisans in the American psychiatric community). Unlike Freud and Jung, he was unconcerned with cultivating disciples in the United States. Unlike Kraepelin, he devoted no time to currying favor with American philanthropists to secure funding for a research institute. Except for writing occasional scientific articles, lecturing, and updating various editions of his psychiatry textbook, he spent the last two decades of his life indulging his passion for the esoteric. This included attending séances and writing dense metaphysical volumes that bore the spirit of German romanticism and, at least to those critics imbued with scientific materialism, the faint taint of vitalism and spiritualism. The creator of schizophrenia lost sight of his creation after it crossed the Atlantic. Or so it seemed.

Then, in late 1929, he visited Massachusetts to spend time with his son, Manfred Bleuler (1903–1994), who was training in Boston under the neurosurgeon Harvey Cushing. Alarmed by the American framing of schizophrenia, both father and son delivered lectures in which they attempted to correct the rampant misrepresentation of Bleuler's original disease concept. In a presentation to the Massachusetts Psychiatric Society on 7 December 1929 Bleuler explicitly differentiated himself from Meyer's "well-known theory of the disease" based on "psychic causes" by claiming that "these psychic mechanisms . . . do not explain the whole disease": "On the whole, schizophrenia seems to be a physical disease with a lingering *course,* which, however, can exacerbate irregularly from some reason unknown to us, into sudden episodes, then get better again."[87]

"Since coming to the United States I have had the valuable experience of realizing that the conceptions of schizophrenia are very different here from those held in our clinic at the Burghölzli," the twenty-six-year-old son told an audience later that same month at the Bloomingdale Hospital in White Plains, New York. "Most European psychiatrists regard the functional theories as insufficient to explain the primary disorder in schizophrenia. The difference of opinion between Americans and Europeans on this point is striking."[88]

American schizophrenia was—and would continue to be—a cloud of unknowing, a mirage on the horizon, something seen but never quite grasped. A wound without flesh.

And what of the personal fate of Emil Kraepelin? It was this giant of German psychiatry, after all, who set our story in motion.

The creator of dementia praecox occupied most of the last two years of his life with efforts to attract American philanthropic funding for the establishment of the independent, multidisciplinary, German Research Institute for Psychiatry (Deutsche Forschungsanstalt für Psychiatrie), housed in its own separate complex of state-of-the-art laboratories for serology, genetics. psychology, neuropathology, biochemistry, and other relevant disciplines. Kraepelin's Institute began formal research in April 1918. He was joined by several of his closest coworkers at Munich University as "senior consultants."[89] A house at Bavariaring 46, donated by James Loeb, an American benefactor, was its only building. But it was disconnected from the University Clinic, where the Institute occupied laboratory space, and from the local hospital in the Schwabing district, where a single psychiatric ward was set aside for research purposes.

Since the end of the war Kraepelin's institute had to share laboratory space and patients ("clinical material") with the University Clinic in Munich. During his last years it was headed by one of his most vocal adversaries, Oswald Bumke (1877–1950), a much younger man with intellectual perspectives of his own. In April 1924 Bumke had succeeded Kraepelin as the chair of psychiatry at Munich University and as director of the University Clinic, positions that Kraepelin had left in 1922 in order to devote his energies to the Institute. The men both respected and despised one another. Bumke would be only too glad to see Kraepelin and his staff move somewhere else.

In October 1923, just months before assuming his positions in Munich as Kraepelin's successor, Bumke gave a lecture in which he directly cast doubt on the reality of dementia praecox as a disease entity. *"What if dementia praecox simply does not exist?"* he asked. Bumke, like his mentor Alfred Hoche, was skeptical of disease concepts in psychiatry. Furthermore, he accused Kraepelin of creating a dogma which blinded psychiatrists to clinical reality: "Our ability to perceive certain connections which are possible according to clinical experience has been blocked for years by the dogma that there are only disease entitites in psychiatry, and that the *'unity'* of these diseases always has to do with *course* and *outcome*." Sounding very much like Adolf Meyer, Bumke said he much preferred the term "schizophrenic reactions."[90] Interestingly, in the last quarter of 1921, just a few months before Kraepelin retired from the university clinic in early 1922, the clinic staff had begun dropping "dementia praecox" as a diagnosis in favor of "schizophrenia." By the end of 1922 "Kraepelin's disease" was no longer diagnosed in the university clinic he had opened in November 1904.[91]

On 8 June 1925, while on an extended visit to the United States with the head of the Institute's serology department, Felix Plaut (1877–1940), Kraepelin went to the headquarters of the Rockefeller Foundation in New York City and formally requested a grant of one million "gold marks" (the equivalent of $250,000) for the erection of a building on land to be donated by the city of Munich.[92] He was turned down by the president of the foundation, George Vincent. But when this refusal was later mentioned to Simon Flexner (1863–1946), the director of the Rockefeller Institute for Medical Research, Flexner advised the board of trustees (of which he was a member) to reconsider. Flexner said that the Rockefeller Foundation should investigate the matter further, "suggesting that the institute might become a training center for American psychiatrists."[93] Thanks to Flexner, who of course was only thinking of how to advance *American* medicine, Kraepelin's dream was once again a possible reality. At a meeting of the board of trustees on 6 November 1925 it was decided that Alan Gregg (1890–1957), a physician who served the Foundation in an advisory capacity for European projects from his office in Paris, should be dispatched to Kraepelin's Institute in Munich to assess the situation.

Alan Gregg's diary for the period he spent in Munich (11–14 November 1925) vividly described the physical, political, and professional tensions faced by Kraepelin and his Institute. After arriving in Munich Gregg went immediately to Kraepelin's office and psychology laboratories at Bavariaring 46 for a series of interviews between "a stiff and stuffy tea." "There is very obviously a marked antipathy between Bumke and Kraepelin in regard to the use of clinical material," Gregg observed. He was astute enough to question Kraepelin about his opinion of the current status of psychiatry, and Kraepelin's response indicated a clear appreciation for the role of biological research in the profession's future, particularly after the development of the Wassermann reaction test for syphilis and advances in endocrinology:

> I questioned K. offhand on any shift that may have taken place in his interests in psychiatry in the last 10 years, and he replied that the development of serology had greatly changed his attitude; he stated that it had been very difficult for him to write the last edition of his book, in view of the great progress made in that field. He mentioned nothing besides serology; he is openly intolerant of Freud and Jung.[94]

For the next year Kraepelin exchanged a flurry of letters and detailed proposals with the Rockefeller Foundation. But the initial surge of hope that Gregg's visit had sparked in him soon gave way to frustration. Rampant postwar inflation in Germany led to requests for greater and greater sums of money. A sum of gold marks equivalent to $400,000, not $250,000, would now be needed. He was also losing valuable staff to institutions in other countries where they could live and work in a financially secure environment. Whereas the initial idea was that Kraepelin's originally requested sum would have been disbursed to him after the February 1926 board meeting, the board members balked and requested that Kraepelin first demonstrate that he could produce supplementary funds from other sources. The board was particularly worried about

Kraepelin's vagueness concerning the source of income that would cover the annual operating costs of the Institute once it was built. Where would this money come from? They agreed on 26 May 1926 to grant his originally requested amount of $250,000 but wanted concrete proof of his other sources of funding to complete and maintain the Institute. No money would cross the Atlantic until then. This was a major disappointment to Kraepelin. He must have wondered if his dream was evaporating before his eyes. But he was resolute. Other than looking forward to a trip to India at the end of the year, attaining funds from the Rockefeller Foundation was clearly uppermost in his mind during the last weeks of his life. Indeed it seems to have been his dying thought.

In late August 1926 Gregg met with Kraepelin for two days at his vacation home on Lago Maggiore in Pallanza, Italy. Kraepelin promised to send Gregg a detailed document accounting for extra funding sources for the proposed Institute by mid-September. But during the second week in September, while still at his Italian villa, Kraepelin became ill with what seemed to be a gastrointestinal ailment. His condition worsened. He returned to Munich, conducted a round of meetings with his colleagues and financial backers, and on 27 September sent the requested information—and another plea for a disbursement of funds—to New York. Three days later he was bedridden, suffering from clear symptoms of heart insufficiency. On 7 October he died. "The end was not easy," said his friend and colleague Felix Plaut. "Kraepelin must have suffered much."[95] He was seventy years old.

An autopsy confirmed what physicians had suspected: a greatly enlarged heart with "advanced Coronasklerose" (coronary sclerosis). On the morning of 9 October 1926 Kraepelin was cremated "with no pomp, no deputations and no speeches; only with flowers and music."[96]

One of Kraepelin's daughters, a physician, wrote a touching letter of gratitude to Alan Gregg a week after her father's cremation:

> Even in the last moments before his death, my father thought of you with the greatest gratitude, and although my father could hardly speak he asked me to tell you how much he was obliged to you. His last words before his passing away were: "Write to Dr. Gregg: my last hope, my last firm hope is that the money for the Experimental Institution will be obtained." I wrote down these words on my note book the very moment he pronounced them; I was afraid to lose a single word of what he told me.[97]

The following month the Rockefeller Foundation approved Kraepelin's request for additional funds, and on 11 February 1927 the first allotment was transferred to Munich. A building was erected. On 15 June 1928 the Institute was formally dedicated. The street alongside the structure was named Kraepelinstrasse, and a marble bust of Emil Kraepelin greeted visitors. The creator of dementia praecox had crossed the Asclepian threshold from mortal to legend.

Dementia praecox would die an official death in the United States only in 1952. In that year the first edition of the American Psychiatric Association's *Diagnostic and Statistical Manual: Mental Disorders* appeared (a volume now often referred to as *DSM-I*).[98] Dementia praecox was no longer recognized as a diagnosis. Instead "schizophrenic reaction" became the newly preferred nomenclature. In 1968 the term "reaction" was dropped.

Neither in the first *DSM* nor in the second edition of 1968 was schizophrenia a syndrome in any sense of the word. The presence or absence of particular signs and symptoms were of no consequence, nor were course or outcome. Schizophrenia was simply a synonym for severe functional impairment, a nonphysical "psychosis" at the end of a unitary continuum reaching back to neurosis and mental health, a label for grossly impaired persons who could not meet the "ordinary demands of life." This thin, deliberately imprecise sketch would be American psychiatry's rationale for rendering a diagnosis of schizophrenia until the publication of *DSM-III* in 1980.[99] In the end, for a time—indeed for a very long time—Adolf Meyer had achieved victory.

Unfortunately he was not alive to experience it. After retiring from the Phipps Psychiatric Clinic in 1940 Meyer continued to teach, deliver invited lectures, and of course write. Despite his prominence in psychiatry, his poor communication skills and vaguely defined jargon never made him a media celebrity. *Time* magazine ridiculed Meyer to an extent in an 18 May 1936 article: "Psychiatry . . . has not grown up into a clean-cut profession. The specialists showed more skill in discovering mental and emotional defects than in remedying them. In particular they seem lost in the woods of psychobiology."[100] The article then fingered Meyer as the creator of the concept. Meyer died in 1950 during an era dominated by a psychogenic theory of mental disease, psychoanalysis, which he had allowed to take root in psychiatry because of its resonances with his own ideas. But by the time of his death Meyer and his "reactions" were acknowledged only as quaint historical precursors to Sigmund Freud and the psychoanalytic theory of the power of the unconscious mind. Except for the names of the three classical forms of the schizophrenic reaction—the paranoid, hebephrenic, and catatonic—Emil Kraepelin and his disease had silently slipped into the underworld.

But history is often cyclic, and sometimes the pendulum swings back to a point where the present resembles the past. Today it is Kraepelin again who is relevant to twenty-first-century narratives of schizophrenia, and Meyer is a ghost. But his words still ring true: "The history of dementia praecox is really that of psychiatry as a whole."[101]

> Perhaps most fundamentally, the act of diagnosis links the
> individual to the social system; it is necessarily a spectacle
> as well as a bureaucratic event. Diagnosis remains a ritual
> of disclosure: a curtain is pulled aside, and uncertainty is
> replaced—for better or worse—by a structured narra-
> tive. . . . Both physician and patient are hostage to this age-
> old ritual. There is an instructive irony in the way in which
> nosological tables can effectively reshape the lives of men
> and women, even when the physician bestowing a particu-
> lar diagnosis is aware of how arbitrary that determination
> may be.
>
> Charles E. Rosenberg,
> *Our Present Complaint* (2007)

The story of the rise and fall of dementia praecox in America is but one
narrow angle of approach to understanding a key transitional period
in American psychiatry, 1896 to 1930 or so, marked by its mystifying
richness of personalities, problems, and professional roles. American
eclecticism was born during this era and defined much of the profession in the twentieth century. To some degree, as Adolf Meyer argued,
this was indeed a pragmatic response to clinical perplexities, especially
asylum conditions such as dementia praecox. During the monotheistic
reign of the Freudians from the 1940s to the 1970s, a period that began
with psychoanalysis and psychosurgery coexisting under the Meyerian
banner of "psychobiology," eclecticism imposed a fragile peace on rivals in the service of the greater goal of restoring maladjusted or un-
productive individuals to society.[1] Biological research and somatic
treatments were always allowed to exist in a skeptical psychogenic cli-
mate. Even Meyer knew such activity was necessary for the prestige of
the profession.

But eclecticism under the Meyerians and Freudians also kept alive
early nineteenth-century habits of medical cognition in American psy-

chiatry that emphasized the unique and the individual over the general and the dimensional over the categorical and openly devalued laboratory research, statistical methods, psychiatric nosology, and the assumption of discrete mental diseases. These attitudes were anachronizing and derationalizing forces that opposed the trajectory of the rest of the American medical professions in the twentieth century. But it wasn't just the elite of the profession that held on to nineteenth-century traditional medical cognition; until forced to do otherwise between 1918 and 1921, most of the superintendents of the more than four hundred institutions for the insane refused to submit annual statistical tables listing the forms of insanity in their populations because of the widespread assumption, based on personal asylum experience, that these maladies were merely situationally transitional moments of symptoms along an incomprehensible and inconstant dimensional concept of "insanity," a unitary psychosis. Madness was madness.

As we have seen, between 1906 and 1911 an elite American framing of dementia praecox emerged from this eclectic stew based on a cluster of ideas: psychogenesis; a "type" comprised of a republic of dissociated maladaptive "reactions" to environmental (biopsychosocial) stressors unique to an individual (hence, each patient was in essence a "type of one"); and a linkage of this morbid condition to a premorbid "prepsychotic" or "shut-in" personality or a "deterioration type," identifiable in shy children and introverted adults. Prevention, effective treatment ("habit training"), and sometimes even cures were promised to the American public. Biological etiologies and pathophysiologies were either flatly denied or set aside.

To the average asylum physician all of this seemed counterintuitive; insanity had long been regarded as organic in some way, and the severe disability exhibited by psychotic patients within asylum walls often seemed quite biological in presentation. Elite discourse eventually adapted to experienced clinical reality. During World War I psychoanalytic physicians chimerized dementia praecox into a neuropsychiatric amalgam of the vegetative nervous system and Freudian mechanisms. Still it was not a "disease" to be specified but a "reaction" to be mulled over ad infinitum, and as such most Americans did not bother themselves with European methods such as the identification of characteristic signs and symptoms, or characteristic courses, or even characteristic outcomes (other than to insist, without quantitative data of their own, that the prognosis was good in many cases). There was a decided lack of interest in the development of these severe psychotic conditions once they had become manifest—the focus was on the unique circumstances of a person's past. In fact attention to the premorbid personality of persons with dementia praecox and schizophrenia would intensify in the 1920s and 1930s. Biographical history, not biological reduction or long-term follow-up study, was the preferred evidential base.

Unfortunately for historians American eclectics kept the term "dementia praecox" for their construction, and then later hid it under the name "schizophrenia," but neither Emil Kraepelin (especially after 1906) nor Eugen Bleuler could honestly say that the Americans were using their European disease concepts. The psychiatric elite either denied or was skeptical of a disease concept of dementia praecox—again, all the while allowing the bulk of laboratory and neuropathological studies and experimental somatic treatments to proceed as if a disease concept was their guide. This American dementia praecox is often neglected in histories of American psychiatry, many of which imply that the Americans adopted Kraepelin's full disease concept, then switched to Bleuler's schizophrenia because it was psychoanalytic, then adopted the *DSM-III* mental disorder of schizophrenia in 1980 to meet the research needs of biological psychiatry. A neat and clear lineage. As the preceding narrative demonstrates, this is false on multiple levels.[2] Instead of direct and uncomplicated reception, which historians love to trace, the Americans engaged in something akin to what the literary scholar Harold Bloom called "misprision," a necessary misreading of prior texts as a precondition for creative endeavors.[3]

Perhaps there can be such as thing as too much creative space, and American eclecticism may have exemplified it. A common language of discourse could not develop. The turn to psychoanalysis by the psychiatric elite by 1940 was an attempt to rectify that problem, but it failed. Tensions within the profession, and between psychiatry and the greater world of scientific biomedicine, were enormous.

This tolerance of ambiguity and paradox did not hold. Rationalizing forces external to psychiatry, unleashed by biomedical research into brain chemistry, psychopharmacology, and genetics in the 1950s and 1960s, eventually tipped the philosophical balance of power from Meyer and Freud back to Kraepelin. In the 1970s "neo-Kraepelinian" physicians constructed a new diagnostic manual, *DSM-III* (1980), with discrete categories of mental disorders and specific diagnostic criteria that would not only serve clinicians but also be the common linguistic and conceptual foundation of comparative research—a first for psychiatry.[4] Biological psychiatry had purged the profession of its eclecticism by the end of the 1980s. Schizophrenia was re-created as brain disease with neurodevelopmental roots, a uterine alembic distillation of genetics and possible environmental factors such as viruses, amoebic parasites, and birth complications. Neurotransmitters were implicated in its pathophysiology. The psychogenic vocabulary of reactions and Freudian mechanisms has now vanished. Neither maladjustments nor mothers are blamed for the illness.[5]

The victory of biological psychiatry has been so pervasive that it is difficult for many of us alive today to imagine a time when things were not so. Nor is there much concern today about whether psychiatry is a legitimate discipline within modern scientific medicine; its transformation into something resembling "applied pharmacology," which the historian Charles E. Rosenberg predicted in 1975, has alleviated the professional insecurities betrayed by book titles such as *Why Psychiatry Is a Branch of Medicine* (1992).[6] Such titles now seem like relics of a bygone era.

The illusive cohesion of our era's biological psychiatry is indeed a stark contrast to the inchoate profession of nervous and mental disease specialists of a century ago. Whether psychiatry remains biological, or perhaps even a branch of medicine, will depend on how effectively it reframes or ignores attempts to reintroduce legitimate observations about the reactive nature of many disorders. Biological psychiatry—by epistemological necessity—ignores the unique individual circumstances or personal context in which symptoms arise. Opening the door (even a crack) to psychosocial interpretations of the origin of common conditions now treated through psychopharmacology rather than psychotherapy is viewed as risky: it might open Pandora's jar. Such heterodox thinking might eventually snowball into a challenge to our era's foundational concept in biological psychiatry: schizophrenia as a brain disease (or diseases). As the story of dementia praecox illustrates, it has certainly happened before. American psychiatrists of the twenty-first century still fear the specter of Adolf Meyer. And they should.[7]

Dementia praecox was created and re-created in an effort to solve fundamental problems—professional, bureaucratic, clinical, scientific, moral, and societal—that are still very much with us. Our schizophrenia is our solution for our time.

This is not to say that dementia praecox and schizophrenia in any of their historical incarnations are "merely" social constructions. Few historians or sociologists would hold to such an extreme view. One thing is certain: when we have the courage to look, and are honest about what we see, all that we ever really find beneath the shedding skins of social construction is personal tragedy. The magnitude of despair wrought by inexplicable madness can never be conveyed by a psychiatric concept, nor in "disease history" books such as this one. The story I told of Bayard Holmes and his mission to save his son comes closest to illustrating the desperation felt by those personally touched by such misfortune. As a ward psychologist in a state hospital in the mid-1980s I lived with the social and personal devastation of schizophrenia on a daily basis. There will never be an adequate vocabulary for such misery. I have a profound sympathy for the physicians, nurses, and psychologists of the past who tried to comprehend, manage, and salvage the mentally ill. I was once one of them.

By placing the history of American psychiatry within the larger currents of the history of medicine we can make some sense out of why American alienists were receptive to Emil Kraepelin and his two great insanities, dementia praecox and manic-depressive insanity. Although the early evangelizing of August Hoch and Adolf Meyer was certainly the catalyst, it would be a mistake to believe it was merely the unquestioned utility and perceived German superiority of Kraepelin's nosology. Nor was it just the fact that diagnosis by prognosis served the bureaucratic needs (and excused the failures) of asylum management, although this was undoubtedly a significant factor. A deeper medical principle at the core of Kraepelin's perspective is what mattered.

Of all the European influences on American medicine and, eventually, psychiatry, the doctrine of disease specificity was the most powerful. In the transition from traditional to modern medicine, to use the historian Edward Shorter's characterizations, a fundamental change in medical cognition took place.[8] By the last third of the nineteenth century American physicians began to adopt the European notion "that diseases can and should be thought of as entities existing outside their unique manifestations in particular men and women," and furthermore that "disease was equated with specificity and specificity with mechanism, all the while decoupling this increasingly ontological conception from idiosyncrasies of place and person."[9] Diseases had typical signs and symptoms, typical courses, typical outcomes and biological mechanisms. Biological mechanisms were identified at autopsy or in the laboratory. Without the eventual adoption of this doctrine, American alienism would never be *psychiatry* in the German medical science sense. It would never have its place in an increasingly rationalized, disease-specified, laboratory-research-driven American medical profession. An awareness of Kraepelin's work arrived at a pivotal, one might say vulnerable, moment.

Emil Kraepelin was first and foremost a physician. He had practical issues with patients to resolve on a daily basis; his writings reflect this. He wrote as a physician *for* other physicians, not for historians. The fact that so little of his work in experimental psychology, his abiding passion, finds its way into the various editions of his textbook is a testament to his desire to be of practical service to fellow physicians. His mosaic-like compilations of the actual statements and behaviors of his patients are stunningly recognizable, even today, to anyone who has worked in inpatient settings with psychotic individuals. They ring true. As Kraepelin well understood, physicians rely on physical signs as well as expressions of mental symptoms. In his dementia praecox, for example, changes in the behavior of the pupils of the eyes could be significant, a clue for other physicians to note along with signs of "mental weakness" or "defect." As the historians Eric Engstrom and Matthias Weber have pointed out, "Kraepelin considered himself much more of a diagnostician than a nosologist."[10]

Whereas he regarded his diagnostic categories as provisional and changed them over time, he could not abdicate the foundational medical premise that one day natural disease entities would be specified for insanity. As early as 1887, in a lecture titled "The Directions of Psychiatric Research" delivered in Dorpat when he was thirty, Kraepelin argued that the doctrine of disease specificity had to be central to psychiatry if it was to be a branch of medicine. For a true "clinical science of mental disorders," disease specificity would be attained if psychiatric research followed a two-step agenda:

Once we have thus carefully and scientifically surveyed all the different forms derived from psychiatric experience, then it will finally be possible, from a higher vantage point, which accounts for not just one but for all clinical symptoms, to comprehend clearly the natural congruity and boundaries of specific disease manifestations. The first and immediate general problem of psychiatry will be resolved once its material has been sorted and grouped by clinical researchers; the resolution of the second, much more important and difficult problem—tracing disease forms back to their pathological origins—needs the systematic co-operation of all the auxiliary sciences. As things now stand, these sciences are, for the most part, still isolated, unconnected with each other and pursuing their own agendas. For the time being, therefore, it will be clinical observation in the strict sense of the word from which we can expect tangible progress in our scientific knowledge.[11]

Kraepelin's program for disease specificity is easily recognizable in the logic of biological psychiatry today. It also expresses, in a general way, the rationale behind the categorical structure of the various editions of the *Diagnostic and Statistical Manual of Mental Disorders,* from its epoch-making third edition of 1980 to its forthcoming fifth edition, which is projected to appear in 2013. In theory these volumes represent steps on the yellow brick road to complete disease specificity. In practice the proliferation of new but increasingly overlapping (comorbid) mental disorders in each succeeding edition has pulled psychiatry in the opposite direction, away from discrete categories and toward a consideration of dimensional diagnosis based on the kinds and severity of signs and symptoms—a possible return to a practice that the Meyerians and Freudians would have recognized. As I write, groups of North American psychiatrists who are involved in the construction of the forthcoming *DSM-5* (no more Roman numerals) are considering a combination of categorical and dimensional methods for diagnosing mental disorders. No longer believing that pouring muddy water from one jug into another makes it any clearer, their new solution is to the break the jugs.[12]

From the intellectual perspective of researchers, a dimensional rating of signs and symptoms might be a better fit with the confusing findings in genetics, which refuse to obey the limits imposed by our diagnostic categories. Indeed genetics research is dissolving the distinction between schizophrenia and bipolar disorder, creating a potential new disease concept that the psychiatrist and noted schizophrenia researcher

E. Fuller Torrey whimsically called "manicdephrenia."[13] Because these constructions are regarded as descendants of the two great psychotic disorders of 1899 an elimination of this categorical dichotomy would fundamentally extract the Kraepelinian episteme from the gut of American psychiatry. This operation is not proposed for *DSM-5*, but for the first time in over a century it is a distinct possibility that Kraepelinian classification will one day entirely disappear.[14]

Of more immediate historical interest is the fact that a convergence of clinical and biological (particularly genetic) evidence has led to the proposed elimination in *DSM-5* of the three classic subtypes of schizophrenia: paranoid, catatonic, and disorganized (formerly hebephrenic). These were of course originally Kraepelin's three subtypes for dementia praecox. This vestige of the nineteenth century will almost certainly disappear in 2013. Given the views expressed by the older Kraepelin in his 1920 essay, "The Manifestations of Insanity," in which the blurring of the boundaries between dementia praecox and manic-depressive insanity betrayed a retreat from strict categorical classification, and his lifelong appreciation for the potential of biological research to bend and break nosology, I imagine that he would welcome these developments.

Although no fans of classification schemes for mental disorders, Meyer and other American eclectics such as Hoch, Jelliffe, and Macfie Campbell might have found a certain validation in the current proposal to add something called "psychosis risk syndrome" to *DSM-5*. Although the precognitive abilities of twenty-first-century psychiatrists may not be any better than those of Meyer's time, this proposal marks a return to the prepsychotic personality concept that served the prophylaxis propaganda of American eclecticism and the mental hygiene movement. Today it serves the pharmaceutical industry by opening up a large new market (primarily adolescents, but also children) for its array of atypical antipsychotic drugs. The proposed disorder also has resonances with Bleuler's "simple schizophrenic" and "latent schizophrenic" characters. This of course is the familiar linkage of a premorbid personality concept to a psychotic disease concept (in this case, schizophrenia) that characterized the American eclectic concept of dementia praecox. It extends the dimension of psychosis backward in time to a point where certain symptoms are just peeking up over the horizon. Time will tell if this proposal proves to be a factor in a dimensional deconstruction of the schizophrenia disease category. The current proposal is problematic, to say the least, and it will be interesting to see if the psychosis risk syndrome (or "attenuated psychosis syndrome") appears in *DSM-5*. The psychiatrist Allen Frances, the chair of the *DSM-IV* Task Force in the 1990s, warns that "this suggestion could lead to a public health catastrophe."[15]

But it is almost certain that distinct categories of mental disorders—certainly at least one for schizophrenia, or a new psychotic disorder merging aspects of schizophrenia and bipolar disorder—will remain as long as psychiatry remains a distinct medical specialty. The reasons for this are many and varied. There are many systemic and practical barriers to pure dimensional diagnosis. Our Moloch of managed mental health care bureaucracies jealously demands categorical diagnoses that resemble those in the rest of medicine. Sliding scales of symptom severity unleashed from their jugs will not translate well into the preexisting system. Thirty years of new clinicians entering the mental health field have been conditioned to see expressions of extreme emotional and behavioral distress as examples of *DSM* categories and believe in the possibility, indeed the reality of specific biological disease processes behind ADHD, major depression, dysthymic disorder, generalized anxiety disorder, and of course the familiar impulse control problems (alcoholism, gambling, shopping, sex, and so on). Since the 1990s the mood disorders—bipolar disorders and major depression—have replaced schizophrenia as the rhetorical flashpoint for critiques of the psychiatric profession as a whole. Separate categories of "well" and "ill," which Freudian dimensional thinking did not separate, once again exist in theory, but the persistence of dimensional cognition in psychiatry is re-erasing this line in its characterization and treatment of mood disorders.[16] Quantification of symptom dimensions may seem logical to researchers, and may seem like a solution to the defects of Meyerian and Freudian eclecticism, but may not translate well into clinical practice. Everyday clinicians may find the dimensional rating of symptoms in an arbitrary quantitative fashion burdensome. (How severely, on a scale of 1 to 4, is this person plagued by hallucinations? By delusions? Mental health workers roll their eyes at such questions.) Indeed over time everyday diagnostic practice, which has always taken place far away from the psychiatric elite and laboratory researchers, may revisit the traditional medicine of centuries past and turn dimensions of the primary symptom into the new disorders.

But as E. E. Southard keenly observed a century ago, consensual agreement on the definition of a symptom term ("psychomotor excitement" or "dementia" in his day, perhaps "bizarre delusions" in ours) is as problematic as specifying the boundaries of a category. The limits of our language are indeed the limits of our world. We continue to have as much difficulty in linguistically characterizing the physically visible patients we encounter today as the alienists and neurologists of a century ago did when trying to make sense of their own patients, the true nature of whom seems so invisible to us. For better or worse we continue to bury their bodies beneath the verbiage of modernity and its hyperreflexive mode of consciousness.[17]

As the story of dementia praecox and schizophrenia reveals, a struggle between categorical and dimensional thinking had characterized not only psychiatry, but also the medical profession, since at least the mid-1800s. Life—biological and psychological—flows most naturally along dimensional paths. As it did in the past, a resurgence of dimensional concepts may lead to a new derationalization of American psychiatry. "Reaction-forms" may make a reappearance. The psychiatry of 2040 might end up resembling that of 1940. But if discrete conceptual boundaries between disorders can dissolve, so can the trust of the American public in psychiatry's claim to be a branch of medicine. Everyday people have no interest in the philosophical distinction between a *DSM* mental disorder and a medical disease concept, especially when the usual treatment they receive for both is medication. But patients want a diagnosis. They want a structured narrative that puts their suffering into a larger context, something that unites them with an imagined community of other souls who are suffering in the same way. Disease concepts *are* the stories they seek.

Kraepelin may rest in peace after all. Natural disease entities in psychiatry are not—yet—in danger of extinction. There are indeed several current *DSM* mental disorders that, many argue, have enough clinical and biological findings hooked to them to resemble the kinds of disease entities commonly found under the jurisdiction of the other medical specialties. In the psychiatry of the twenty-first century these include schizophrenia, bipolar I disorder, and a severe endogenous form of depression that is increasingly known as "melancholia."[18] As for the hundreds of other mental disorders available in the current edition of *DSM-IV-TR* (2000), collapsing many of them into dimensions of signs and symptoms might become, for the current generation of psychiatrists, one of those seductive paradigm shift temptations of the mind to which flesh is heir.

Dementia praecox was the vehicle through which American psychiatry reentered general medicine. It descended into American asylums from the Valhalla of superior German medicine and presented American alienists with a divine gift: its first truly specifiable disease concept. Despite Meyer's misgivings, it arrived in 1896 as one of Kraepelin's "metabolic disturbances"—a truly medical condition—and as an asylum insanity par excellence it fit naturally into the autointoxication paradigm that had already structured the logic of asylum laboratory research in America. In one form or another, from endocrine dysfunction to neurohumoral (neurotransmitter) imbalance, laboratory specifications of dementia praecox and schizophrenia would never lose their metaphoric affinity with humoral dyscrasias. The waxing and waning of psychosis lent itself naturally to notions of fluidity, whether as currents of electrons or of chemicals, and defied rational treatments to alter its course.

Even when reframed as a psychogenic reaction by the literary elites of the twentieth century, the physical reality of hundreds of thousands of inexplicably psychotic individuals confined within state hospital walls, many disabled for decades, made it impossible to deny that a catastrophic *medical* problem needed to be solved. The problem needed a name— and dementia praecox and schizophrenia were chosen for those persons deemed the most irredeemable. The fate of the American psychiatric profession, indeed its very identity became linked to the legitimacy conferred upon it by the existence of this disease concept. The profession and the psychosis were—are—inseparable. This was the true meaning behind Meyer's observation that the history of dementia praecox is the history of psychiatry.

For more than a century dementia praecox and schizophrenia have been the principal concepts that have kept American psychiatry tethered to scientific medicine. A Meyerian or Freudian psychiatry could have flourished forever in private clinics and consulting rooms well outside the jurisdiction of the American medical profession, but the failure of the eclectics to solve the social and medical problem of the institutionalized mentally ill kept American psychiatry from reverting into a nineteenth-century therapeutic sect. Biological psychiatry, which had always existed in one form or another in the United States since the late 1880s, was all that was left to deal with the legacy of asylum alienism. Philanthropic and government funding for biomedical research in psychiatry logically targeted dementia praecox and schizophrenia above all other mental disorders throughout the twentieth century. Somatic treatments, from chemical or electric shock and psychosurgery to pharmacotherapy, have all imposed a disproportionate therapeutic discipline on individuals with these two diagnoses. There could have been no modern medical science of American psychiatry in the twentieth century without dementia praecox. There can be no biological psychiatry in the twenty-first century without schizophrenia.

NOTES

Introduction

1. Paul R. Baker, *Stanny: The Gilded Life of Stanford White* (New York: Free Press, 1989), 321–322; Paula Uruburu, *American Eve: Evelyn Nesbit, Stanford White, the Birth of the "It" Girl and the Crime of the Century* (New York: Riverhead Books, 2008), 151.

2. E. R. Pinta, "Examining Harry Thaw's 'Brain-Storm' Defense: APA and ANA Presidents as Expert Witnesses in a 1907 Trial," *Psychiatric Quarterly,* 79 (2008): 83–89. See also his self-published expansion of this article, *Expert Testimony in the Harry K. Thaw "Brain-Storm" Defense: Concepts of Temporary Insanity in a 1907 Trial* (Columbus, OH: E. R. Pinta, 2008).

3. This short reenactment of the murder is included in the Public Broadcasting System's documentary, *American Experience: Murder of the Century* (1995), written and produced by Carl Charlson.

4. See Peter Conrad, *The Medicalization of Society: On the Transformation of Human Conditions into Treatable Disorders* (Baltimore: The Johns Hopkins University Press, 2007). The tension between "medicalization" and "de-medicalization" has been identified as the primary theme underlying scholarship in the history of medicine. See John C. Burnham, *What Is Medical History?* (Cambridge, UK and Malden, MA: Polity Press, 2005), 6–9.

5. "Shift by Jerome Gives Thaw Hope: Day Spent in Attack on the 'Brain Storm' Theory of the Experts," *New York Times,* 5 March 1907.

6. F. A. Mackenzie, *The Trial of Harry Thaw* (London: Geoffrey Bles, 1928), 191–192.

7. Emil Kraepelin, *Psychiatrie: Ein Lehrbuch für Studirende und Aerzte. Funfte, vollständig umgearbeitete Auflage* (Leipzig: J.A. Barth, 1896); Emil Kraepelin,

Psychiatrie: Ein Lehrbuch für Studirende und Aerzte. Sechste, vollständig umgearbeitete Auflage (Leipzig: J.A. Barth, 1899). For context, see also G. E. Berrios and R. Hauser, "The Early Development of Kraepelin's Ideas on Classification: A Conceptual History," *Psychological Medicine* 18 (1988): 813–821; David Healy, Margaret Harris, Fiona Farquhar, Stefanie Tschinkel, and Joanna Le Noury, "Historical Overview: Kraepelin's Impact on Psychiatry," *European Archives of Psychiatry and Clinical Neuroscience* 258 (Suppl.) (2008): 18–24.

8. J. T. W. Rowe, "Is Dementia Praecox the 'New Peril' in Psychiatry?," *American Journal of Insanity* 63 (1907): 385–393. See also the earlier British alarm in Connally Norman, "Dementia Praecox," *British Medical Journal* 2 (1904): 972–976.

9. Eugen Bleuler, "Die Prognose der Dementia Praecox— Schizophreniegruppe," *Allgemeine Zeitschrift für Psychiatrie* 65 (1908): 436–464.

10. "Shocker," *Time,* 20 December 1948, 44–52; Krin Gabbard and Glen O. Gabbard, *Psychiatry and the Cinema* (Chicago: University of Chicago Press, 1987), 68–72, 77–80.

11. The most recent review of these issues is David Fraguas, "Problems with Retrospective Studies of the Presence of Schizophrenia," *History of Psychiatry* 20 (2009): 61–71. The position that schizophrenia is a disease of recent historical origin has prominent proponents: E. Fuller Torrey, *Schizophrenia and Civilization* (New York: Jason Aronson, 1980); E. Fuller Torrey and Judy Miller, *The Invisible Plague: The Rise of Mental Illness from 1750 to the Present* (New Brunswick, NJ: Rutgers University Press, 2002); Edward Shorter, *A History of Psychiatry: From the Era of the Asylum to the Age of Prozac* (New York: Wiley, 1997), 62–63.

12. German E. Berrios, Rogelio Luque, and José M. Villagrán, "Schizophrenia: A Conceptual History," *International Journal of Psychology and Psychological Therapy* 3 (2003): 112, 111. See also G. E. Berrios, "Schizophrenia: A Conceptual History," in *New Oxford Textbook of Psychiatry,* ed. Michael Gelder, Juan Lopez-Ibor, and Nancy Andreasen (Oxford: Oxford University Press, 2000), 1:567–571.

13. Charles E. Rosenberg, *Our Present Complaint: American Medicine, Then and Now* (Baltimore: The Johns Hopkins University Press, 2007), 30. Rosenberg employs the term "medicalization" in a broader sense than its usual function in sociology.

   The voices of dementia praecox patients are often recorded in a fragmentary manner in hospital records and clinical archives. For an example of a case history of dementia praecox (not included in this volume), the reader is referred to Richard Noll, "Styles of Psychiatric Practice,

1906–1925: Clinical Evaluations of the Same Patient by James Jackson Putnam, Adolf Meyer, Emil Kraepelin and Smith Ely Jelliffe," *History of Psychiatry* 10 (1999): 145–189. An exceptionally vivid account of the case of this same patient, Stanley McCormick, told through the biography of his wife, can be found in Armond Fields, *Katharine Dexter McCormick: Pioneer for Women's Rights* (Westport, CT: Praeger, 2003).

14. For an exemplary sociological analysis of elites in the organized world of nervous and mental disease work in a period of pivotal professional and scientific transition in American medicine, see Andrew Delano Abbott, "The Emergence of American Psychiatry, 1880–1930," PhD diss., University of Chicago, 1982. This extensively researched and cogently argued study deserves much wider attention than it has received. Indeed, it is an unsung classic in the history of American psychiatry and is an essential starting point for any scholar. Through sociological analysis Abbott answered many questions of interest to historians. Much of my discussion in the text is framed by his insights.

15. R. Tandon, M. S. Keshavan, and H. A. Nasrallah, "Schizophrenia, Just the Facts: What We Know in 2008. Part 1: Overview," *Schizophrenia Research* 100 (2008): 4, 11. As the historian Sander Gilman recognized, "*Schizophrenia* is still a label in search of a structure." Sander L. Gilman, "Constructing Schizophrenia as a Category of Mental Illness," in *History of Psychiatry and Medical Psychology,* ed. Edwin R. Wallace IV and John Gach (New York: Springer, 2008), 461. The psychiatrist Allen Frances, the chief editor of *DSM-IV* in 1994 and its text revision in 2000, recently stated, "There may eventually turn out to be twenty or fifty or two hundred kinds of 'schizophrenia.' As it stands now the definition and boundaries of schizophrenia are necessarily arbitrary . . . The more we learn about 'schizophrenia' the more it resembles a heuristic, the less it resembles a disease." Allen Frances, "DSM in Philosophyland: Curiouser and Curiouser," *Association for the Advancement of Philosophy and Psychiatry Bulletin* 17(2) (2010): 4. Schizophrenia in the twenty-first century is still a diagnosis that lacks validity as a specific disease entity. The same lack of validity is true for its defining symptoms, such as "delusions" and "hallucinations." See Joseph M. Pierre, "Deconstructing Schizophrenia for *DSM-V*: Challenges for Clinical and Research Agendas," *Clinical Schizophrenia and Related Psychoses* 2 (2008): 166–174. If there can be such a thing as an official policy statement on American psychiatry's view of schizophrenia as a biological disease or diseases, see the four-stage "neurodevelopmental model" articulated by a prominent official of the National Institute of Mental Health, Thomas R. Insel, "Rethinking Schizophrenia," *Nature* 468 (11 November 2010): 187–193. The neurodevelopmental

model has been the dominant framing of schizophrenia in the United States since 1986.

16. Gerald N. Grob, *Mental Illness and American Society, 1875–1940* (Princeton: Princeton University Press, 1983), 36; Gerald N. Grob, "Rediscovering Asylums: The Unhistorical History of the Mental Hospital," in *The Therapeutic Revolution: Essays in the Social History of American Medicine,* ed. Morris J. Vogel and Charles E. Rosenberg (Philadelphia: University of Pennsylvania Press, 1979), 142.

17. "Phipps Interested in Thaw: Prisoner's Case Is Said to Have Influenced Steel Man's Donation," *New York Times,* 16 June 1908.

18. Allan McLane Hamilton, *Recollections of an Alienist, Personal and Professional* (New York: George H. Doran, 1916), 401.

19. See, for example, Simon Flexner and James Thomas Flexner, *William Henry Welch and the Heroic Age of American Medicine* (New York: Viking Press, 1941), 348–350. For recent journalistic retrospectives on the architectural planning and founding of the Phipps Psychiatric Clinic, see Anne Bennett Swingle, "Where a Mind Could Find Itself Again," *Hopkins Medical News* (Winter 2003) and Janet Farrar Worthington, "When Psychiatry Was Very Young," *Hopkins Medicine* (Winter 2008) in the "past issues" archives of this Johns Hopkins alumni publication at http://esgweb1.nts.jhu.edu/hmn/.

20. In Germany eighteen university psychiatric clinics were established between the late 1870s and 1914. Unlike the larger rural asylums, where the emphasis was on custodial care and treatment, the university clinics were created to be acute, high-volume, short-term care "transit stations" that emphasized the professional training of medical students and psychiatrists as well as the promotion of scientific research, especially laboratory research. They were either quasi-independent institutions (such as those founded in Heidelberg in 1878 and Munich in 1904, where Kraepelin worked in succession from 1891 to his death in 1926), separate wards in large urban hospitals, or wards in some rural asylums. On the history of university psychiatric clinics in Imperial Germany to the year 1914, see Eric J. Engstrom, *Clinical Psychiatry in Imperial Germany: A History of Psychiatric Practice* (Ithaca, NY: Cornell University Press, 2003). The 1913 founding of the Phipps Clinic at Johns Hopkins punctuates the relative backwardness of an American psychiatry that was at least four decades behind developments in German scientific medicine.

1. The World of the American Alienist, 1896

1. The standard works that document this transition are William G. Rothstein, *American Physicians in the 19th Century: From Sects to Science* (Balti-

more: The Johns Hopkins University Press, 1985); Kenneth M. Lud-
merer, *Learning to Heal: The Development of American Medical Education*
(Baltimore: The Johns Hopkins University Press, 1985); Paul Starr, *The
Social Transformation of American Medicine* (New York: Basic Books, 1982);
Thomas Neville Bonner, *Becoming a Physician: Medical Education in Britain,
France, Germany and the United States, 1750–1945* (Baltimore: The Johns
Hopkins University Press, 1995); John Harley Warner, "The Fall and Rise
of Professional Mystery: Epistemology, Authority and the Emergence of
Laboratory Medicine in Nineteenth-Century America," in *The Laboratory
Revolution in Medicine,* ed. Andrew Cunningham and Perry Williams
(Cambridge: Cambridge University Press, 1992), 110–141; John Harley
Warner, *The Therapeutic Perspective: Medical Practice, Knowledge, and Identity
in America, 1820-1885* (Cambridge, MA: Harvard University Press, 1986)
None of these works discusses the training and practice of alienists as part
of its larger story of the history of American medicine. For a perspective on
changing doctor-patient dyads, see Edward Shorter, *Doctors and Their Patients: A Social History* (New York: Simon and Schuster, 1985).

2. An energetic and accessible narrative of the origins and significance of
   the Johns Hopkins Medical School can be found in John M. Barry, *The
   Great Influenza: The Story of the Deadliest Pandemic in History* (New York:
   Penguin books, 2004), 11–87.

3. "Though an accurate account is impossible to attain at this late date, the
   author believes on the basis of fragmentary records that no less than fifteen thousand American medical men—students, young physicians,
   older practitioners—undertook some kind of serious study in a German
   university between 1870 and 1914." Thomas Neville Bonner, *American
   Doctors and German Universities: A Chapter in International Intellectual Relations, 1870–1914* (Lincoln: University of Nebraska Press, 1963), 23. According to Bonner, "Even Sigmund Freud was involved at one time in an
   English language course for Americans in Vienna" (96).

4. See Bayard Taylor Holmes, "Is it Desirable and Practicable in Medical
   Schools to Teach Methods of Investigation in Medical Literature?," *Medical News* (Philadelphia) 63 (1893): 171–173; Bayard Holmes, "The Neglect of Medical Literature," *American Medicine* 15 (1909): 175.

5. Abraham Flexner, *Medical Education in the United States and Canada: A
   Report to the Carnegie Foundation for the Advancement of Teaching* (New
   York: Carnegie Foundation for the Advancement of Teaching, 1910). For
   context and a summary of the report's main findings, see Ludmerer,
   Learning to Heal, 166–190.

6. The historian John Harley Warner made this point well: "It is unmis-
   takable that the laboratory functioned as a force of elitism. . . . The

laboratory provided the material and cognitive basis for an elitist epistemology and a regrounding of medicine on a decidedly privileged body of
knowledge accessible to only a small proportion of Americans. It entailed
privileged knowledge rooted in a privileged epistemology that to most
patients made medical knowledge increasingly a mystery" ("The Fall and
Rise," 140–141). Elsewhere, Warner (*The Therapeutic Perspective,* 91) described the transition from a notion of disease based on the "disruption of
a natural imbalance to a deviation from fixed norms" that accompanied
the rise of the laboratory, thereby leading to a change in therapeutics. His
distinction forms the basis of my discussion. However, it should be noted
that Warner used the term "specificity" to refer to the earlier, traditional
notion of disease and treatment, whereas I follow other scholars (such as
Charles Rosenberg) in using the term "disease specificity" to refer to the
new concept of disease that arose in Europe in the latter half of the nineteenth century. The French physician Armand Trousseau (1801–1867)
was noted for his use of the term in this latter sense: "The principle of
specificity dominates all medicine." See Karl Menninger, *The Vital Balance: The Life Process in Mental Health and Illness* (New York: Viking Press,
1963), 30.

7. The only difference between regular physicians from AMA training
   schools and homeopaths was the materia medica of the homeopaths,
   which the regulars regarded as quackery. Homeopaths shunned older techniques such as bloodletting, blistering, and, later, the use of sedative
   drugs for the treatment of insanity. The eclectic sect in medicine relied
   on botanical remedies and drugs.

8. Rothstein, *American Physicians,* 344–345.

9. Starr, *The Social Transformation of American Medicine,* 109.

10. On the epistemological basis of causes of disease in early nineteenth-
    century practical medicine, see K. Codell Carter, *The Rise of Causal Con-
    cepts of Disease: Case Histories* (Hants, England: Ashgate, 2003), 10–23.

11. For a discussion of the asylum reform movement led by neurologists
    and charity workers between 1874 and 1884, see Barbara Sicherman, *The
    Quest for Mental Health in America, 1880–1917* (New York: Arno Press,
    1980), 12–77; Bonnie Ellen Blustein, "'A Hollow Square of Psychologi-
    cal Science': American Neurologists and Psychiatrists in Conflict," in
    *Madhouses, Mad-Doctors, and Madmen: The Social History of Psychiatry in the
    Victorian Era,* ed. Andrew Scull (Philadelphia: University of Pennsylva-
    nia Press, 1981), 241–271. Also useful are Jacques M. Quen, "Asylum
    Psychiatry, Neurology, Social Work and Mental Hygiene: An Explor-
    atory Study in Interprofessional History," *Journal of the History of the Be-
    havioral Sciences* 13 (1977), 3–11; Edward M. Brown, "Neurology's Influ-

ence on American Psychiatry: 1865–1915," in *History of Psychiatry and Medical Psychology: With An Epilogue on Psychiatry and the Mind-body Relation,* ed. Edwin R. Wallace and John Gach (New York: Springer, 2008), 519–531.

12. S. Weir Mitchell, "Address before the Fiftieth Annual Meeting of the American Medico-Psychological Association," in *Proceedings of the American Medico-Psychological Association Annual Meeting* (Utica, NY: American Medico-Psychological Association, 1894), 102.

13. Louis Casamajor, "Notes for an Intimate History of Neurology and Psychiatry in America," *Journal of Nervous and Mental Disease* 98 (1943): 603.

14. Weir Mitchell, "Address," 102, 108, 110. For the response the following year (June 1895) by the president of the AMPA, see Edward Cowles, "The Advancement of Psychiatry in America," *American Journal of Insanity* 10 (1896): 364–386.

15. See the discussion by Gerald Grob, "Adolf Meyer on American Psychiatry in 1895," *American Journal of Psychiatry* 119 (1963): 1135–37; Gerald Grob, *Mental Illness and American Society, 1975–1940* (Princeton: Princeton University Press, 1983), 39–41.

16. For a detailed case study of the intertwined roles of the asylum and moral treatment, see Nancy Tomes, *The Art of Asylum-Keeping: Thomas Story Kirkbride and the Origins of American Psychiatry* (Philadelphia: University of Pennsylvania Press, 1994). See also the well-illustrated discussions in Lynn Gamwell and Nancy Tomes, *Madness in America: Cultural and Medical Perceptions of Mental Illness before 1914* (Ithaca, NY: Cornell University Press, 1995), 37–118; Carla Yanni, *The Architecture of Madness: Insane Asylums in the United States* (Minneapolis: University of Minnesota Press, 2007), 17–50.

17. Richard Dewey, "Early Days and Experiences in Psychiatry, 1870–1900," *Medical Life* 35 (1928): 97. See also his *Recollections of Richard Dewey: Pioneer in American Psychiatry* (Chicago: University of Chicago Press, 1936).

18. William Alanson White, *The Autobiography of a Purpose* (Garden City, NY: Doubleday, Doran, 1938), 39.

19. James M. Keniston, "Recollections of a Psychiatrist," *American Journal of Insanity* 72 (1916): 465.

20. Andrew Delano Abbott, "The Emergence of American Psychiatry, 1880–1930," PhD diss., University of Chicago, 1982, 54, 57. Abbott's reconstruction of the profession and career paths of assistant physicians in asylums on 49–62 is unparalleled in the literature of the history of American psychiatry. The most vivid and detailed memoir of an assistant physician in an asylum is Victor R. Small, *I Knew 3000 Lunatics* (New York: Farrar

and Rinehart, 1935). See also Hardie Albright, *All the Living: A Play in Three Acts. Based on the Book "I Knew 3000 Lunatics" by Victor R. Small* (New York: Samuel French, 1938).

21. N. Emmons Paine, "Psychiatry and the Homeopathic Medical Colleges," in *Transactions of the World's Congress of Homoeopathic Physicians and Surgeons, Chicago Ill., May 29 to June 3, 1893,* ed. Pemberton Dudley (Philadelphia: Sherman, 1894), 937–944. Psychiatric training in medical schools and university associations with mental hospitals would only gain ascendancy after 1914, and until then psychiatry remained largely "in isolation" from the rest of the medical profession, according to Franklin G. Ebaugh and Charles A. Rymer, *Psychiatry in Medical Education* (New York: Commonwealth Fund, 1942), 19.

22. Grob, "Adolf Meyer," 1141. The problem persisted until well into the next century. The neurologist and psychiatrist Louis Casamajor remarked in 1943, "Until fairly recently, the mental hospitals drew their doctors from the lower tenth of the medical school classes. This is not true today" ("Notes for an Intimate history," 600).

23. Paine, "Psychiatry," 941. For a view of what the patients of homeopathic asylums were administered instead of sedatives, see the chapter on the "compendium of materia medica" for the treatment of mental disorders in Selden Haines Talcott, *Mental Diseases and Their Modern Treatment* (New York: Boericke and Runyon, 1901), 264–341. Homeopathic institutional care of the insane is unfortunately underrepresented in two excellent surveys: John S. Haller Jr., *The History of Homeopathy: The Academic Years, 1820–1935* (London: Informa Healthcare, 2005); John S. Haller Jr., *The History of American Homeopathy: From Rational Medicine to Holistic Health Care* (New Brunswick, NJ: Rutgers University Press, 2009).

24. Selden H. Talcott, "Hahnemann and His Relations to Psychological Medicine," *American Homoeopathist* 24 (1898): 28–34. See also George Allen, "The Situation at Middletown," *North American Journal of Homoeopathy* 40 (1892): 772. It should be remembered that despite his generous philanthropic efforts to establish regular scientific medicine in the twentieth century, John D. Rockefeller preferred irregular homeopathic physicians.

25. Weir Mitchell, "Address," 103.

26. George Weisz, *Divide and Conquer: A Comparative History of Medical Specialization* (Oxford: Oxford University Press, 2006), 98. See also the directory *Medical and Surgical Register of the United States* (Detroit: R. L. Polk, 1896).

27. This is based on the estimates in the charts for 1850 to 1930 provided in Abbott, "The Emergence," 146–149. Most alienists (647) were in federal,

state, county, or municipal asylums for the insane, 6 in institutions for epileptics, 33 in asylums or "colonies" for the feebleminded, and 58 in mostly one-man, family-run private sanitariums. As for physicians in private specialty practice (mostly "nerve specialists" or neurologists), there were none in 1865, 15 in 1870, 55 in 1880, and 130 in 1895. In 1895 private practitioners made up an estimated 15 percent of the profession, but expanded rapidly as asylum physicians began to migrate from the asylums after 1900, challenging the traditional jurisdiction of neurologists over the treatment of the neuroses. In 1870 90 percent of all physicians who treated nervous and mental disorders were in government institutions for the insane, a proportion dropping to 78 percent in 1880, 77 percent in 1890, 69 percent in 1900, and 59 percent in 1910—all during a period in which many new state hospitals had opened. By 1920 only 49 percent of physicians who treated nervous and mental diseases were in institutions for the insane, and 33 percent were in private practice.

28. See Walter E. Barton, *The History and Influence of the American Psychiatric Association* (Washington, DC: American Psychiatric Press, 1987). One of the earliest uses of the term "psychiatrist" to refer to an American asylum physician can be found in G. Alder Blumer, "The Coming of Psychasthenia," *Journal of Nervous and Mental Disease* 33 (May 1906): 338. World War I seemed to be the turning point, with the term "psychiatrist" quickly becoming the accepted term for the profession by the early 1920s.

29. *Proceedings of the American Medico-Psychological Association Annual Meeting* (Utica, NY: American Medico-Psychological Association, 1896), 1–27.

30. For narrative purposes I shall refer to asylum physicians as male, as the vast majority of them were. I hope the reader will forgive me for taking this liberty. However, there were indeed a small number of female asylum physicians who tended female patients. They were paid less than male asylum physicians and, given the barriers to career advancement within the walls of these institutions, they therefore tended to have shorter lengths of employment. See Constance M. McGovern, "Doctors or Ladies? Women Physicians in Psychiatric Institutions, 1872–1900," *Bulletin of the History of Medicine* 55 (1981): 88–107.

31. These particular details, as well as a few others that follow, were taken from a chapter describing common "accidents among the insane" in one of the first training manuals for attendants and nurses who worked in asylums. See William D, Granger, *How to Care for the Insane: A Manual for Nurses* (New York: G. P. Putnam's Sons, 1898), 71–84. For descriptions of what conditions might be like within a typical asylum, especially those which might deviate from the ideal, see John S. Billings and Henry

M. Hurd, *Suggestions to Hospital and Asylum Visitors* (Philadelphia: Lippincott, 1895).

32. White, "Autobiography, 50.

33. Edward J. Kempf, "The Unsane Treatment of Our Insane Patients," in *Edward J. Kempf: Selected Papers,* ed. Dorothy Clarke Kempf and John C. Burnham (Bloomington: Indiana University Press, 1974), 14.

34. Richard W. Fox, *So Far Disordered in Mind: Insanity in California 1870–1930* (Berkeley: University of California Press, 1978), 37.

35. Grob, "Adolf Meyer," 1139–40.

36. Adolf Meyer, "Report from Kankakee (1896)," in *The Collected Papers of Adolf Meyer.* Vol. 2: *Psychiatry,* ed. Eunice E. Winters (Baltimore: The Johns Hopkins Press, 1951), 50.

37. See Lawson G. Lowrey, "On the Indexing of Case Records—An Analysis of the Methods Used at the Danvers State Hospital," *Bulletin of the Massachusetts Commission on Mental Disorders* 2 (April 1918): 311. Abandoning the case books in favor of individual case files was not only practical from clinical and bureaucratic perspectives, but also necessary for larger research purposes. At Danvers, one of the few innovative places that became a dual clinical and research institution under the leadership of Superintendant Charles W. Page, the case book system was discontinued in 1903. For the adoption of the loose-leaf and individual case file system in general hospitals, see Stanley Joel Reiser, "Creating Form out of Mass: The Development of the Medical Record," in *Transformation and Tradition in the Sciences: Essays in Honor of I. Bernard Cohen,* ed. Everett Mendelsohn (Cambridge, MA: Harvard University Press, 1984), 307–310.

38. Adolf Meyer, "The Treatment of the Insane (1894)," in *The Collected Papers,* 2:45.

39. Sidney Ringer and Harrington Sainsbury, "Sedatives," in *A Dictionary of Psychological Medicine,* ed. Daniel Hack Tuke (Philadelphia: P. Blakiston, 1892), 2:1128–47. This last point was well made by David Healy, *The Creation of Psychopharmacology* (Cambridge, MA: Harvard University Press, 2002), 37–75.

40. George Allen, "Some Statistical Facts Concerning Insanity," in Dudley, *Transactions,* 972. The story of American homeopathic alienists still needs to be told. For an introductory discussion of the homeopathic sect in psychiatry, with reference to its practice in the Lehigh Valley (Allentown, Bethlehem, Easton) area of Pennsylvania, see Abbott, "The Emergence," 368–370, 373–403.

41. Bayard Taylor Holmes, "The Laboratory for Psychiatry," in *The Friends of the Insane, The Soul of Medical Education, and Other Essays* (Cincinnati: Lancet-Clinic Publishing, 1911), 138. As a point of comparison between

asylums and other medical inpatient institutions, see the description of the routine laboratory analysis of the urine and the blood of patients in two general hospitals in 1900 and 1925, which seem to have been of little direct clinical or therapeutic relevance but which legitimized the image of the physician as a man or woman of science, in Joel D. Howell, *Technology in the Hospital: Transforming Patient Care in the Early Twentieth Century* (Baltimore and London: The Johns Hopkins University Press, 1995). The conduct of urinalysis and blood counts in general hospitals, especially when repeated, signaled that the institution was providing a continuous monitoring model of patient care—something which asylums for the insane and state hospitals were often accused of not doing. Hence, the lack of laboratory technologies in asylums was increasingly interpreted as patient neglect, even though such tests could lead to no medical benefit for the patient.

42. Kempf, "Unsane Treatment," 19. Beginning in 1901 patients at the Manhattan State Hospital East on Ward's Island were placed in tents due to extreme overcrowding in the buildings. Some tents were designated for tuberculosis patients. See C. Floyd Haviland, "Tent Life for the Tuberculosis Insane," *Proceedings of the American Medico-Psychological Association* 16 (1902): 289–291. At the same institution twenty individuals—"Most of these patients were very stupid and demented"—were put in a separate tent to see if they would improve. Apparently they did. See Arthur D. Wright, "Tent Life for the Demented and Uncleanly," *Proceedings of the American Medico-Psychological Association* 16 (1902): 281.

43. Granger, *How to Care for the Insane,* 23. For examples of asylum life in two New York asylums, including a discussion of the roles of attendants, see Ellen Dwyer, *Homes for the Mad: Life inside Two Nineteenth-Century Asylums* (New Brunswick, NJ: Rutgers University Press, 1987). For a factually grim depiction of the difficult working conditions of nurses and attendants at one state hospital between 1902 and 1917 see Gerald N. Grob, *The State and the Mentally Ill: A History of the Worcester State Hospital in Massachusetts, 1830–1920* (Chapel Hill, NC: University of North Carolina Press, 1966), 319–328. Social historians will find much of interest in the testimonies of the superintendant, physicians, nurses, attendants and support staff in *Report of the Special Committee on Investigation of the Government Hospital for the Insane, with Hearings May 4—December 13, 1906, and Digest of the Testimony. U.S. Congress (59th) House Reports, December 3, 1906—March 4, 1907, Volumes 3 and 4* (Washington, D.C.: Government Printing Office, 1907). The 2251 pages of this report provide the most detailed information available about the inner life of an American asylum of that era.

44. Grob, *Mental Illness,* 26.
45. This was the typical response the young Adolf Meyer received from his colleagues and attendants at Kankakee and Worcester when attempting to institute reforms. See Grob, "Adolf Meyer," 1140–41.

2. Adolf Meyer Brings Dementia Praecox to America

1. Meyer wrote this in a letter to Henry H. Donaldson, who was then the head of the biology program at Clark University in Worcester, Massachusetts. Barbara J. Betz, "Adolf Meyer: Youth and Young Manhood 1866–1896. Part III, Chapters X through XIII," *American Journal of Social Psychiatry* 1 (1981): 33.
2. The reign of a third of a century is offered by Barbara Sicherman, "Adolf Meyer (1866–1950): Profile of A Swiss-American Psychiatrist," *Swiss-American Historical Society Newsletter* 5 (December 1969): 2; and a reign of 1895 to 1940 is posited by one of his former colleagues at the Phipps Clinic, Theodore Lidz, "Adolf Meyer and the Development of American Psychiatry," *American Journal of Psychiatry* 123 (1966): 321. Despite (or perhaps because of) the considerable amount of personal documents that he left behind, there is no book-length biography of Meyer. Biographical information can be found in the articles cited in this chapter as well as in the introductions to the various sections of Meyer's writings in Alfred Lief, ed., *The Commonsense Psychiatry of Dr. Adolf Meyer* (New York: McGraw-Hill, 1948). Although he was originally from Switzerland, Swiss scholars have shown little interest in Meyer because he wrote primarily in English and he was difficult to comprehend, let alone translate. See U. H. Peters, "Adolf Meyer und die Bezeihung zwischen deutscher und amerikanischer Psychiatrie," *Fortschrift für Neurologie und Psychiatrie* 58 (1990): 332–338. Meyer's reforms at Worcester are chronicled by Gerald N. Grob, *The State and the Mentally Ill: A History of Worcester State Hospital in Massachusetts, 1830–1920* (Chapel Hill, NC: University of North Carolina Press, 1966), 263–319. A recent work which will define Meyer studies for the next generation is Susan D. Lamb, "Pathologist of the Mind: Adolf Meyer, Psychobiology and the Phipps Psychiatric Clinic at the Johns Hopkins Hospital, 1908–1917 (PhD diss., The Johns Hopkins University, 2010).
3. See the entry on Meyer in Edward Shorter, *A Historical Dictionary of Psychiatry* (Oxford: Oxford University Press, 2005), 177–178. On the even longer influence of Meyer in Britain, see Michael Gelder and Hugh Freeman, "Adolf Meyer (1866–1950)," in *A Century of Psychiatry,* ed. Hugh Freeman (Barcelona: Mosby, 1999), 103–106. A sympathetic treatment of Meyer's influence on American psychiatry can be found in Jack Press-

man, *Last Resort: Psychosurgery and the Limits of Medicine* (Cambridge: Cambridge University Press, 1998), 1–18.

4. Thomas Bonner, *American Doctors and German Universities: A Chapter in International Intellectual Relations 1870–1914* (Lincoln: University of Nebraska Press, 1963), 139.

5. Betz, "Adolf Meyer . . . Part III," 38.

6. The English translation caused a similar public frenzy when it appeared three years later. See Max Nordau, *Degeneration* (New York: D. Appleton, 1895). On the similar concerns of a Swiss contemporary of Meyer's, Carl Gustav Jung, see Richard Noll, "Max Nordau's *Degeneration*, C. G. Jung's Taint," *Spring* 55 (1993): 1–12. For the influence of degeneracy theory in medicine, psychiatry, and culture, see J. Edward Chamberlin and Sander L. Gilman, eds., *Degeneration: The Dark Side of Progress* (New York: Columbia University Press, 1985); Daniel Pick, *Faces of Degeneration: A European Disorder, c. 1848–c. 1918* (Cambridge: Cambridge University Press, 1989); Ian Dowbiggin, *Inheriting Madness: Professionalization and Psychiatric Knowledge in Nineteenth Century France* (Berkeley: University of California Press, 1991); Elof Axel Carlson, *The Unfit: A History of a Bad Idea* (Cold Spring Harbor, NY: Cold Spring Harbor Press, 2001). The "original sin" quote is from George Drinka, *The Birth of Neurosis: Myth, Malady and the Victorians* (New York: Simon and Schuster, 1984), 53. On the whole, degeneration theory was not a major topic of discussion in American psychiatry after the late 1890s. The role of degeneration in producing dementia praecox is hardly mentioned in the hundreds of articles published on this subject between 1900 and 1920, with most (still only a handful) appearing only after the 1910 creation of the Eugenics Records Office.

7. See Adolf Meyer, "A Review of the Signs of Degeneration and of Methods of Registration," *American Journal of Insanity* 52 (1895): 344–363.

8. Betz, "Adolf Meyer . . . Part III," 34.

9. Ibid., 38.

10. Ibid., 33, 36, 37.

11. Edward Shorter, *A History of Psychiatry: From the Era of the Asylum to the Age of Prozac* (New York: Wiley, 1997), 92.

12. Adolf Meyer, "The Bridge between Parent and Scientist (1938)," in *The Collected Papers of Adolf Meyer*. Vol. 4, *Mental Hygiene,* ed. Eunice Winters (Baltimore: The Johns Hopkins University Press, 1952), 378.

13. Adolf Meyer, "British Influences in Psychiatry and Mental Hygiene (1933)," in *The Collected Papers of Adolf Meyer*. Vol. 3, *Medical Teaching,* ed. Eunice Winters (Baltimore: The Johns Hopkins University Press, 1951), 404.

14. Betz, "Adolf Meyer . . . Part III," 38.

15. Adolf Meyer, "Thirty-five Years of Psychiatry in the United States and Our Present Outlook (1928)," in *The Collected Papers of Adolf Meyer.* Vol. 2, *Psychiatry,* ed. Eunice Winters (Baltimore: The Johns Hopkins Press, 1951), 7.

16. Eunice E. Winters, "Adolf Meyer's Two and a Half Years at Kankakee. May 1, 1893–November 1, 1895," *Bulletin of the History of Medicine* 40 (1966): 441.

17. For a general discussion of this method, see W. F. Bynum, *Science and the Practice of Medicine in the Nineteenth Century* (Cambridge: Cambridge University Press, 1994).

18. The rise and fall of this neuropathology-driven "first biological psychiatry" is vividly chronicled in Edward Shorter, *A History of Psychiatry,* 69–112.

19. Winters, "Adolf Meyer's Two and a Half Years," 446.

20. Ibid., 444.

21. Adolf Meyer, "Report From Kankakee," (1895), in *Collected Papers,* 2:50.

22. Winters, "Adolf Meyer's Two and a Half Years," 449.

23. Meyer, "British Influences," 419.

24. Winters, "Adolf Meyer's Two and a Half Years," 453.

25. Some alienists cited at least nine different diagnostic categories: "The generally recognized mental diseases, as late as 1895, included the following types:—mania, melancholia, dementia, imbecility, idiocy, general paresis, chronic delusional insanity or paranoia and senile insanity." James V. May, *Mental Diseases: A Public Health Problem* (Boston: Richard G. Badger, Gorham Press, 1922), 223–224. However, each of these terms had multiple modifiers (acute, chronic, etc.).

26. William Alanson White, *The Autobiography of a Purpose* (Garden City, NY: Doubleday, Doran, 1938), 53.

27. These included the various editions of the following volumes, listed here according to their first American editions: Thomas S. Clouston, *Clinical Lectures on Mental Diseases* (Philadelphia: Henry C. Lea's Son, 1884); Henry Maudsley, *Physiology and Pathology of Mind* (New York: Appleton, 1867); W. R. Gowers, *A Manual of Nervous Diseases* (Philadelphia: Blakiston, Son, 1888); Daniel Hack Tuke, *A Dictionary of Psychological Medicine,* 2 vols. (Philadelphia: P. Blakiston, Son, 1892). The various editions of the following works by these American neurologists were also in common usage: Charles L. Dana, *A Textbook of Nervous Disease* (New York: William Wood, 1892); Edward C. Spitzka, *Insanity: Its Classification, Diagnosis, and Treatment. A Manual for Students and Practitioners of Medicine* (New York: Birmingham, 1883). Textbooks by American authors that would be influential between 1900 and 1920, such as that by A. Church and Frederick

Peterson, and one by Moses Allan Starr, began appearing only in 1899. For an analysis of the knowledge transfer from European to American specialists in nervous and mental diseases up to the year 1910, after which the influence of European texts in American medical schools disappeared, see Andrew Delano Abbott, "The Emergence of American Psychiatry, 1880–1930," PhD diss., University of Chicago, 1982, 304–338.

28. For historical background on the *Einheitspsychose* concept, see G. E. Berrios and D. Beer, "Unitary Psychosis Concept," in *A History of Clinical Psychiatry: The Origin and History of Psychiatric Disorders,* ed. German Berrios and Roy Porter (London: Athlone Press, 1995), 312–335. As a formal psychiatric concept it largely spread to American asylum physicians and neurologists through the translation of the influential 1861 second edition of the textbook of Wilhelm Griesinger (1817–1868), *Mental Pathology and Therapeutics,* 2nd ed., trans. C. L. Robertson and J. Rutherford (New York: William Wood, 1882). Few American alienists of the generation of the 1890s mentioned Griesinger's book, although it certainly influenced the preceding generation, including figures such as Edward Cowles (see Chapter 4). In Griesinger's era the idea of a unitary psychosis (a single disease of insanity) matched the prominent belief that the brain functioned in a holistic manner. Convincing evidence of the localization of function in the brain would not be accepted until after about 1871 or 1872. After this time Griesinger's famous dictum "Mental disease is brain disease" would be reinterpreted to support the notion of separate and specific mental diseases that may involve separate and specific brain structures and functions. Based on analysis of the topics of articles on mental disease published in the American periodical literature, the shift to an acceptance of disease specificity among members of the psychiatric elite occurred only after 1910: "Most mental disease periodical writing in both Europe and America in the years before 1910 concerned 'insanity,' the general category, rather than the specific diseases analyzed here" (Abbott, "The Emergence of American Psychiatry," 328–329). Later Meyerian and Freudian psychiatrists were particularly attracted to a dimensional approach to diagnosis, and an underappreciated book that was devoted to a return to the unitary concept of mental illness in the mid-twentieth century is Karl Menninger, *The Vital Balance: The Life Process in Mental Health and Illness* (New York: Viking, 1963). Menninger reviews the history of the unitary concept and offers a remarkably complete and astute appendix (pages 419–489) that traces the history of psychiatric classification.

29. Adolf Meyer to August Hoch, handwritten letter on the stationary of the Worcester Lunatic Hospital, 15 October 1896, Adolf Meyer Collection,

Box I/1725/2, Alan Mason Chesney Archives, Johns Hopkins University, Baltimore. Press, 1966).

3. Emil Kraepelin

1. My biographical material on Emil Kraepelin are derived from the following sources: the classic text translated by Eric J. Engstrom, Wolfgang Burgmair, and Matthias M. Weber, "Emil Kraepelin's 'Self-Assessment': Clinical Autobiography in Historical Context," *History of Psychiatry* 13 (2002): 89–119; Emil Kraepelin, *Memoirs,* ed. Hanns Hippius, Gerd Peters, and Detlev Ploog, trans. J. Rubin (Berlin: Springer Verlag, 1987). Both autobiographical documents by Kraepelin were found among the personal papers he left behind in Munich at the time of his death; they were published more than half a century later. Also useful is Jacques M. Quen, "Introduction to the English Edition," in Emil Kraepelin, *Psychiatry: A Textbook for Students and Physicians.* Vol. 1, *General Psychiatry* (1899), trans. Helga Metoui (Canton, MA: Science History Publications, 1990), vii–xxii. American readers should also be aware that Kraepelin is pronounced "krep-LEEN," with a Germanic roll of the "r."

2. Edward Shorter, *A History of Psychiatry: From the Era of the Asylum to the Age of Prozac* (New York: Wiley, 1997), 100.

3. Kraepelin, *Memoirs,* 57–58.

4. Engstrom et al., "Self-Assessment," 109–110.

5. Ibid., 92.

6. Kraepelin, *Memoirs,* 3.

7. Ibid., 6, 7.

8. Ibid., 11.

9. Ulrich Müller, Paul C. Fletcher, and Holger Steinberg, "The Origin of Pharmacopsychology: Emil Kraepelin's Experiments in Leipzig, Dorpat and Heidelberg (1882–1892)," *Psychopharmacology* 184 (2006): 132.

10. Kraepelin, *Memoirs,* 19.

11. Ibid., 21. On the scientific activities of Kraepelin during his years in Leipzig, see the following: Holger Steinberg, *Kraepelin in Leipzig: Eine Begegnung von Psychiatrie und Psychologie* (Bonn: Psychiatrie-Verlag, 2001); Holger Steinberg and Ulrich Müller, "Emil Kraepelin 1882/1883 in Leipzig und seine frühen pharmacopsychologischen Arbeiten im Lichte der aktuellen Forschung," in *200 Jahre Psychiatrie an der Universität Leipzig: Personen und Konzepte,* ed. Matthias C. Angemeyer and Holger Steinberg (Berlin: Springer, 2005). The correspondence between Kraepelin and Wundt can be found in Holger Steinberg, ed., *Briefwechsel zwischen Wilhelm Wundt und Emil Kraepelin: Zeugnis einer jahrzehntelangen Freundschaft* (Bern: Huber, 2002).

12. Kraepelin, *Memoirs*, 26.

13. On Kraepelin's activities in Lebus and Dresden, see the following works by Holger Steinberg and Matthias C. Angermeyer: "Der Aufenthalt Emil Kraepelins an der schlesischen Provinzial-Irrenanstalt Lebus," *Fortschrift für Neurologie und Psychiatrie* 70 (2002): 252–258; "Emil Kraepelin's Years at Dorpat as Professor of Psychiatry in Nineteenth-Century Russia," *History of Psychiatry* 12 (2001): 297–327.

14. This is the opinion of Ulrich Müller et al., "The Origin of Pharmacopsychology," 131. While in Heidelberg Kraepelin summarized the research he conducted in Dorpat in a monograph: Emil Kraepelin, *Über die Beinflussung einfacher psychischer Vorgänge durch einige Arzneimittel* (Jena: Fischer, 1892). After the publication of this monograph he no longer explored the influence of drugs on psychological processes. The essential source for Kraepelin's years in Dorpat is Wolfgang Burgmair, Eric J. Engstrom, and Matthias M. Weber, eds., *Emil Kraepelin*. Vol. 4, *Kraepelin in Dorpat, 1886–1891* (Munich: Belleville, 2003).

15. Kraepelin, *Memoirs*, 46.

16. The major publications by Kraepelin and his associates can be found in Wolfgang Burgmair, Eric J. Engstrom, and Matthias Weber, et al., eds., *Emil Kraepelin*. Vol. 5, *Kraepelin in Heidelberg, 1891–1903* (Munich: Belleville, 2005). Indispensible is Paul Hoff, *Emil Kraepelin und die Psychiatrie als klinische Wissenschaft* (Berlin: Springer, 1994), especially his discussion of the evolution of the dementia praecox concept in Kraepelin's works (112–126).

17. German E. Berrios, "Die Gruppirung der psychischen Krankheiten . . . Part III, by Karl Kahlbaum (1863) (Classic Text No. 25; introduction and translation)," *History of Psychiatry* 7 (1996): 167. For Kahlbaum's influence on Kraepelin and Carl Wernicke (1848–1905), who devised a competing approach to the insanities in the 1890s, see Mario Lanczik, "Karl Ludwig Kahlbaum (1828–1899) and the Emergence of Psychopathological and Nosological Research in German Psychiatry," *History of Psychiatry* 3 (1992): 53–58. Short biographies of Kahlbaum and Hecker can be found in Abdulla Kraam, "Karl Ludwig Kahlbaum, by Dr. Ewald Hecker (1899) (Classic Text No. 73; introduction and translation)," *History of Psychiatry* 19 (2008): 77–85; Abdullah Kraam and German E. Berrios, "Ewald Hecker (1843–1909), by Karl Wilmanns (Classic Text No. 52; introduction and translation)," *History of Psychiatry* 13 (2002): 455–465.

18. Karl Kahlbaum, *Die Gruppirung der psychischen Krankheiten und die Eintheilung der Seelenstörungen* (Danzig: A. W. Kafemann, 1863).

19. See German E. Berrios, "The Clinico-Diagnostic Perspective in Psychopathology, by K. Kahlbaum (1878) (Classic Text No. 70; introduction and translation)," *History of Psychiatry* 18 (2007): 231–245.

20. Karl Kahlbaum, *Die Katatonie, oder das Spannungsirresein* (Berlin: Hirschwald, 1874).
21. Abdullah Kraam, " 'Hebephrenia. A Contribution to Clinical Psychiatry,' by Dr. Ewald Hecker in Görlitz (1871) (Classic Text. No. 72; introduction and translation, Part 1)," *History of Psychiatry* 20 (2009): 96–97. See also Abdullah Kraam, " 'On the Origin of the Clinical Standpoint in Psychiatry,' by Dr. Ewald Hecker in Görlitz (1871) (Classic Text no. XX; introduction and translation)," *History of Psychiatry* 15 (2004): 345–360. Although Kahlbaum and Hecker worked closely together for ten years, and despite their good personal relationship, in a June 1889 lecture (published the following year) Kahlbaum made it a point to remind the world that it was he, not his younger disciple, who first identified and named hebephrenia, and that it was he who had provided Hecker with his own case material. See G. E. Berrios and A. Kraam, " 'On Heboïdophrenia,' by Director. Dr. Kahlbaum in Görlitz (1890)," (Classic Text no. 50; introduction and translation)," *History of Psychiatry* 13 (2002): 197–208.
22. Kraam, "Hebephrenia," 93
23. Kraepelin, *Memoirs,* 60–61. Scholars have commented on Kraepelin's original diagnostic cards and have cast doubt on his contention that his conclusions followed his data. On this, see Volker Roelcke, "Biologizing Social Facts: An Early 20th Century Debate on Kraepelin's Concepts of Culture, Neurasthenia, and Degeneration," *Culture, Medicine and Psychiatry* 21 (1997): 383–403. For a review of the debate on Kraepelin's diagnostic cards, see Hannah S. Decker, "The Psychiatric Works of Emil Kraepelin: A Many-Faceted Story of Modern Medicine," *Journal of the History of the Neurosciences* 13 (2004): 267–272. For a challenge to Kraepelin's claim that insights followed research, see Eric J. Engstrom and Matthias M. Weber, "Kraepelin's 'Diagnostic Cards': The Confluence of Clinical Research and Preconceived Categories," *History of Psychiatry* 8 (1997): 375–385.
24. Kraepelin, *Memoirs,* 59. Leon Daraszkiewicz, *Über Hebephrenie, inbesondere deren schwere Form* (Dorpat: H. Laakmann, 1892).
25. Heinrich Schüle, *Klinische Psychiatrie: Specielle Pathologie und Therapie der Geisteskrankheiten. Dritte völlig umgearbeitete Auflage* (Leipzig: F. and W. Vogel, 1886), 14, 250, 451–452, 477; Arnold Pick, "Über primäre Demenz (so. Dementia praecox) in jugendlichen Alter," *Praeger mediziniche Wochenschrift* 16 (1891): 312–315. On the priority issue, see German E. Berrios, Rogelio Luque, and José M. Villagrán, "Schizophrenia: A Conceptual History," *International Journal of Psychology and Psychological Therapy* 3 (2003): 111–140. For a discussion of Morel's use of the term in 1852 and 1860, see Ian Dowbiggin, "Back to the Future: Valentin Magnan, French Psychiatry, and the Classification of Mental Diseases, 1885–1925," *Social*

History of Medicine 9 (1996): 383–408. Kraepelin prominently listed Schüle's 1886 edition in the introduction of his own work: Emil Kraepelin, *Psychiatrie: ein kurzes Lehrbuch für Studirende und Aerzte. Zweite, vollständig umgearbeitete Auflage* (Leipzig: Abel, 1887), 3.

26. See Edward Shorter, *A Historical Dictionary of Psychiatry* (Oxford: Oxford University Press, 2005), 268.

27. Kraepelin, *Memoirs*, 68.

28. Adolf Meyer, "Thirty-five Years of Psychiatry in the United States and Our Present Outlook (1928)," in *The Collected Papers of Adolf Meyer. Vol. 2, Psychiatry*, ed. Eunice Winters (Baltimore: Johns Hopkins Press University, 1951), 6.

29. Adolf Meyer, "Emil Kraepelin, M.D. 1856–1926 (1926)," in *The Collected Papers of Adolf Meyer. Vol. 3, Medical Teaching*, ed. Eunice Winters (Baltimore: The Johns Hopkins University Press, 1951), 523.

30. Engstrom et al., "Self-Assessment," 101.

31. Emil Kraepelin, *Psychiatrie: Ein Lehrbuch für Studirende und Aerzte, Fünfte, vollständig Auflage* (Leipzig: Verlag von Johann Ambrosias Barth, 1896), v, my translation.

32. Eric Engstrom, *Clinical Psychiatry in Imperial Germany* (Ithaca, NY: Cornell University Press, 2003), 144. Engstrom placed more weight on proximal, social, material, and bureaucratic determinants of Kraepelin's classification system than on Kraepelin's claims about the unbiased scientific accuracy of the conclusions he drew from his research data. Doubt is therefore cast on Kraepelin's claims about the correspondence of his diagnostic categories with actual, real, natural disease entities. In his discussion Engstrom argued, "Kraepelin's influential classification of psychiatric disorders was a derivative of this new economy of clinical research" (146). In other words, it was a perfect fit for the specific bureaucratic needs of the operation of the Heidelberg clinic in the 1890s. After moving to Munich and opening a new university clinic in November 1904, Kraepelin and his colleagues acknowledged in their first annual report that they were very conscious of the fact that they were on uncertain ground when diagnosing dementia praecox in patients who were under observation for only a short time. See Robert Gaupp's comments in the "Dementia praecox" section in *Jahresbericht über die Königliche Psychiatrische Klinik in München für 1904 und 1905* (Munich: J.F. Lehmanns Verlag, 1907), 38.

33. See ibid., 123–127. I am indebted to Eric Engstrom for clarifying my communication of this point when this book was still in manuscript form.

34. In 1878 Karl Kahlbaum made the point that these four ancient forms of insanity were not diseases but just clusters of symptoms: "A fundamental

principle of modern clinical psychopathology can be formulated out of these observations, namely, that the known forms of mental disorder are just symptom-clusters or general psychological states . . . and by themselves cannot be considered as autonomous conditions or lead to any specific diagnosis" (Berrios, "The Clinico-Diagnostic Perspective," 236).

35. William Alanson White, *The Autobiography of A Purpose* (Garden City, NY: Doubleday, Doran, 1938), 54.

36. Emil Kraepelin, "Dementia Praecox," in *The Clinical Roots of the Schizophrenia Concept: Translations of Seminal European Contributions on Schizophrenia,* ed. John Cutting and Michael Shepherd (Cambridge: Cambridge University Press, 1987), 13. This selection from Kraepelin is the first English translation of his section on dementia praecox in the fifth edition of *Psychiatrie,* and it is from pages 426–441 of the original German edition.

37. Kraepelin, "Dementia Praecox," 19, 20–21.

38. Ibid., 21–24.

39. Adolf Meyer, "Book Review," *American Journal of Insanity* 53 (October 1896): 298–302. Rather than footnoting every quote from this short review by Meyer, the reader should assume they they can all be found in the same source.

4. The American Reception of Dementia Praecox and Manic Depressive Insanity, 1896–1905

1. See Adolf Meyer, "Special Reports of the Medical Department, Worcester Lunatic Hospital, 1898," in *The Collected Papers of Adolf Meyer.* Vol. 2. *Psychiatry,* ed. Eunice Winters (Baltimore: The Johns Hopkins University Press, 1951), 62–67; State Board of Lunacy and Charity of Massachusetts, *Twentieth Annual Report of the State Board of Lunacy and Charity of Massachusetts, January 1899* (Boston: Wright and Potter, 1899), 75–76.

2. Meyer, "Special Reports," 63, 66.

3. Lawrence C. Kolb and Leon Roizon, *The First Psychiatric Research Institute: How Research and Education Changed Practice* (Washington, DC: American Psychiatric Press, 1993), 40.

4. The biographical material on Hoch that follows, including descriptions of his personality, comes from Adolf Meyer, "August Hoch, M.D., 1868–1919," *Archives of Neurology and Psychiatry* 2 (1919): 573–576; Adolf Meyer, "August Hoch, M.D., 1868–1919," *Journal of Nervous and Mental Disease* 50 (1919): 510–512; Kolb and Roizon, *The First Psychiatric Research Institute,* 39–46.

5. Ludwig Hirt, *The Diseases of the Nervous System: A Text-Book for Physicians and Students,* trans. August Hoch with the assistance of Frank R. Smith,

introduction by William Osler (New York: D. Appleton, 1893). The only psychiatric topics discussed by Hirt are the "neuroses" of neurasthenia, epilepsy, and hysteria and their hypnotic treatment. The insanities are not addressed.

6. Details of the life and career of Edward Cowles, his hiring of August Hoch, and the establishment of the laboratory at McLean are based on the information provided in S. B. Sutton, *Crossroads in Psychiatry: A History of the McLean Hospital* (Washington, DC: American Psychiatric Press, 1986), 111–165. The "most solid friendship of Hall's later life" was that with Cowles, according to Dorothy Ross, *G. Stanley Hall: The Psychologist as Prophet* (Chicago: University of Chicago Press, 1972), 160–161.

7. G. Stanley Hall, "Laboratory of the McLean Hospital, Somerville, Mass.," *American Journal of Insanity* 51 (1895): 362–363. These details about Hoch's activities are from a report by Edward Cowles about the McLean laboratory in response to a request for information on a circular dated 24 September 1894 and sent from a Brown University professor. Sections of it were published in French translation in E. B. Delabarre, "Les Laboratoires de Psychologie en Amerique," *L'Année Psychologique* 1 (1894): 209–255. Hall possessed the complete report and used it as the basis of his January 1895 article. On Mosso and his "ergograph" of 1890, see Camillo Di Giulio, Franca Daniele, and Charles M. Tipton, "Angelo Mosso and Muscular Fatigue: 116 Years after the First Congress of Physiologists," *Advances in Physiology Education* 30 (2006): 51–57.

8. Hall, "Laboratory," 363.

9. This is according to an unacknowledged source in Sutton, *Crossroads,* 114.

10. Charles Beard, *A Practical Treatise on Nervous Exhaustion (Neurasthenia), Its Symptoms, Nature, Sequences, Treatment* (New York: William Wood, 1880). The literature on neurasthenia in the late nineteenth century and early twentieth is of considerable size, but a primary reference of value is F. G. Gosling, *Before Freud: Neurasthenia and the American Medical Community, 1870–1910* (Chicago: University of Illinois Press, 1987). See also Edward Shorter, *From Paralysis to Fatigue: A History of Psychosomatic Illness in the Modern Era* (New York: Free Press, 1991).

11. This census capacity statistic for the McLean Asylum in 1887 is from Sutton, *Crossroads,* 121. A journalistic account of the elite nature of the McLean Hospital can be found in Alex Beam, *Gracefully Insane: The Rise and Fall of America's Premiere Mental Hospital* (New York: Public Affairs, 2001).

12. According to Cowles, "Neurasthenia is a morbid condition of the nervous system, and its underlying characteristics are excessive weakness,

and irritability or languor, with mental depression and weakened attention. . . . Neurasthenia may be regarded as the initial term of many nervous disorders having a varied etiology." Edward Cowles, *Neurasthenia and Its Mental Symptoms. The Shattuck Lecture, 1891. Read before the Massachusetts Medical Society, June 9, 1891* (Boston: David Clapp and Son, 1891), 2. See also Edward Cowles, "The Laboratories of the McLean Hospital for Research in Pathological Psychology and Biochemistry," in *The Institutional Care of the Insane in the United States and Canada*, vol. 2, ed. Henry Hurd (Baltimore: The Johns Hopkins University Press, 1916), 621; Adolf Meyer, "Thirty-Five Years of Psychiatry in the United States and Our Present Outlook," *American Journal of Psychiatry* 8 (1929): 8–9. A summary of his views can also be found in Kenneth Levin, "Edward Cowles on Neurasthenia," *McLean Hospital Journal* 2 (1977): 167–176.

13. See the references to his original ideas from publications in the early 1890s in Cowles, "The Laboratories of the McLean Hospital," 618–636.

14. The Harvard neuropathologist Elmer E. Southard referred to Cowles as the leading alienist of the past quarter century in his June 1919 presidential address to the American Medico-Psychological Association. See E. E. Southard, "Cross-Sections of Mental Hygiene, 1844, 1869, 1894," *American Journal of Insanity* 76 (1919): 107.

15. Cited in Cowles, "The Laboratories of the McLean Hospital," 623. The original observation in French appears in Delabarre, "Les Laboratoires," 235.

16. The descriptions of the laboratory and its equipment are from Hall, "Laboratory," 359–360.

17. August Hoch and Emil Kraepelin, "Über die Wirkung der Theebestandtheile auf körperliche und geistige Arbeit," *Psychologische Arbeiten* 1 (1895): 378–488. This was published as a separate offprint by William Engelmann of Leipzig later that same year.

18. August Hoch, "On Certain Studies with the Ergograph," *Journal of Nervous and Mental Disease* 28 (1901): 620–628. For his summary of the work of others between 1895 and 1903, see also August Hoch, "A Review of Some Psychological and Physiological Experiments Done in the Connection with Mental Diseases," *Psychological Bulletin* 1 (1904): 241–257.

19. See the biographical sketch "Dr. William Noyes" in Henry Hurd, ed., *The Institutional Care of the Insane in the United States and Canada*, vol. 4 (Baltimore: The Johns Hopkins University Press, 1918), 465.

20. August Hoch, "Kraepelin on Psychological Experimentation in Psychiatry," *American Journal of Insanity* 52 (1896): 387–396. This was a summary of Emil Kraepelin, "Der psychologische Versuch in der Psychiatrie," *Psychologische Arbeiten* 1 (1895): 1–97.

21. Hoch, "Kraepelin," 391–392.

22. Ibid., 387, 388, 393–394. I am indebted to Eric Engstrom for pointing out to me that Kraepelin increased his emphasis on the importance of the role of the premorbid personality in the eighth edition of his textbook, which appeared in four volumes between 1909 and 1915. On Kraepelin's linkage, indeed the diagnostic primacy, of the destruction of the core intellectual functions of the personality to dementia praecox in 1913, see the discussion in Paul Hoff, *Emil Kraepelin und die Psychiatrie als klinische Wissenschaft* (Berlin: Springer-Verlag, 1994), 124–125.

23. August Hoch, "Nerve-Cell Changes in Somatic Diseases. A Preliminary Consideration," *American Journal of Insanity* 55 (1898): 240.

24. Edward Shorter, *A History of Psychiatry: From the Era of the Asylum to the Age of Prozac* (New York: Wiley, 1997), 109.

25. See Sutton, *Crossroads,* 146, 150–152. In a paper published in 1910 the neuropathologist Elmer E. Southard quoted extensively from a letter he received from Cowles in response to a question about the origin of the clinic or case conference method, attributing its first use in the United States in 1889 to Cowles. See Elmer E. Southard, "The Laboratory Work of the Danvers State Hospital, Hawthorne, Massachusetts, with Especial Relation to the Policy Formulated by Dr. Charles Whitney Page. Superintendent, 1888–1898, 1903–1910," in *Danvers State Hospital Laboratory Papers: Charles Whitney Page Series* (Boston: W. M. Leonard, 1910, 24–25.

26. Adolf Meyer, "August Hoch, M.D., 1868–1919," *Archives of Neurology and Psychiatry* 2 (1919): 574.

27. August Hoch, "On Changes in the Nerve Cells of the Cortex in a Case of Acute Delirium and a Case of Delirium Tremens," *American Journal of Insanity* 54 (1898): 593.

28. Edward Cowles, "Progress in the Clinical Study of Psychology," *Proceedings of the American Medico-Psychological Association Annual Meeting* 6 (1899): 116.

29. Ibid., 114.

30. Edward Cowles, "Annual Report (Eighty-fourth) of the Superintendent of the McLean Hospital," in *Eighty-Eighth Annual Report of the Trustees of the Massachusetts General Hospital. Including the General Hospital in Boston, the McLean Hospital and the Convalescent Home in Waverly. 1901* (Boston: Barta Press, 1902), 198. In his report Cowles admitted, "The development of the method of clinical conferences, with the introduction of the teachings of Kraepelin, were reinforced by Dr. Hoch's second visit to Heidelberg in 1897" (194).

31. Cowles, "Progress," 126–127.

32. August Hoch, "On the Clinical Study of Psychiatry," *Proceedings of the American Medico-Psychological Association Annual Meeting* 7 (1900): 326.

This paper was also published in the *American Journal of Insanity* 57 (1900): 281–295.

33. For a summary of "psychological research in psychiatric settings" during this period, see Josef Brozek, *Explorations in the History of Psychology* (Lewisburg, PA: Bucknell University Press, 1984), 207–228. For a contemporary description of a short-lived (September 1897 to 1899) psychology lab at the asylum in Kankakee, Illinois, see William Krohn, "Laboratory Psychology as Applied to the Study of Insanity," *Psychiater* 1 (1898): 49–66. August Hoch, who had assumed his new position as chief of the New York State Psychiatric Institute on 1 February 1910, continued his biographical research into premorbid personality types and, in 1912 and 1913, attempted to replicate Kraepelin's pharmacopsychologic "model psychosis" paradigm. Without ever identifying the drugs, nor publishing his results, he abandoned this Kraepelinian line of work. See Lawrence C. Kolb and Leon Roizin, *The First Psychiatric Institute: How Research and Education Changed Practice* (Washington, DC: American Psychiatric Press, 1993), 42. After Hoch resigned from the Institute on 1 October 1917 experimental psychological research within the Institute and with institutionalized populations elsewhere was sporadic until the 1930s. From 1930 until his death in 1962, Carney Landis (1897–1962) revived experimental psychological research at the New York State Psychiatric Institute, but like many of the other researchers who had come from academic backgrounds, especially from biomedical research, he was skeptical of psychoanalysis. This led to decades of warfare between psychoanalytic clinicians on the one side, and biological researchers and experimental psychologists on the other. See David Zubin and Joseph Zubin, "From Speculation to Empiricism in the Study of Mental Disorders: Research at the New York State Psychiatric Institute in the First Half of the Twentieth Century," *Annals of the New York Academy of Sciences* 294 (1977): 104–135. For the first use of psychological research methods to establish research diagnostic criteria for studying schizophrenia, see R. L. Cautin, "David Shakow and Schizophrenia Research at the Worcester State Hospital: The Roots of the Scientist-Practitioner Model," *Journal of the History of the Behavioral Sciences* 44 (2008): 219–237; David Shakow, "The Worcester State Hospital Research on Schizophrenia (1927–1946), *Journal of Abnormal Psychology Monograph* 80 91972): 67–110.

34. The first phrase is from Nathan G. Hale Jr., *Freud and the Americans: The Beginnings of Psychoanalysis in the United States, 1876–1917* (Oxford: Oxford University Press, 1971), 71–97. The second phrase is from Shorter, *A History of Psychiatry*, 99–109.

35. Silke Feldmann, "Die Verbreitung der Kraepelinischen Krankheitslehre
im deutschen Sprachraum zwischen 1893 und 1912 am Beispiel der Dementia Praecox," PhD diss., Justus-Liebig-Universität, Giessen, Germany,
2005, 5. The summary of criticisms aimed at Kraepelin by his German
colleagues is drawn from this useful dissertation. In articles published in
1906 and 1912, Alfred Hoche sharply criticized Kraepelin's claim that
there were "natural disease entities" that could be specified, mocking it as
a "hunt after a phantom." Instead the clinical phenomena of mental disorder were best regarded as "symptom-complexes" that were neither symptoms of a specific disease nor evidence for underlying natural disease entities, as postulated by Kraepelin. In addition to the sections on Hoche in
Feldmann's dissertation, see T. R. Denning and G. E. Berrios, "Introduction to 'The Significance of Symptom-Complexes in Psychiatry' by Alfred
Hoche [1912]," (Classic Text No. 7), *History of Psychiatry* 2 (1991): 329–333;
G. E. Berrios and T. Dening, "Alfred Hoche and DSM-III-R," *Biological
Psychiatry* 29 (1991): 93–95; and especially Volker Roelcke, "Naturgege-
bene Realität oder konstrukt? Die debate über die 'Natur' der Schizophrenie, 1906 bis 1932," *Fundamanta Psychiatrica* 2 (2000): 44–53. Hoche's critique was known and mentioned in passing in the writings of American
authors such as Adolf Meyer, August Hoch, E. E. Southard, Smith Ely
Jelliffe, and Charles Macphie Campbell, but Hoche's "symptom-complex"
idea was not discussed in detail and played no apparent role in the evolution of the American framing of dementia praecox. Oswald Bumke completed his *Habilitation* under Hoche, a massive volume documenting the
scientific literature on disturbances in the behavior of the pupils of the eyes
in nervous and mental disorders, including dementia praecox: Oswald
Bumke, *Die Pupillenstörungen bei Geistes- und Nervenkrankheiten* (Jena: G.
Fischer, 1904). On Bumke see G. W. Schimmelpenning, "Oswald Bumke
(1877–1950): His Life and Work," *History of Psychiatry* 4 (1993): 483–497;
Hanns Hippius, Hans-Jürgen Möller, Norbert Müller and Gabriele
Neundörfer-Kohl, *The University Department of Psychiatry in Munich: From
Kraepelin and His Predecessors to Molecular Psychiatry* (Heidelberg: Springer,
2008), 111–133; Oswald Bumke, *Erinnerungen und Betrachtungen. Der Weg
eines Deutschen Psychiaters* (Munich: Richard Pflaum-Verlag, 1952). Just
prior to replacing Kraepelin in Munich, in October 1923 Bumke said at a
conference, "*What if dementia praecox simply does not exist?* . . . if we let go of
the idea that dementia praecox is a disease entity, and speak instead of
schizophrenic reactions which might be elicited in different ways, the
whole picture will immediately become clearer." Per Dalen, "'The Dissolution of Dementia Praecox' by Oswald Bumke [1924] (classic Text No.
13), trans. and introduction, *History of Psychiatry* 4 (1993): 137.

36. Alexander Bernstein, "Ueber die Dementia praecox," *Allgemenie Zeitschrift für Psychiatrie* 60 (1903): 569.

37. Emil Kraepelin, "Zur Diagnose und Prognose der Dementia Praecox," *Allgemenie Zeitschrift für Psychiatrie* 56 (1899): 254–263.

38. The literature on this phenomenon is unwieldy and relentless. As a single cogent source on this topic I recommend Hannah S. Decker, "How Kraepelinian Was Kraepelin? How Kraepelinian Are the Neo-Kraepelinians?—From Emil Kraepelin to DSM-III," *History of Psychiatry* 18 (2007): 337–360. *DSM-III* of 1980 and its successors are not, strictly speaking, proposing a nosology in the medical sense because there is no explicit claim that the diagnostic categories represent natural disease entities.

39. Sutton, *Crossroads,* 150–151.

40. These passages are from the most recent English translation of Kraepelin's 1899 sixth edition of *Psychiatrie:* Emil Kraepelin, *Psychiatry: A Textbook for Students and Physicians,* vol. 2, ed. with an introduction by Jacques Quen, trans. Sabine Ayed (Canton, MA: Science History Publications, 1990), 103.

41. Ibid., 120.

42. Ibid., 121. With each new edition of his textbook, the number of pages devoted to dementia praecox expanded significantly. In the fifth edition of 1896, dementia praecox was described in 39 pages; in the sixth edition of 1899, 78 pages; in the seventh edition of 1904, 105 pages; in the eighth edition of 1913, 305 pages, taking up most of volume 3.

43. Ibid., 137.

44. Ibid., 139.

45. Ibid., 154. Kraepelin's speculation about chemical damage to the cortex was informed by his interest in the research on "inner secretions" (later, "hormones") conducted in the early 1890s. He was not speaking of neurotransmitters here; the concept did not exist. The transmission of impulses from one part of the brain to another was assumed by many to be electrical, not chemical, in Kraepelin's lifetime. At the risk of lapsing into presentism, I should note that endocrinological research provided a direct and important analogical bridge that led to the much later verification of chemical neurotransmitters in the brain. Following the 1921 discovery by Otto Loewi (1873–1961) of a substance in the peripheral nervous system, later identified as acetylcholine, "neurohormones" and "neurohumors" were terms applied to the proposed internal secretions of nerve cells. Indeed the term "neurotransmitter" did not come into use until the 1960s, only after the revolutionary decade between 1955 and 1965, when the "electrical brain" became the "chemical brain." See Eliot Valenstein, *The War of the Soups and the Sparks: The Discovery of Neu-*

rotransmitters and the Dispute over How Nerves Communicate (New York: Columbia University Press, 2005).

46. David Healy et al., "Historical Overview: Kraepelin's Impact on Psychiatry," *European Archives of Psychiatry and Clinical Neuroscience* 258 (2008): 18. For background on Kraepelin's other great insanity, see K. Trede, P. Salvatore, C. Baethge, A. Gerhard, C. Maggini, and R. J. Baldessarini, "Manic-Depressive Illness: Evolution in Kraepelin's Textbook, 1883–1926," *Harvard Review of Psychiatry* 13 (2005): 155–178; and especially Paul Hoff, *Emil Kraepelin und die Psychiatrie als klinische Wissenschaft* (Berlin: Springer-Verlag, 1994), 97–111.

47. See the illuminating discussion of these points in David Healy, *Mania: A Short History of Bipolar Disorder* (Baltimore: Johns Hopkins University Press, 2008), 74–77, 135–160. I am indebted to David Healy for a personal communication in which he pointed out the relative slowness with which manic-depressive insanity was received in Britain.

48. This point is illustrated in in Richard Noll, "The Blood of the Insane," *History of Psychiatry* 17 (2006): 412n1. To give just one example: only six neuropathological studies of manic-depressive illness of any significance appeared in print between 1899 and 1988, and the modern era of neuropathological studies of mood disorders began only in 1998, according to P. J. Harrison, "Is Any of This Real? The Word from the Grave," in *Bipolar Disorder: The Upswing in Research and Treatment,* ed. C. McDonald, K. Schultze, R. M. Murray, and M. Tohen (London: Taylor and Francis, 2005). See also Frederick K. Goodwin and Kay Redfield Jamison, *Manic-Depressive Illness: Bipolar Disorders and Recurrent Depression,* 2nd ed. (Oxford: Oxford University Press, 2007).

49. Hoch, "On the Clinical Study of Psychiatry," 331. According to Meyer, "This group is the best-founded entity of the Heidelberg school." Adolf Meyer, "A Review of Recent Problems in Psychiatry [1904]," in *The Collected Papers,* 2:348.

50. Hurd, *The Institutional Care of the Insane,* 2:111.

51. Meyer, "Thirty-Five Years," 13.

52. Charles W. Page, "Superintendent's Report," in Board of Trustees, Connecticut Hospital for the Insane, *Report of the Connecticut Hospital for the Insane to the Governor for the Two Years Ended September 30, 1900* (Middletown, CT: Pelton and King, 1900), 8–9.

53. Board of Trustees, *Connecticut Hospital for the Insane,* 32.

54. The information about Henry Smith Noble relies on his biographical sketch in Hurd, *The Institutional Care of the Insane,* 4:464–465.

55. Henry S. Noble, "Dementia Praecox," *Yale Medical Journal* 7 (1900–1901): 287–292. Noble's article appeared in a 1901 issue. See also Richard Noll,

"The American Reaction to Dementia Praecox, 1900," *History of Psychiatry* 15 (2004), 127–128.

56. Noble, "Dementia Praecox," 287–288.

57. This second point is raised by numerous critics throughout the twentieth century, including, to some extent, Adolf Meyer. It is also raised in an unpublished thesis: Atsu Greg Winchell, "The Era of Prognosis and Prophylaxis: The Reception of Dementia Praecox in North America, 1896–1910," Master's thesis, York University, Toronto, 1991.

58. Noble, "Dementia Praecox," 292.

59. Adolf Meyer, "Albert M. Barrett, M.D. 1871–1936," *Archives of Neurology and Psychiatry* 36 (1936): 613.

60. Emil Kraepelin, *Clinical Psychiatry,* translated, adapted and abridged by Allan Ross Diefendorf (New York: Macmillan, 1902); Emil Kraepelin, *Clinical Psychiatry,* translated, adapted and abridged by Allan Ross Diefendorf (New York: Macmillan, 1907). These translations of Kraepelin's sixth and seventh editions of *Psychiatrie,* respectively, remained the standards in the English language. For the next fifteen years after Diefendorf's first translation appeared, there were few other English-language sources for Kraepelin's actual words on dementia praecox. One was a brief article from 1901 containing a translation of Kraepelin's description of dementia praecox in the sixth edition of 1899 by Albert E. Brownrigg, an assistant physician at the New Hampshire State Hospital in Concord. The second was a chapter on dementia praecox in the authorized translation of Kraepelin's lectures on clinical psychiatry by a British psychiatrist, Thomas Johnstone. In 1919 an English translation appeared of Kraepelin's new reformulations of dementia praecox and manic-depressive insanity, published in German in the 1913 third volume of the eighth edition of *Psychiatrie.* See Albert E. Brownrigg, "A General View of Dementia Praecox: Translated from the German of Kraepelin," *American Journal of Insanity* 58 (1901): 121–132; Emil Kraepelin, *Lectures on Clinical Psychiatry,* trans. and ed. Thomas Johnstone (London: Bailliere, 1904). This latter book was a translation of Emil Kraepelin, *Einführung in die Psychiatrische Klinik: Dreissig Vorlesungen* (Leipzig: Barth, 1901).

61. Although he embedded the information in a lecture delivered in March 1897 with more general themes, Meyer attempted to educate his American colleagues about Kraepelin and dementia praecox in Adolf Meyer, "A Short Sketch of the Problems of Psychiatry," *American Journal of Insanity* 53 (1896–1897): 538–549.

62. F. X. Dercum, "A Clinical Classification of Insanity," *Journal of Nervous and Mental Disease* 38 (1901): 502, 505.

63. William Pickett, "A Study of the Insanities of Adolescence," *Journal of Nervous and Mental Disease* 38 (1901): 453–454.

64. The three similar versions by Gershom H. Hill are "Dementia Praecox," *Proceedings of the American Medico-Psychological Association* 7 (1900): 282–290; "Dementia Praecox," *American Journal of Insanity* 57 (1900): 319–324; "Dementia Praecox," *Transactions of the Iowa State Medical Society* 18 (1900): 299–308. The following year he published a different, much more polished article under the same title: Gershom H. Hill, "Dementia Praecox," *Medical Age* 19 (1901): 526–533.

65. Benjamin F. Gue, *The History of Iowa from the Earliest Times to the Beginning of the Twentieth Century*. Vol. 4, *Iowa Biography* (New York: Century History, 1903), 131.

66. See Gershom H. Hill, "A Review of the Pathological Work in the Hospital for the Insane in Independence, Iowa," *Proceedings of the American Medico-Psychological Association* 8 (1901): 272–274. He presented this paper at the annual meeting in June 1901.

67. Hill, "Dementia Praecox" (1901), 529.

68. Hill, "Dementia Praecox," *Proceedings*, 290.

69. Ibid., 288.

70. Board of Trustees, Bellevue and Allied Hospitals, *Nomenclature of Diseases and Conditions and Rules for the Recording and Filing of Histories for Bellevue and Allied Hospitals* (New York: Martin B. Brown Press, 1903), 32.

71. David Kennedy Henderson, *The Evolution of Psychiatry in Scotland* (Edinburgh: E. & S. Livingstone, 1964), 158. Henderson was an intern and then an assistant physician at the New York Psychiatric Institute from 1908 to 1911.

72. State of New York, State Commission in Lunacy, *Seventeenth Annual Report, October 1, 1904 to September 30, 1905* (Albany: Brandow Printing, 1906), 920.

73. State of New York, State Commission in Lunacy, *Sixteenth Annual Report, October 1, 1903 to September 30, 1904* (Albany: Brandow Printing, 1905), 768. This report contains separate annual reports for Manhattan State Hospital East and West. The statistical tables for each reflect pre-Kraepelinian diagnostic categories. Superintendent Dent of the West branch noted in his narrative that the staff had been trying to apply the concepts of Kraepelin for the past three years but were having difficulty converting from the old terms to the new. However, on page 802 he noted that the 290 new admissions during the fiscal year that would have fit the diagnosis of dementia praecox constituted 31.8 percent of the total. Manic-depressive insanity is not mentioned.

74. State of New York, State Commission in Lunacy, Seventeenth Annual Report, 915.

75. Ibid., 916.

76. See the table representing the percentage distribution of psychoses of first admission to state hospitals for the years 1922, 1926, 1930, 1935, and 1940 in Gerald Grob, *Mental Illness and American Society, 1875–1940* (Princeton: Princeton University Press, 1983), 192.

77. Charles E. Rosenberg, *The Trial of the Assassin Guiteau: Psychiatry and Law in the Gilded Age* (Chicago: University of Chicago Press, 1968), 248.

78. Adolf Meyer, "Discussion of Cooperation between the State Hospitals and the Institute [1904]," in *The Collected Papers,* 2:124.

79. Clarence B. Farrar, "Dementia Praecox in France with some References to the Frequency of This Diagnosis in America," *American Journal of Insanity* 62 (1905): 269, 267. Farrar based his charts on published annual reports, all of which reflect fiscal years, not calendar years. The annual report for the 1896–97 fiscal year at the Worcester Lunatic Hospital—the exact period and place where Meyer was diagnosing dementia praecox for the first time anywhere in North America—lists the combined cluster of disorders of periodical insanity, circular insanity, and maniacal and depressed states as more prevalent. But beginning in 1898 (except for the year 1900, in which there was a virtual tie) dementia praecox dominated Meyer's institution. McLean Hospital introduced dementia praecox and depressive-maniacal insanity in its 1899 annual report, but the latter diagnosis remained far more prevalent in all subsequent annual reports. At the Boston Insane Hospital dementia praecox was introduced in 1902 but was diagnosed far less often than old categories of diseases such as the various manias and melancholias and circular insanity. However, in 1905 dementia praecox rose in admission numbers to almost overtake these mood disorders. Manic-depressive insanity was still not employed as a diagnosis at this institution in 1905. Two institutions in New York State, the Bloomingdale Asylum and the Utica State Hospital, still used pre-Kraepelinian concepts. The institutions where dementia praecox dominated admissions from its first year of introduction were the Connecticut Hospital for the Insane in Middletown (1898), the Manhattan State Hospital, West (1904), and two Massachusetts institutions, the Danvers Insane Hospital (1903) and the Taunton Insane Hospital (1903).

80. See Jules Christian, "Dementia Praecox: A Contribution to the Study of Hebephrenia," *American Journal of Insanity* 58 (1901): 239. The article originally appeared in 1899 in the *Annales Medico-Psychologique.* It describes twenty-eight case histories of patients with hebephrenia, a disease that Christian prefers to call dementia praecox but that is also synonymous with "juvenile dementia" and "idiocy" (217–218).

81. Adolf Meyer said this at a meeting of all the superintendents of state hospitals in the State of New York in December 1903. Adolf Meyer,

"Discussion of the Cooperation between the State Hospitals and the Institute [1904]," in *The Collected Papers,* 2:136.

82. See the frequency tables in Emil Kraepelin, *Psychiatrie: Ein Lehrbuch für Studirende und aertze. Achte, vollständig umgearbeitete Auflage, I. Band* (Leipzig: Barth, 1908), 527. In 1942 Meyer characterized these, and similar tables in a later edition of *Psychiatry,* as "remarkably frank and telling." See Adolf Meyer, "General Historical Fragments on the Neurological and Psychiatric Specialties," in *The Collected Papers of Adolf Meyer.* Vol. 1, *Neurology,* ed. Eunice Winters (Baltimore: The Johns Hopkins University Press, 1950), 314.

83. See Stewart Paton, *Psychiatry: A Textbook for Students and Physicians* (Philadelphia: J. P. Lippincott, 1905). For context, see C. B. Farrar, "I Remember Stewart Paton," *American Journal of Psychiatry* 117 (1960): 160–162. For a description of some possible English-language sources in British publications that some American alienists may have had access to, see R. M. Ion and M. D. Beer, "The British Reaction to Dementia Praecox, 1893–1913. Part I," *History of Psychiatry* 13 (2002): 285–304. Kraepelin's ideas also appeared in translations of foreign works, many of which were obscure a century ago and remain so today, as for example a work that originally appeared in French: Joseph Rogues de Fursac, *Manual of Psychiatry,* ed. and trans. Joseph Collins (New York, 1905).

84. J. T. W Rowe, "Is Dementia Praecox the 'New Peril' in Psychiatry?," *American Journal of Insanity* 63 (1907): 385–393. This article is based on a presentation Rowe made in Boston in June 1906.

5. The Lost Biological Psychiatry

1. This literature on the sociology of science is large, and many of its contributions are well known to scholars. Although I have kept an interpretive framework for the narrative in this text to a minimum, all of the following have shaped my perspective: Ludwig Fleck, *Genesis and Development of a Scientific Fact,* trans. Fred. Bradley and Thaddeus J. Treen, with a foreword by Thomas S. Kuhn (Chicago: University of Chicago Press, 1979), originally published in German in 1935; Georges Canguilhem, *The Normal and the Pathological,* trans. Carolyn R. Fawcett, with an introduction by Michel Foucault (New York: Zone Books, 1991), originally published in French in 1966; Georges Canguilhem, *A Vital Rationalist: Selected Writings from Georges Canguilhem,* ed. François Delaporte, translated by Arthur Goldhammer (New York: Zone Books, 1994); Paul Thagard, *How Scientists Explain Diseases* (Princeton: Princeton University Press, 1999); Ian Hacking, *The Social Construction of What?* (Cambridge, MA: Harvard University Press, 2000); Allan V. Horwitz, *Creating*

Mental Illness (Chicago: University of Chicago Press, 2002); Allan V. Horwitz and Jerome C. Wakefield, *The Loss of Sadness: How Psychiatry Transformed Normal Sorrow into Depressive Disorder* (Oxford: Oxford University Press, 2007); David Healy, *Mania: A Short History of Bipolar Disorder* (Baltimore: The Johns Hopkins University Press, 2008); Peter Conrad, *The Medicalization of Society: On the Transformations of Human Conditions into Treatable Disorders* (Baltimore: The Johns Hopkins University Press, 2007); Alexander Rosenberg, *Instrumental Biology or the Disunity of Science* (Chicago: University of Chicago Press, 1994); John Dupré, *The Disorder of Things* (Cambridge, MA: Harvard University Press, 1993); Charles E. Rosenberg, *Our Present Complaint: American Medicine, Then and Now* (Cambridge, MA: Harvard University Press, 2007); Gerald N. Grob and Allan V. Horwitz, *Diagnosis, Therapy and Evidence: Conundrums in Modern American Medicine* (New Brunswick, NJ: Rutgers University Press, 2010).

2. The best—but imperfect—source of descriptions of alienist-patient social interactions can be found in the large literature of autobiographical accounts. See Gail A. Hornstein, "Appendix: Bibliography of First-Person Narratives of Madness in English (Fourth Edition)," in *From Madness to Mental Illness: Psychiatric Disorder in Western Civilization,* ed. Greg Eghigian (New Brunswick, NJ: Rutgers University Press, 2009), 421–452.

3. Emil Kraepelin, *Psychiatry: A Textbook for Students and Physicians, Volume 2,* ed. with an introduction by Jacques Quen, trans. Sabine Ayed (Canton, MA: Science History Publications, 1990), 110.

4. Ibid.

5. William Rush Dunton Jr., "Some Points in the Diagnosis of Dementia Praecox," *American Journal of Insanity* 9 (1902–1903): 55, 57. This same paper was published the following year under the same title in *Medical Reports of the Sheppard and Enoch Pratt Hospital* 1 (1903): 77–85. He reported another case of dementia praecox with this same physical sign elsewhere: William Rush Dunton Jr., "Report of a Case of Dementia Praecox Insanity in Children and Adolescents," *American Journal of Medical Sciences* 123 (1902): 109–115.

6. Dunton, "Some Points," 54–55, 60, 58, 60.

7. William Rush Dunton Jr., "Report of a Case of Dementia Praecox with Autopsy," *American Journal of Insanity* 59 (1903): 427–439; William Rush Dunton Jr., "Report of a Second Case of Dementia Praecox with Autopsy," *American Journal of Insanity* 60 (1904): 761–775.

8. William Rush Dunton Jr., "Note on the Mechanical Irritability of the Facial Nerve in Dementia Praecox," *American Medicine* 10 (1905): 94.

9. An assistant physician at Danvers State Hospital claimed that 78 percent of the 241 dementia praecox patients he examined had a bluish tint to

their hands, and that it seemed to him that the "grade of cyanosis" might carry prognostic significance. See William Burgess Cornell, "Cyanosis in Dementia Praecox," *Journal of the American Medical Association* 12 (12 December 1912): 2208–9. Others claimed that a series of 115 dementia praecox patients all exhibited eye symptoms (enlarged pupils, negative sensory reflex, negative Piltz reflex, and so on) "not found in any other psychosis," which were due to an intestinal autointoxication process. See H. H. Tyson and L. Pierce Clark, "Preliminary Report on the Significance of the Ocular Signs and Symptoms of Dementia Praecox as Observed in a Series of 115 Consecutive Cases," *American Journal of Insanity* 64 (1907–1908): 563–573. See also L. Pierce Clark, "The Eye Syndrome of Dementia Praecox," *Journal of Nervous and Mental Disease* 35 (1908): 708–713. On the observable physical signs indicative of the vegetative nervous system in dementia praecox patients, or "schizophrenics" (an early use of this term), see Smith Ely Jelliffe, "The Vegetative Nervous System and Dementia Praecox," *New York Medical Journal,* 26 May 1917, 968–971.

10. Dunton, "Report of a Second Case," 775. Dunton published more papers on dementia praecox than any other American author between 1900 and 1912. See also the following by William Rush Dunton Jr.: "The Forms of Dementia Praecox," *Proceedings of the American Medico-Psychological Association* 14 (1907): 247–256; "The Cyclic Forms of Dementia Praecox," *Proceedings of the American Medico-Psychological Association* 16 (1909): 107–118; "Predementia Praecox," *Journal of the American Medical Association* 59 (21 December 1912): 2206–7. See also William Burgess Cornell, "A Study of the Auto and Somatopsychic Reaction in Four Cases of Dementia Praecox," *Proceedings of the American Medico-Psychological Association* 16 (1909): 475–482.

11. Elmer E. Southard, "The Mind Twist and the Brain Spot Hypotheses in Psychopathology and Neuropathology," *Psychological Bulletin* 11 (1914): 117–130.

12. See D. Riesman, "Deceased Diseases," *Annals of Medical History* 8 (1936): 160–167. On the rise of bacterial, serological, and chemical tests and their technologies, all important in the investigation of autointoxication theories, see Stanley Joel Reiser, *Medicine and the Reign of Technology* (Cambridge: Cambridge University Press, 1981), 122–143. In the opinion of two prominent American neuropathologists, not shared by other American physicians at the time, one variant of the autointoxication hypothesis had been rejected by 1915: "On the whole, the hypothesis of gastrointestinal autointoxication as a cause of mental disorder is not now regarded as well grounded." E. E. Southard and M. M. Canavan, "Note on the Relation of Somatic (Non-Neural) Neoplasms to Mental Disease," in State

Board of Insanity and the State Institutions for Mental Disease and Defect, Commonwealth of Massachusetts, *Collected Contributions, Third Series, 1915* (Boston: Wright and Potts, 1916), 246.

13. One of the best treatments of this "discontinuity" in the history of medicine can be found in K. Codell Carter, *The Rise of Causal Concepts of Disease* (Hants, England: Ashgate, 2003), 62–128.

14. Theodore Deeke, "On the Germ-Theory of Disease," *American Journal of Insanity* 24 (1874): 443–463. On Deeke, see Adolf Meyer, "Thirty-Five Years of Psychiatry in the United States and Our Present Outlook," *American Journal of Psychiatry* 8 (1928): 3.

15. See Merriley Borrell, "Organotherapy, British Physiology, and the Discovery of Internal Secretions," *Journal of the History of Biology* 9 (1976): 235–268; R. B. Welbourn, "Endocrine Diseases," in *Companion Encyclopedia of the History of Medicine,* ed. William F. Bynum and Roy Porter (London: Routledge, 1993), 1:484–511.

16. Hermann Senator, "Über ein Fall von Hydrothionamie und über Selbstinfektion durch abnorme Verdauungsvorgänge," *Berliner klinische Wochenschrift* 5 (1868): 254; Hermann Senator, "Über Selbstinfektion durch abnorme Zersetzungsvorgänge und ein dadurch bedingtes (dyskrasisches) Coma (Kussmaulscher Symptomenkomplex des 'diabetischen Coma')," *Zeitschrift für klinische Medizin* 7 (1884): 7–8.

17. Charles Jacques Bouchard, *Leçons sur les auto-intoxications dans les maladies* (Paris: F. Sauy, 1887); A. Conrepois, "The Clinician, Germs and Infectious Diseases: The Example of Charles Bouchard in Paris," *Medical History* 46 (2002): 197–220.

18. Charles Jacques Bouchard, *Lectures on Auto-Intoxication in Disease of Self-Poisoning of the Individual,* trans. Thomas Oliver (Philadelphia: F. A. David, 1894), 14.

19. E. Regis and F. A. Chevalier-Lavaure, "Auto-Intoxication in Mental Disease," *Medical Week* 11 (1893): 373.

20. Bouchard, *Lectures,* xi.

21. D. E. Jacobson, "Über Autointoxikationspsychosen," *Allgemeine Zeitschrift für Psychiatrie* 51 (1895): 379–406; Albert E. Sterne, "Toxicity as an Etiology of Nervous Disease," *Journal of the American Medical Association* 2 (1895): 103–106; Francis X. Dercum, "Address on Mental Diseases," *Journal of the American Medical Association* 24 (1895): 937–938.

22. Julius von Wagner-Jauregg, "Über Psychosen auf Grundlage gastrointestinaler Autointoxication," *Wiener klinische Wochenschrift* 10 (1896): 164–170.

23. Veronika Jahn, *Die gastrointestinalen Autointoxikationspsychosen des späten 19. Jahrhunderts* (Zurich: Juris Druck, 1975).

24. For an example of the variety of approaches to the autointoxication hypothesis prior to Starling's "hormone" concept, see C. A. Ewald, "Die Autointoxication," *Berliner klinische Wochenschrift* 37 (1900): 133–136, 166–170. The characterization of the Endocrine Society as a "sect" is from Andrew Delano Abbott, "The Emergence of American Psychiatry, 1880–1930," PhD diss., University of Chicago, 1982, 253. On the history of the organization, see Hans Lisser, "The Endocrine Society: The First Forty Years," *Endocrinology* 80 (1967): 5–28. For the tradition of endocrine psychiatry in the twentieth century, with specific reference to its characterization of mood disorders such as depression, see Edward Shorter and Max Fink, *Endocrine Psychiatry: Solving the Riddle of Melancholia* (New York: Oxford University Press, 2010).

25. Emil Kraepelin, Psychiatrie: Ein Lehrbuch für Studirende und Aertze. Fünfte, vollständig umgearbeitete Auflage, I. Band (Leipzig: J. A. Barth, 1896), 36–37.

26. Ibid., 439; Emil Kraepelin, "Dementia Praecox," in *The Clinical Roots of the Schizophrenia Concept: Translations of Seminal European Contributions on Schizophrenia,* ed. John Cutting and Michael Shepherd (Cambridge: Cambridge University Press, 1987), 23.

27. Kraepelin, *Psychiatry* (1990), 154.

28. Emil Kraepelin, *Psychiatrie: Ein Lehrbuch für Studirende und Ärztze. Achte, vollständig umgearbeitete Auflage, III. Band, II. Teil. Klinische Psychiatrie* (Leipzig: J. A. Barth, 1913), 931.

29. Emil Kraepelin und Johannes Lange, *Psychiatrie: Ein Lehrbuch für Studirende und Ärztze. Neunte, vollständig umgearbeitete Auflage. II. Band.* (Leipzig: J. A. Barth, 1927), 22. Kraepelin's speculations in 1896–1926 about a possible autotoxic etiology for dementia praecox were also traced by Paul Hoff, *Emil Kraepelin und die Psychiatrie als klinische Wissenschaft* (Berlin: Springer-Verlag, 1994), 117, 119, 123, 125.

30. Wilhelm Weygant, "Critical Comments on the Psychology of Dementia Praecox," in Cutting and Shepherd, *Clinical Roots,* 47–48. The original is Wilhelm Weygant, "Kritische Bemerkungen zur Psychologie der Dementia Praecox," *Monatsschrift für Psychiatrie und Neurologie* 22 (1907): 289–301. His famous monograph on the mixed states in manic-depressive insanity is Wilhelm Weygant, *Über die Mischzustande des manisch-depressive Irreseins* (Munich: Verlag von J. F. Lehmann, 1899). An English translation of this seminal paper in psychiatry is Paul Salvatore et al., "Weygandt's *On the Mixed States of Manic-Depressive Insanity:* A Translation and a Commentary on Its Significance in the Evolution of the Concept of Bipolar Disorder," *Harvard Review of Psychiatry* 10 (2002): 255–275.

31. Carl Gustav Jung, *The Psychology of Dementia Praecox,* trans. A. A. Brill (New York: Nervous and Mental Disease Publishing, 1936), 89. An earlier English translation by Frederick W. Peterson and A. A. Brill under the same title appeared in 1909 as part of the Nervous and Mental Disease Monograph Series (No. 3). The original German work is Carl Gustav Jung, *Über die Psychologie der Dementia praecox: Ein Versuch* (Halle, 1907).

32. Eugen Bleuler, *Dementia Praecox, or the Group of Schizophrenias,* trans. Joseph Zinkin (New York: International Universities Press, 1950), 34.

33. Silvia B. Sutton, *Crossroads in Psychiatry: A History of the McLean Hospital* (Washington, DC: American Psychiatric Press, 1986), 159.

34. Lawrence C. Kolb and Leon Roizin, *The First Psychiatric Institute: Research and Education Changed Practice* (Washington, DC: American Psychiatric Press, 1993), xv.

35. For the story of this extraordinary chapter in the history of American laboratory medicine, see the chapter on Van Gieson in Kolb and Roizin, *The First Psychiatric Institute,* 7–19. For a vivid discussion of Van Gieson's fall, see Ian Robert Dowbiggin, *Keeping America Sane: Psychiatry and Eugenics in the United States and Canada 1880–1940* (Ithaca, NY: Cornell University Press, 1997), 50–58.

36. See Ira Van Gieson, "Remarks on the Scope and the Organization of the Pathological Institute of the New York State Hospitals, Part II: The Toxic Basis of Neural Diseases," *State Hospitals Bulletin* 1 (1896): 407–488. Van Gieson, who appreciated the psychological side of human nature, nonetheless considered the insanities a subset of neurological diseases. His sudden elevation to prominence in psychiatry led to a discussion of his autointoxication hypotheses at the annual meeting of the American Medico-Psychological association in May 1897. See C. K. Clarke, "General Questions of Auto-Infection" and the following "Discussion," in *Proceedings of the American Medico-Psychological Association at the Fifty-Third Annual Meeting held in Baltimore, May 11–14, 1897* (Utica, NY: American Medico-Psychological Association, 1897), 150–157, 166–173.

37. Ira Van Gieson, "Notes and Comment," *American Journal of Insanity* 54 (1897–1898): 618.

38. Phillip Schaffer, "Otto Folin (1867–1934)," *Journal of Nutrition* 52 (1954): 7. See also Phillip Anderson Schaffer, "Otto Folin, 1867–1934: A Biographical Memoir," in *The National Academy of Sciences Biographical Memoirs* (Washington, DC: National Academy of Sciences, 1954), 27:47–82. This latter memoir contains a complete bibliography of Folin's works as well as a more detailed description of the chemical substances he searched for in the urine of the insane. The 1902 case study that served as the only qualified success for Folin's researches into the metabolism of the insane

is Otto Folin and Philip Schaffer, "On Phosphate Metabolism," *American Journal of Physiology* 7 (1902): 135–140. On the evolution of urinalysis in American medicine, and a mention of Folin's contributions, see Joel D. Howell, *Technology in the Hospital: Transforming Patient Care in the Early Twentieth Century* (Baltimore: The Johns Hopkins University Press, 1995), 69–102.

39. Schaffer, "Otto Folin (1867–1934)," *Journal of Nutrition*, 8–9.

40. Otto Folin, "Some Metabolism Studies with Special Reference to Mental Disorders," *American Journal of Insanity* 61 (1904–1905): 328.

41. Ibid., 299–300.

42. Ibid., 364.

43. John C. Whitehorn, "A Century of Psychiatric Research in America," in *One Hundred Years of Psychiatry,* J. K. Hall, Gregory Zilboorg, and Henry Alden Bunker (New York: Columbia University Press, 1944), 169.

44. Eugene F. McCampbell, "A Study of the Metabolism in Five Cases of Dementia Praecox," *Columbus Medical Journal* 28 (November 1904): 481–491, 546–557.

45. Lewis C. Bruce, "Clinical and Experimental Observations on Katatonia," *Journal of Mental Science* 49 (1903): 614–628. This laboratory study of dementia praecox may be the first in the British literature. Bruce examined the blood of these subjects and found correlations of psychotic symptoms with the number and nature of the white blood cells. Another alienist in Scotland who held to an autotoxic theory of dementia praecox was W. Ford Robertson. In his view dementia praecox was characterized by an inherited vulnerability to certain bacterial infections. See, for example, W. Ford Robertson, *Therapeutic Immunization in Asylum and General Practice* (New York: William Wood, 1921), 37.

46. For other studies that analyzed the urine of dementia praecox patients in a search for possible autotoxic processes, see the paper by the (then) director of the Clinical Laboratory of the Sheppard and Enoch Pratt Hospital, Francis M. Barnes, Jr., "A Study of the Metabolism of Two Atypical Cases Related to the Dementia Praecox Group," *American Journal of Insanity* 65 (1909): 591–605; Giacomo Pighini and Giuseppe Statuti, "Metabolism in Dementia Praecox," *American Journal of Insanity* 67 (1910–1911): 299–316; Ellison I. Ross, "The Source of Urinary Indol-Acetic Acid in Two Dementia Praecox Patients," *Archives of Internal Medicine* 12 (1913): 231–235, and his publication the following year of a study that examined both urine and feces, "Metabolism in Dementia Praecox," *Archives of Internal Medicine* 13 (1914): 889–903; Ellison L. Ross, "Some Forms of Urinary Nitrogen Affected by the Administration of Desiccated Thyroid to Dementia Praecox Patients," *Archives of Internal Medicine* 12 (1913): 746–750;

A. F. Wussow, "Metabolism Studies in Dementia Praecox," *Institute Quarterly* 4 (1913–1914): 71–81.

47. Blood: H. D. Purdum and R. E. Wells, "Dementia Praecox: A Composite History of Two Hundred Cases with Blood Findings in Fifty Cases," *Journal of the American Medical Association,* 4 July 1908, 34–36; Francis M. Barnes, "A Clinical Study with Blood Examinations of Two Atypical Cases Related to the Dementia Praecox Group," *American Journal of Insanity* 65 (1909): 559–591; Ellen Corson White and S. D. W. Ludlum, "The Differentiation between Dementia Praecox and Depressive States by So-called Biologic Blood-Tests," *Journal of the American Medical Association* 54 (4 June 1910): 1868; R. E. Wells, "Artificial Increase of Eosinophile Cells in Dementia Praecox," *Journal of the American Medical Association* 54 (22 January 1910): 284–285; Max A. Bahr, "Wasserman Reaction in Dementia Praecox," *Illinois Medical Journal* 25 (1914): 245–254; J. B. Rogers, "A Brief Study of the Blood Picture in Some Forms of Psychosis," *Iowa Medical Journal* 20 (1914): 594–598; H. W. Keatley and R. M. Bobbit, "Report of Five Cases of Dementia Praecox Treated by Nuclein Solution (Lundvall's Formula)," *West Virginia Medical Journal,* December 1914, 193–194.

Thyroid gland: Randolph Winslow, "Partial Thyroidectomy in Dementia Praecox," *Journal of the American Medical Association* 55 (3 October 1910): 1195–96.

Cerebrospinal fluid: G. H. H. Smith, "A Bacteriological Examination of the Cerebrospinal Fluid in Dementia Praecox," *Archives of Neurology and Psychiatry Pathological Laboratory* 4 (1909): 244–246.

Brain chemistry: W. Koch, "Chemical Study of the Brain in Cases of Dementia Praecox," *Journal of Experimental Medicine* 13 (1911): 301–307.

Ductless glands: F. X. Dercum and A. G. Ellis, "An Examination of the Ductless Glands in Eight Cases of Dementia Praecox," *Journal of Nervous and Mental Disease* 40 (1913): 73–90.

Lymph node abnormalities: Haven Emerson, "Note on the Incidence of Status Lymphaticus in Dementia Praecox," *Archives of Internal Medicine* 14 (1914): 881–882.

Thymus and pituitary glands: S. D. W. Ludlum, "The Thymus and Pituitary in Dementia Praecox as Physiological Characteristics in Insanity," *Transactions of the College of Physicians of Philadelphia* 37 (1915): 77–81; Beverley R. Tucker, "Pituitary Disturbance in Its Relation to the Psychoses of Adolescence," *Journal of the American Medical Association* 71 (13 August 1918): 330–333.

Optic neuritis and eye-movement abnormalities: Hayward G. Thomas, "Optic Neuritis and the Color Fields in the Diagnosis of Syphilis, Neurasthenia, Hyperthyroidism, Dementia Praecox, Manic-Depressive Insanity, and Third Generation Syphilis," *American Journal of Insanity* 72 (1915–1916): 59–91. One of the most modern and consistently cited experimental psychology studies of dementia praecox and manic-depressive illness was one that compared these clinical groups with normal controls in their ability to conduct what we today would call "smooth-pursuit eye movements." See Allan Ross Diefendorf and Raymond Dodge, "An Experimental Study of the Ocular Reactions of the Insane from Photographic Records," *Brain* 31 (1908): 451–489. In the late twentieth century such abnormalities were found in some persons with schizophrenia. See L. Erlenmeyer-Kimilng, "Biological Markers for the Liability to Schizophrenia," in *Biological Perspectives of Schizophrenia,* ed. H. Helmschen and F. Hein (New York: Wiley, 1987).

Saliva: John Albert Marshall, "The Salivary Factor and Its Relation to Dental Caries and Immunity in Dementia Praecox and Epilepsy," *American Journal of Physiology* 40 (1916): 1–11.

Fundus oculi: Clinton T. Cooke, "The Appearance of the Fundus Oculi in General Paresis, Manic Depressive Insanity and Dementia Praecox," *Ophthalmology* 13 (1916–1917): 34–42.

Shape and movement of hands: F. W. Langdon, "Biologic Aspects of Dementia Praecox," *American Journal of Insanity* 73 (1917): 681–692. Langdon, the medical director of the Cincinnati Sanitorium and a professor of psychiatry at the University of Cincinnati, noted the "simian" or ape-like hands of dementia praecox patients. His paper was a eugenic call to action.

Review articles on autointoxication and endocrinopathy: Milton A. Harrington, "The Endocrine Glands in Dementia Praecox," *State Hospitals Quarterly* 4 (1918): 183–190; H. I. Gosline, "Newer Conceptions of Dementia Praecox Based on Unrecognized Work," *Journal of Laboratory and Clinical Medicine* 2 (1917): 691–707; G. Dunlop Robertson, "The Catatonic Type of Dementia Praecox: The Genesis of the Auto-Intoxication in the Catatonic Types of Dementia Praecox, from an Hereditarily Transmitted Defective Biochemistry," *Journal of Mental Science* 61 (1915): 392–412.

It should be noted that the publications reviewed in this note are primarily from the period 1900–1920. This is a largely forgotten literature that was not included in the summary of research on dementia praecox between 1920 and 1935 in Nolan D. C. Lewis, *Research in Dementia Praecox (Past Attainments, Present Trends and Future Possibilities)* (New York: National Committee for Mental Hygiene, 1936).

48. Dunton, "The Forms of Dementia Praecox," 247.

49. R. O. Woodman, "Some Considerations of Insanity," *Medical Century* 14 (1906): 330. Woodman was a physician at the State Homeopathic Hospital in Middletown, New York.

50. C. Macfie Campbell, "A Modern Conception of Dementia Praecox: With Five Illustrative Cases," *Proceedings of the American Medico-Psychological Association* 16 (1909): 399.

51. William Alanson White, "Etiology of Dementia Praecox," *Journal of the American Medical Association* 46 (1906): 1519–21.

52. F. X. Dercum, "The Heboid-Paranoid Group (Dementia Praecox): Clinical Relations and Nature," *American Journal of Insanity* 62 (1906): 541–559. On Dercum, see C. W. Burr, "Memoir of Francis X. Dercum," *Transactions of the College of Physicians of Philadelphia* 54 (1932): 65–71; T. B. Throckmorton, "Francis X. Dercum: Physician, Teacher and Philosopher," *Journal of Nervous and Mental Disease* 96 (1942): 529–541.

53. See Roy Hoskins, *The Biology of Schizophrenia* (New York: Norton, 1946). See also Nolan D. C. Lewis, *Constitutional Factors in Dementia Praecox, with Particular Attention to Circulatory System and Some of the Endocrine Glands* (New York: Nervous and Mental Disease Publishing, 1923). For a larger context, see Richard Noll, "The Blood of the Insane," *History of Psychiatry* 17 (2006): 395–418; Richard Noll, "Kraepelin's 'Lost Biological Psychiatry'? Autointoxication, Organotherapy and Surgery for Dementia Praecox," *History of Psychiatry* 18 (2007): 301–320. A full account of Hoskins's schizophrenia research program still needs to be written, but a brief treatment can be found in David Shakow, "The Worcester State Hospital Research on Schizophrenia (1927–1946)," *Journal of Abnormal Psychology Monograph* 80 (1972), 67–110.

54. A. von Wasserman, A. Neisser, and C. Bruck, "Eine serodiagnostische Reaktion bei Syphilis," *Deutsche medizinische Wochenschrift* 32 (1906): 745–746. See also Felix Plaut, *The Wasserman Sero-Diagnosis of Syphilis in Its Application to Psychiatry,* trans. Smith Ely Jelliffe and Louis Casamajor (New York: Journal of Nervous and Mental Disease Publishing, 1909), originally published in German in 1907. For the story of how neurosyphilis became a scientific "fact," see Fleck, *Genesis and Development.* The original report of the discovery of the syphilis spirochete in the brains of paretics was H. Noguchi and J. W. Moore, "A Demonstration of *Treponema pallidum* in the Brain of Cases of General Paralysis," *Journal of Experimental Medicine* 17 (1913): 232–238.

55. This is my rephrasing of a famous sentence by Ludwig Fleck: "How does one define syphilis and set up a blood test, so that after some experience almost any research worker will be able to demonstrate a relation between them to a degree that is adequate in practice?" (Fleck, *Genesis and Development,* 98). For a description of the blood tests available at the beginning of the twentieth century, see Howell, *Technology in the Hospital,* 169–190.

56. H. Much and W. Holzmann, "Eine Reaktion im Blute von Geisteskran-ken," *Münchner mediziner Wochenschrift* 56 (1909): 1001–9. See also "Test-ing Insanity in the Laboratory. Two German Physicians Think They Have Found a Way to Diagnose Certain Forms. Call It Psycho-reaction. Reports Have Been Made on 151 Cases. Its Efficiency Is Doubted Here," *New York Times,* 1 August 1909, 16.

57. J. G. Fitzgerald, "Immunity in Relation to Psychiatry," *American Journal of Insanity* 67 (1911): 693.

58. August Fauser, "Zur Frage des Vorhandenseins spezifischer Schutzfer-mente im Serum vom Geisteskranken," *Münchner mediziner Wochenschrift* 11 (18 March 1913): 584–586; August Fauser, "Pathologische-serologische Befunde bei Geisteskrankheiten auf Grund der Abhaldenschen Anschau-ung und Methodik," *Allgemeine Zeitschrift für Psychiatrie und psychisch-gerichtliche Medizin* 70 (31 May 1913): 841–849; August Fauser, "Die Se-rologie in der Psychiatrie: Rückblicke und Ausblicke," *Münchner mediziner Wochenschrift* 60 (9 September 1913): 1984–89.

59. Emil Abderhalden, *Die Schutzfermente des tierischen Organismus* (Berlin: Springer, 1912); Emil Abderhalden, *Die Abwehrfermente des tierischen Or-ganismus,* 3rd ed. (Berlin: Springer, 1913); Emil Abderhalden, *Defensive Ferments of the Animal Organism,* translation of the third German edition (New York: William Wood, 1914).

60. Emil Abderhalden, "Ausblicke über die Verwertbarkeit der Ergebnisse neu-rer Forschungen auf dem Gebeite des Zellstoffwechsels zur Lösung von Fragestellungen auf dem Gebeite der Pathologie des Nervensystems," *Deutsche medizinische Wochenschrift* 48 (28 November 1912): 2252–55.

61. August Fauser, "Einige Untersuchungsergebnisse und klinische Aus-blicke auf Grund der Abderhaldenschen Anschauungen und Methodik," *Deutsche medizinische Wochenschrift* 52 (26 December 1912): 2446–51.

62. A. M. Harvey, "Pioneer American Virologist—Charles E. Simon," *The Johns Hopkins Medical Journal* 142 (1978): 161–186.

63. Charles E. Simon, "The Abderhalden-Fauser Reaction in Mental Dis-eases with Special Reference to Dementia Praecox," *Journal of the Ameri-can Medical Association* 62 (30 May 1914): 1703.

64. Simon, "The Abderhalden-Fauser," 1702.

65. The 1913–1914 controversy in the German scientific literature over Abderhalden's concept of "defensive ferments" and his methods for detect-ing them is well-chronicled in M. Kaasch, "Sensation, Irrtum, Betrug?—Emil Abderhalden und die geschichte der Abwehrfermente," *Acta Historica Leopoldina* 36 (2000): 168–178. For an American critique, see D. D. Van Slyke, M. Vinograd-Villchur, and J. Losee, "The Abderhalden Reaction," *Journal of Biological Chemistry* 23 (1915): 377–389.

66. In an article published in the 14 May 1998 issue of *Nature* two German scholars accused Emil Abderhalden of outright fraud rather than incompetence. See Ulrich Deichmann and Benno Müller-Hill, "The Fraud of Abderhalden's Enzymes," *Nature* 393 (1998): 109–111. The issue of error versus fraud was explored more evenly in Kaasch, "Sensation, Irrtum, Betrug."

67. Cited in Deichmann and Müller-Hill, "The Fraud," 110.

68. In 1897 Alzheimer published an article in which he reported a "pathological neuroglia fiber formation" that had been limited to certain areas in a patient with katatonia. Although he said nothing about dementia praecox in this article, catatonia at that time was in the same group of diseases with dementia praecox and dementia paranoides. See Alois Alzheimer, "Beitrage zur pathologischen anatomie der Hirnrinde und zur anatomischen Grundlagen der Psychosen," *Monatsschrift für Psychiatrie und Neurologie* 2 (1897): 82–120.

69. The mortality rate for those who were stricken with dysentery was 23.1 percent (thirty-six patients). See the ten reports published by the staff in the *Boston Medical and Surgical Journal* 61 (11 November 1909): 679–714.

70. Frederick P. Gay, *The Open Mind: Elmer Ernst Southard, 1876–1920* (Chicago: Normandie House, 1938), 241. See Elmer E. Southard and Frederick P. Gay, "The Significance of Bacteria Cultivated from the Human Cadaver: A Study of 100 Cases of Mental Disease, with Blood and Cerebrospinal Fluid Cultures and Clinical and Histological Correlations," *Zentralblatt für Bakteriologie* 55 (1910): 117–133; Elmer E. Southard and Myrtelle Canavan, "Bacterial Invasion of the Blood and the Cerebrospinal Fluid by Way of Mesenteric Lymph Nodes: A Study of Fifty Cases of Mental Disease," *Boston Medical and Surgical Journal* 163 (1910): 202–209; Elmer E. Southard and Myrtelle Canavan, "Second Note on Bacterial Invasion of the Blood and Cerebrospinal Fluid by Way of Lymph Nodes: Findings in Bronchial and Retroperitoneal Lymph Nodes," *Boston Medical and Surgical Journal* 167 (1912): 109–113; Elmer E. Southard and Myrtelle Canavan, "Bacterial Invasion of the Blood and Cerebrospinal Fluid by Way of Lymph-Nodes, Findings in Lymph-Nodes Draining the Pelvis," *Journal of the American Medical Association* 61 (1913): 1526–1528; Elmer E. Southard and Myrtelle Canavan, "The Significance of Bacteria Cultivated from the Human Cadaver: A Second Series of One Hundred Cases of Mental Disease, with Blood and Cerebrospinal Fluid Cultures and Clinical and Histological Correlations," *Journal of Medical Research* 31 (1914–1915): 339–365.

71. Gay, *The Open Mind,* 52–53, 315–316. Gay's biography is the standard treatment of Southard, but his years as director of the Boston Psycho-

pathic Hospital (June 1912–May 1919) are discussed throughout Eliza-
beth Lunbeck, *The Psychiatric Profession: Knowledge, Gender and Power in
Modern America* (Princeton: Princeton University Press, 1994). See also L.
Vernon Briggs, *History of the Psychopathic Hospital, Boston, Massachusetts*
(Boston: Wright and Potter, 1922).

72. Gay, *The Open Mind*, 263–264, 242.

73. See E. E. Southard, "General Psychopathology," *Psychological Bulletin* 12
(1915): 245–273; E. E. Southard, "General Psychopathology," *Psychological Bulletin* 13 (1916): 229–257; E. E. Southard, "General Psychopathology," *Psychological Bulletin* 14 (1917): 193–215; E. E. Southard, "General
Psychopathology," *Psychological Bulletin* 16 (1919): 187–199.

74. E. E. Southard, "The Mind Twist and Brain Spot Hypotheses in
Psychopathology and Neuropathology," *Psychological Bulletin* 11 (1914):
117–130.

75. Ibid., 129.

76. Ibid., 121.

77. Gay, *The Open Mind*, 200.

78. Ibid., 246.

79. See Clarence O. Cheney, "A Review of Reported Brain Changes in Dementia Praecox," *State Hospital Quarterly* 4 (1918): 325–356. This is an
excellent review of the findings in the American, German, and French
literatures, but he devoted the largest portion of his paper to a sharp critique of Southard's work. Between Dunton's 1903 and 1904 autopsy reports and 1920 there were only a few scattered neuropathological studies
of dementia praecox contributed by Americans to the medical literature:
Henry A. Cotton, "Fatty Degeneration of the Cerebral Cortex in the
Psychoses, with Special Reference to Dementia Praecox," *Journal of Experimental Medicine* 22 (1915): 492–516; Mary Elizabeth Morse, "Tha-
lamic Gliosis in Dementia Praecox," *American Journal of Insanity* 72 (1915–
1916): 103–121; Mary Elizabeth Morse, "The Histopathology of the
Autonomic Nervous System in Certain Somatic and Organic Nervous
Diseases," *Journal of Nervous and Mental Disease* 45 (1917): 23–25; Charles
B. Dunlap, "Preliminary Suggestions for a Study of the Pathological
Anatomy of Dementia Praecox," *State Hospital Quarterly* 4 (1918): 52–58;
Eva Rawlings, "The Histopathologic Findings in Dementia Praecox,"
American Journal of Insanity 76 (1920): 263–287; Lawson Gentry Lowrey, "A
Note on a Certain Anomaly of Gyration in Brains of the Insane," *American
Journal of Insanity* 77 (1920–1921): 87–211. There may be others, but these
were the publications that specifically targeted dementia praecox in some
way. See also the English translation by Henry Cotton of Alois Alzheimer,
"The Present Status of Our Knowledge of the Pathological History of the

Cortex in the Psychoses," *American Journal of Insanity* 70 (1913): 175–205. The first appearance of a truly modern neuropathological study of dementia praecox, in the scientific sense, with a matched group of normal controls, is Charles B. Dunlap, "Dementia Praecox: Some Preliminary Observations on Brains from Carefully Selected Cases, and a Consideration of Certain Sources of Error," *American Journal of Psychiatry* 3 (1924): 403–421. On Dunlap, see the many references to the man and his work in Kolb and Roizin, *The First Psychiatric Institute*. See also George H. Kirby, "The New York Psychiatric Institute and Hospital: A Sketch of Its Development from 1895 to 1929," *Psychiatric Quarterly* 4 (1930): 151–167.

80. Gay, *The Open Mind*, 228.

81. Southard is credited for being the first to express this idea (in 1915) by P. J. Harrison, "The Neuropathology of Schizophrenia Diseases: Historical Aspects and Present Knowledge," *Brain* 122 (1999): 593–624.

82. E. E. Southard and J. B. Ayer Jr., "Dementia Praecox, Paranoid: Associated with Bronchiestic Lung Disease and Terminated by Brain Abscesses (Micrococcus catarrhalis)," *Boston Medical and Surgical Journal* 159 (1908): 890–895; E. E. Southard, "A Study of the Dementia Praecox Group in Light of Certain Cases Showing Anomalies or Scleroses in Particular Brain Regions," *American Journal of Insanity* 67 (1910): 119–176; E. E. Southard, "A Series of Normal Looking Brains in Psychopathic Subjects," *American Journal of Insanity* 69 (1913): 689–704; E. E. Southard, "Anatomical Findings in the Brains of Manic-Depressive Subjects," *Proceedings of the American Medico-Psychological Association* 21 (1914): 237–274; E. E. Southard, "On the Direction of Research as to the Analysis of Cortical Stigmata and Focal Lesions in Certain Psychoses," *Transactions of the Association of American Physicians* 29 (1914): 651–673; E. E. Southard, "On the Topographical Distribution of Cortex Lesions and Anomalies in Dementia Praecox with Some Account of Their Functional Significance," *American Journal of Insanity* 71 (1914–15): 383–403; E. E. Southard, "Advantages of a Pathological Classification of Nerve Cells, with Remarks on Tissue Decomplication as Shown in the Cerebral and Cerebellar Cortex," *Transactions of the Association of American Physicians* 30 (1915): 531–546; E. E. Southard, "Dissociation of Parenchymatous (Neuronic) and Interstitial (Neurologia) Changes in the Brains of Certain Psychopathic Subjects, Especially in Dementia Praecox," *Transactions of the Association of American Physicians* 31 (1916): 293–310; E. E. Southard and M. M. Canavan, "The Stratigraphical Analysis of Finer Cortex Changes in Certain Normal-Looking Brains in Dementia Praecox," *Journal of Nervous and Mental Disease* 45 (1917): 97–129; E. E. Southard and M. M. Canavan, "Notes on the Relation of Dementia Praecox to Tuberculosis," *Journal of*

Nervous and Mental Disease 48 (1918): 193–200; E. E. Southard, "Non-Dementia Non-Praecox: A Note on the Advantages of Mental Hygiene of Extirpating a Term," *Journal of Nervous and Mental Disease* 50 (1919): 251–252; E. E. Southard, "On the Focality of Microscopic Brain Lesions Found in Dementia Praecox," *Archives of Neurology and Psychiatry* 1 (1919): 172–192; Southard, "The Mind Twist."

83. The full text of this lecture was never published in his lifetime. The quote and the full text is found in Richard Noll, " 'Non-Dementia Non-Praecox: Note on the Advantages to Mental Hygiene of Extirpating a Term,' by E. E. Southard [1919] (Classic Text No. 72)," *History of Psychiatry* 18 (2007): 495. A similar conclusion was reached the year before by Southard's arch critic, Clarence O. Cheney, in "A Review of Reported," 354–355.

84. See E. E. Southard, "The Laboratory Work of the Danvers State Hospital, Hawthorne, Massachusetts, with Especial Relation to the Policy Formulated by Dr. Charles Whitney Page, Superintendant, 1888–1898, 1903–1910," in *Danvers State Hospital Laboratory Papers, 1910: Charles Whitney Page Series* (Boston: W. M. Leonard, 1910), 26.

85. See the discussion of the Danvers index, and an admission of the "halt" of a separate statewide project, in Southard's report as state pathologist in 1914 in *Sixteenth Annual Report of the State Board of Insanity of the Commonwealth of Massachusetts for the Year Ending November 30, 1914* (Boston: Wright and Potter, 1915), 233–234. Also see the brief note E. E. Southard, "A Frequency List of Mental Symptoms Found in 17,000 Institutional Psychopathic Subjects (Danvers State Hospital, Massachusetts)," *Journal of Nervous and Mental Disease* 43 (January 1916): 56–57. The Danvers index of symptoms was described in detail by its (then) pathologist, Lawson G. Lowrey, "On the Indexing of Case Records.—An Analysis of the Methods Used at the Danvers State Hospital," *Bulletin of the Massachusetts Commission on Mental Diseases* 2 (April 1918): 311–315. Lowrey later became prominent at the Boston Psychopathic Hospital. On the multiple uses of the card index technique at Danvers, see Charles Whitney Page, *The Care of the Insane and Hospital Management* (Boston: W. M. Leonard, 1912), 149–155.

86. On Barrett, see Adolf Meyer, "In Memoriam: Albert M. Barrett, M. D. (1871–1936)," *American Journal of Psychiatry* 93 (1936): 495–500; Horace William Davenport, *Not Just Any Medical School: The Science, Practice, and Teaching of Medicine at the University of Michigan, 1850–1941* (Ann Arbor: University of Michigan Press, 1999), 282–285. It should be noted that as American psychiatry strove to participate in the laboratory revolution that was rapidly transforming medical training and practice in the United

States from the 1880s to the 1920s, the locations of such work began as outgrowths of pathology laboratories in asylums, then became situated in separate institutions—research institutes and the dual-purpose psychopathic hospitals.

87. E. E. Southard and H. W. Mitchell, "Melancholia with Delusions of Negation: Three Cases with Autopsy," *Journal of Nervous and Mental Disease* 35 (1908): 300–314; E. E. Southard and H. W. Mitchell, "Clinical and Anatomical Analysis of 23 Cases of Insanity Arising in the Sixth and Seventh Decades, with Especial Relation to the Incidence of Arteriosclerosis and Senile Atrophy and to the Distribution of Cortical Pigments," *Proceedings of the American Medico-Psychological Association* 15 (1908): 179–224. As sole author E. E. Southard published "On the Somatic Sources of Somatic Delusions," *Journal of Abnormal Psychology* 7 (1912–1913): 326–339; "The Association of Various Hyperkinetic Symptoms with Partial Lesions of the Optic Thalamus," *Journal of Nervous and Mental Disease* 41 (1914): 617–639; "Data Concerning Delusions of Personality, with a Note on the Association of Bright's Disease and Unpleasant Delusions," *Journal of Abnormal Psychology* 10 (1915): 241–262; "A Comparison of Mental Symptoms Found in Cases of General Paresis with and without Coarse Brain Atrophy," *Journal of Nervous and Mental Disease* 42 (1916): 204–216. Later collaborative efforts that made use of the Danvers symptom index are as follows: E. E. Southard and A. S. Tepper, "The Possible Correlation between Delusions and Cortex Lesions in General Paresis," *Journal of Abnormal Psychology* 8 (1913): 259–275; E. E. Southard and Earl D. Bond, "Clinical and Anatomical Analysis of 25 Cases of Mental Disease Arising in the Fifth Decade, with Remarks on the Melancholia Question and Further Observations on the Distribution of Cortical Pigments," *Proceedings of the American Medico-Psychological Association* 20 (1913): 265–314; E. E. Southard and M. M. Canavan, "Notes on the Relation of Somatic (Non-Neural) Neoplasms to Mental Disease," *Interstate Medical Journal* 22 (1915): 738–751. This final paper with Canavan was reprinted in State Board of Insanity and the State Institutions for Mental Disease and Defect, *The Commonwealth of Massachusetts: Collected Contributions, Third Series, 1915* (Boston: Wright and Potter, 1916), 243–257.

88. H. I. Gosline, "Report of the Pathologist," in *Eighty-Fourth Annual Report of the Trustees of the Worcester State Hospital for the Year Ending November 30, 1916* (Boston: Wright and Potter, 1917), 18. See also H. I. Gosline's remarks in S. M. Bunker, "A Psychiatric Index for Facilitating the Study of Previous Records," *Archives of Neurology and Psychiatry* 8 (1922): 325.

89. E. E. Southard, "Report of the Pathologist," in *Fourteenth Annual Report of the State Board of Insanity, the Commonwealth of Massachusetts, for the Year*

Ending November 30, 1912 (Boston: Wright and Potter, 1913), 39. Southard was assisted in this bibliographical search for new symptoms by J. S.
Van Teslaar, a physician who would go on to publish many psychoanalytic articles later in his career. At Danvers state funds were used to employ a "Miss A. Mallett," who also worked directly under Southard's
supervision. See E. E. Southard, "Report of the Pathologist," in *Sixteenth
Annual Report of the State Board of Insanity of the Commonwealth of Massachusetts for the Year Ending November 30, 1914* (Boston: Wright and Potter,
1915), 233.

90. E. E. Southard and M. M. Canavan, "Notes on the Relation of Somatic
(Non-Neural) Neoplasms to Mental Disease," in State Board of Insanity
and the State Institutions for Mental Disease and Defect, *The Commonwealth of Massachusetts: Collected Contributions, Third Series, 1915* (Boston:
Wright and Potter, 1916), 252–253. Only Southard, a neuropathologist,
seems to have seriously regarded the perspective of Carl Wernicke (1848–
1905) among prominent American alienists. Wernicke is known for his
argument that specific psychotic symptoms could be linked to specific
areas of brain localization. He believed all mental disturbances were the
psychological effects of underlying disorders in the functioning of the
nervous system, particularly the cerebral cortex. Like Adolf Meyer in
America, Wernicke argued that it would be premature to define specific
disease entities in psychiatry and therefore was a critic of Kraepelin's
clinical method and premature assumption of natural disease entities.
The three categories of delusions are from a volume that Southard knew
well, Carl Wernicke, *Grundriß der Psychiatrie in klinischen Vorlesungen,
zweite Auflage* (Leipzig: Georg Thieme, 1906). The first edition of this
work appeared in 1900. For background, see Mario Lanczik and Gundolf
Keil, "Carl Wernicke's Localization Theory and Its Significance for the
Development of Scientific Psychiatry," *History of Psychiatry* 2 (1991):
171–180.

91. Southard, "Report," in *Sixteenth Annual Report*, 233. But Southard understood the transition that American psychiatry was trying to make:
"On the whole, however, while psychiatry is in a fluid state, I am inclined to preach autonomy in the different institutions, with integration
where possible. In going over old records one often runs across some
scheme devised *con amore* by somebody and used more or less faithfully
by assistants for a few months or even years. Then the wind blows from a
new direction."

92. E.E. Southard, "Diagnosis Per Exclusionem in Ordine: General and
Psychiatric Remarks," *Journal of Laboratory and Clinical Medicine* 4 (1918):
31–54.

93. S. M. Bunker, "A Psychiatric Index for Facilitating the Study of Previous Records," *Archives of Neurology and Psychiatry* 8 (1922): 324.
94. M. M. Canavan, *Elmer Ernest Southard and His Parents: A Brain Study* (Cambridge, MA: Privately printed by the University Press, 1925), 12–13.
95. Ibid., 13.
96. Ibid., 14.

6. The Rise of the Mind Twist Men, 1903–1913

1. C. K. Clarke, "Dementia Praecox," *British Medical Journal* 2 (1906): 756.
2. A comprehensive comparative study of the international reception of Kraepelin is lacking, due in no small part to the small secondary literature. In their special Kraepelin issue of the journal *History of Psychiatry,* guest editors Eric J. Engstrom and Matthias M. Weber cited the "dire need for more research on the transmission and dissemination of Kraepelin's teachings," noting the "anachronistic" and presentist flavor of so much of the discussion of Kraepelin's work in recent decades. See Eric J. Engstrom and Matthias M. Weber, "Introduction to Special Issue. Making Kraepelin History: A Great Instauration?," *History of Psychiatry* 18 (2007): 267–273. For the German critique of dementia praecox, which started in 1898, see Silke Feldmann, "Die Verbreitung der Kraepelinischen Krankheitslehre im deutschen Sprachraum zwischen 1893 und 1912 am Beispiel der Dementia praecox," PhD diss., Justus-Liebig-Universität, Giessen. A similar backlash also seems to have started (or at least reached a boiling point) in Britain and France in 1904. For British viewpoints see Connolly Norman, "Dementia Praecox," *British Medical Journal* (1904): 972–975; J. C. McConaghey, "Adolescent Insanity: A Protest against the Use of the Term 'Dementia Praecox,'" *Journal of Mental Science* 51 (1905): 340–348; and especially the later critique by A. R. Urquhart, "Dementia Praecox," *Journal of Mental Science* 54 (1908): 661–668, in which he also argues for a return to the term "adolescent insanity" that had been proposed by the British psychiatrist Thomas Clouston in 1873. The best summary of British views can be found in the two-part study by R. M. Ion and M. D. Beers, "The British Reaction to Dementia Praecox 1893–1913, Part I," *History of Psychiatry* 13 (2002): 285–304, and "Part II," 419–431. For an American observation of the controversy on the French scene, see Clarence B. Farrar, "Dementia Praecox in France with Some References to the Frequency of This Diagnosis in America," *American Journal of Insanity* 62 (1905): 257–282. For another summary of French views, see A. V. Parant, "Letter from France: The Question of Dementia Praecox in France," *American Journal of Insanity* 59 (1905): 501–509. Some aspects of the reception of Kraepelinian classification in France between 1899 and 1920 are further elaborated in Ian Dowbiggin, "Back to the

Future: Valentine Magnan, French Psychiatry, and the Classification of Mental Diseases, 1885–1925," *Social History of Medicine* 9 (1996): 383–408; Jean Garrabé, *Histoire de la Schizophrénie* (Paris: Seghers, 1992), 41–56. While Garrabé focuses on the criticisms of Jules Christian (1840–1907) and Wladimir Serbski (1858–1917), the reception of Kraepelin in France was much more nuanced. Missing from this book is any mention of the strong criticisms by the Paris alienist Evariste Marandon de Montyel (1851–1908), who, along with Serbski, rejected dementia praecox as a specific disease entity, and the more congenial acceptance of Kraepelin by Constance Pascal (1877–1937), who accepted not only Kraepelin's disease but also its possible autotoxic etiology. See the brief discussion of the French reception of Kraepelin in G. E. Berrios and R. Hauser, "Kraepelin: Clinical Section—Part II," in *A History of Clinical Psychiatry: The Origin and History of Psychiatric Disorders,* ed. German Berrios and Roy Porter (London: Athlone Press, 1995), 285. Kraepelin's reception in Spain was somewhat less contentious, according to José Javier Plumed Domingo, "The Introduction of the Concept of Dementia Praecox in Spain, 1902–1919," *History of Psychiatry* 19 (2008): 433–453. Dementia praecox and other creations of Kraepelin seem to have made their way to Japan in 1901. In that year a physician who studied under Kraepelin in Heidelberg, Shŭzŏ Kuré, returned to Japan and was instrumental in establishing Kraepelin's classification system around 1911. In 1937 Bleuler's schizophrenia was introduced as "mind-splitting-disease." Both dementia praecox and schizophrenia were apparently received with little controversy. At present the only literature on this appears to be in Japanese. See the English-language abstract for Y. Okada, "How Did Japanese Psychiatrists Receive Conceptions of Dementia Praecox and Schizophrenia?," *Nippon Ishigaku Zasshi* 42 (1996): 3–27.

3. See the glowing biographical account of Sachs by Adolf Meyer, "Historical Fragments on the Neurological and Psychiatric Specialties: Factors and Results in an Eminent Medical and Specifically Neurological Career [1942]," in *The Collected Papers of Adolf Meyer.* Vol. 1, *Neurology,* ed. Eunice E. Winters (Baltimore: The Johns Hopkins University Press, 1950), 287–323. Meyer certainly knew how to return a favor. See also Bernard Sachs, "Annual Address: Advances in Neurology and Their Relation to Psychiatry," *Proceedings of the American Medico-Psychological Association at the Fifty-Third Annual Meeting Held in Baltimore, May 11–14, 1897* (Utica, NY: American Medico-Psychological Association, 1897), 132–149.

4. Bernard Sachs, "Dementia Praecox," *Journal of Nervous and Mental Disease* 32 (June 1905): 355, 358.

5. See the chapter on cognitive impairment in German E. Berrios, *The History of Mental Symptoms: Descriptive Psychopathology Since the Nineteenth Century* (Cambridge: Cambridge University Press, 1996), 172–207.

6. G. Alder Blumer, "The History and Use of the Term Dementia," *Proceedings of the American Medico-Psychological Association Annual Meeting* 13 (1906): 216–217. In addition to the German terms translated as "deterioration process," "mental weakness," and "defect" that Blumer correctly points out were used by Kraepelin to describe the terminal state of dementia praecox, by 1896 Kraepelin also used a term for a specific clinical sign he found in all forms of dementia praecox, *Zerfahrenheit,* which might be translated as "distraction," "dilapidation," or "incoherence." See U. H. Peters, "Hommage an Kraepelin zu seinem 150. Geburtstag— Zerfahrenheit: Kraepelins spezifisches Symptom für Schizophrenie," *Fortschrift für Neurologie und Psychiatrie* 74 (2006): 656–664.

7. J. T. W. Rowe, "Is Dementia Praecox the 'New Peril' in Psychiatry?," *American Journal of Insanity* 63 (1907): 387.

8. C. K. Clarke, "The Relationship of Psychiatry to General Medicine," *Bulletin of the Ontario Hospitals for the Insane* 2 (1909): 7–8.

9. See the memoir of what the former McLean Hospital physician called "the remarkable septenate," in Earl D. Bond, "Seven Years of Awakening, 1906–1913," *American Journal of Psychiatry* 116 (1959): 110–113.

10. Rather than list a series of representative articles, I urge the reader to access the online service of the *New York Times Historical Index* and conduct a search for "dementia praecox."

11. Charles E. Rosenberg, *The Trial of the Assassin Guiteau: Psychiatry and Law in the Gilded Age* (Chicago: University of Chicago Press, 1968), ix.

12. Hamilton had also testified at Guiteau's trial (see ibid., 171–172), as well as at the trial for Leon Czolgoz, who assassinated President William McKinley. See also his autobiography, Allan McLane Hamilton, *Recollections of an Alienist, Personal and Professional* (New York: George H. Doran, 1916).

13. F. A. Mackenzie, *The Trial of Harry Thaw* (London: Geoffrey Bles, 1928), 169, 175–176. Mackenzie seems to have relied on a transcript of the proceedings rather than newspaper articles (as is the case in other books), but other scholars have tried to locate this transcript without success. The best sources for the psychiatric aspects of the Thaw trial are the recent works of Emil R. Pinta, M.D., an emeritus faculty member of the Department of Psychiatry of the Ohio State University. See E. R. Pinta, "Examining Harry Thaw's 'Brain-Storm' Defense: APA and ANA Presidents as Expert Witnesses in a 1907 Trial," *Psychiatric Quarterly* 79 (2008): 83–89. See also his self-published expansion of this article, *Expert Testimony in the Harry K. Thaw "Brain-Storm" Defense: Concepts of Temporary Insanity in a 1907 Trial* (Columbus, Ohio: E. R. Pinta, 2008). Also useful is Martha Merrill Umphrey, "'Dementia Americana': Harry K. Thaw,

the Unwritten Law, and Narratives of Responsibility," PhD diss., University of Michigan, 2000; Martha Merrill Umphrey, "Dialogics of Legal Meaning: Spectacular Trials, the Unwritten Law, and Narratives of Criminal Responsibility," *Law and Society Review* 33 (1999): 393–423.

14. Pinta, *Expert,* 8, 10–11.

15. See Janet A. Tighe, "'What's in a Name?': A Brief Foray into the History of Insanity in England and the United States," *Journal of the American Academy of Psychiatry and the Law* 33 (2005): 252–258; Janet A. Tighe, "'Be It Ever So Little': Reforming the Insanity Defense in the Progressive Era," *Bulletin of the History of Medicine* 57 (1983): 397–441.

16. The Evans quote is cited from the 13 February 1907 edition of the *New York Times* in Pinta, *Expert,* 19. See the discussion of the reception of "brain storm," and its previous usages, on 20–21.

17. "Shift by Jerome Gives Thaw Hope: Day Spent in Attack on the 'Brain Storm' Theory of the Experts," *New York Times,* 5 March 1907, 8.

18. Pinta, *Expert,* 18.

19. Mackenzie, *The Trial,* 191.

20. Charles G. Hill, "Presidential Address," *American Journal of Insanity* 64 (1907): 1–8.

21. A comprehensive analysis of the content of the psychiatric literature of that era supports the timing of this acceptance of disease specificity by many in the American psychiatric elite. "Most mental disease periodical writing in both Europe and America in the years before 1910 concerned 'insanity,' the general category, rather than the specific diseases." Andrew Delano Abbott, "The Emergence of American Psychiatry, 1880–1930," PhD diss., University of Chicago, 1982, 328–329. See also E. E. Southard, "The Margin of Error in the Diagnosis of Mental Disease: Based on a Clinical and Anatomical Review of 250 Cases Examined at the Danvers State Hospital, Massachusetts, 1904–1908," in *Danvers State Hospital Laboratory Papers, 1910: Charles Whitney Page Series* (Boston: W. M. Leonard, 1910), 32.

22. Frank H. Bowlby and James Hendrie Lloyd, *Wharton and Stille's Medical Jurisprudence.* Vol. 1, *Mental Unsoundness* (New York: Lawyers' Co-Operative Publishing, 1905), 846–856.

23. John J. Reese and Henry Leffmann, *Medical Jurisprudence and Toxicology,* 8th ed. (Philadelphia: P. Blakiston, 1911).

24. Clarence A. Lightner, "Administering Justice—The Medical Prepossession," *Michigan Law Review* 17 (1918–1919): 673.

25. Pinta, *Expert,* 34.

26. Adolf Meyer, "Aims and Plans of the Pathological Institute for the New York State Hospitals (1902)," in *The Collected Papers of Adolf Meyer.* Vol. 2,

Psychiatry, ed. Eunice E. Winters (Baltimore: The Johns Hopkins University Press, 1951), 95. See also Nathan G. Hale Jr., *Freud and the Americans: The Beginnings of Psychoanalysis in the United States, 1876–1917* (New York: Oxford University Press, 1971), 160.

27. Meyer, "Aims and Plans," 96.

28. See the chapter on Meyer in Lawrence C. Kolb and Leon Roizin, *The First Psychiatric Institute: How Research and Education Changed Practice* (Washington, DC: American Psychiatric Press, 1996), 21–37.

29. Adolf Meyer, "Report of the Pathological Institute of the New York State Hospitals, 1903," in *The Collected Papers,* 2:116.

30. Ibid.

31. Adolf Meyer, "Discussion of Cooperation between the State Hospitals and the Institute (1904)," in *The Collected Papers,* 2:131.

32. Adolf Meyer, "Movement for a Change in Statistics (1905)," in *The Collected Papers*, 2:132–133, 140–144.

33. Ibid., 146.

34. Charles T. La Moure, "A Study of the Statistics of the New York State Hospitals for 1913, with Special Regard to Statistics Regarding Dementia Praecox," *Boston Medical and Surgical Journal* 173 (11 November 1915): 745.

35. George H. Kirby to Adolf Meyer, 20 January 1906, Adolf Meyer Collection (hereafter AMC), I/2110/2, Alan M. Chesney Medical Archives, The Johns Hopkins Medical Institutions.

36. Kirby to Meyer, 26 February 1906, AMC. Another disciple of Meyer's, the Scottish psychiatrist David K. Henderson, went to Munich in September 1911 after leaving his post at the Institute, where he had worked under Meyer from 1908 to 1911. He wrote to Meyer about similar disappointments: "I have just had the first week of the post-graduate course and have found it both interesting and disappointing. Kraepelin's clinics are extremely good in their way. He presents the cases very concisely but in a very cut-and-dried way, and seems to base his diagnosis almost entirely on the symptom picture. Very little weight seems to be laid on the previous constitution of the individual, and even a slight analysis does not seem to be attempted. The case histories I have seen are rather meager, and not nearly so good as the average at Ward's Island." He wrote that he and another American, Henry A. Cotton, were "working in Alzheimer's laboratory": "[Alzheimer] stands a long time in the laboratory every day, comes to each one individually, and is very instructive, and very genial. I like him very much." David K. Henderson to Adolf Meyer, 29 October 1911, AMC.

In his memoirs Henderson described Alzheimer as "the dominating personality" in the Munich clinic. "He was a man of magnificent physique, over six feet tall, broad-shouldered, deliberate in movement and speech, very dignified. His face scarred with deep saber cuts must have been a constant reminder of his student days." He also described Kraepelin as he appeared in 1911: "Emil Kraepelin was a more formidable type of man. He was thick-set, bullet-headed, intensely serious, a total abstainer from alcohol and tobacco, and very determined and decided in his views. His appearance was more that of a prosperous industrialist than of a world-renowned professional man." David Kennedy Henderson, *The Evolution of Psychiatry in Scotland* (Edinburgh: E. & S. Livingstone, 1964), 173.

37. G. H. Kirby, "The Psychiatric Clinic at Munich, with Notes on Some Clinical Psychological Methods," *Medical Record* 70 (1906): 991. On Kirby's life and work at the Institute, see Kolb and Roizin, *The First Psychiatric Institute,* 47–58. Kirby was director of the Institute from 1917 to 1931. During this time he published the guidelines for examining patients that Meyer had been passing out in typewritten form since 1905 or so. See George H. Kirby, *Guides for History Taking and Clinical Examination of Psychiatric Cases* (Utica, NY: State Hospitals Press, 1921).

38. Clarence P. Oberndorf, *A History of Psychoanalysis in America* (New York: Grune and Stratton, 1953), 85. Oberndorf, who was at the Manhattan State Hospital in 1909, seemed immune to Meyer's mystique. He observed that where "Meyer's grasp seemed wanting was in the correlation of a wealth of laboriously ascertained facts with the meaning of the clinical picture that the patient presented. Facts without theory, just as theory without facts, are not enough" (84).

39. John Gach, "Culture and Complex: On the Early History of Psychoanalysis in America," in *Essays in the History of Psychiatry: A Tenth Anniversary Supplementary Volume to the* Psychiatric Forum, ed. Edwin R. Wallace and Lucius C. Pressley (Columbia, SC: Wm. S. Hall Psychiatric Institute, 1980). The standard history of psychoanalysis in America in the early twentieth century is Hale, *Freud and the Americans.* See also John Chynoweth Burnham, *Psychoanalysis and American Medicine, 1894–1918: Medicine, Science and Culture.* Psychological Issues, Monograph 20. (New York: International Universities Press, 1967).

40. On these greater forces in American intellectual life, see Hale, *Freud and the Americans;* Burnham, *Psychoanalysis.* Also useful are Barbara Sicherman, *The Quest for Mental Health in America* (New York: Arno Press, 1980); Eric Caplan, *Mind Cures and the Birth of Psychotherapy* (Berkeley: University of California Press, 1998).

41. Adolf Meyer, "An Attempt at Analysis of the Neurotic Constitution (1903)," in *The Collected Papers,* 2:323.

42. Ibid., 329.

43. Adolf Meyer, "Arrest of Development in Adolescence (1903)," in *The Collected Papers*, 2:419.

44. Adolf Meyer, "Remarks on Habit Disorganizations in the Essential Deteriorations, and the Relation of Deterioration to the Psychasthenic, Neurasthenic, Hysterical and Other Constitutions (1905)," in *The Collected Papers*, 2:428.

45. Adolf Meyer, "Fundamental Conceptions of Dementia Praecox (1906)," in *The Collected Papers*, 2:436.

46. Adolf Meyer, "What Do Histories of Cases of Insanity Teach Us Concerning the Preventive Mental Hygiene During the Years of School Life? (1908)," in *The Collected Papers of Adolf Meyer*. Vol. 4, *Mental Hygiene*, ed. Eunice E. Winters (Baltimore: The Johns Hopkins University Press, 1952), 342.

47. The privately printed collection of case histories is Adolf Meyer and George Kirby, "Notes of Clinics in Psychopathology," in *The Collected Papers*, 2:139–223. See also Kirby's advocacy of Meyer's psychogenic etiology of dementia praecox in George H. Kirby, "The Influence of Environment on the Insane with Special Reference to the Functional Psychoses," *State Hospitals Bulletin* 1 (1909): 511–544. Kirby demonstrates explicitly that Meyer and his circle were consciously opposed to an American psychiatry based on the model of the other medical sciences and their project of disease specificity: "In our present state of knowledge it seems more profitable to think merely of mental reaction types, displacing from the center of interest the distraction bother about special disease processes" (517).

48. Michael Osnato, "A Critical Review of the Pathogenesis of Dementia Praecox in Its Relation to the Borderline Psychoses," *Neurological Bulletin: Clinical Studies of Nervous Diseases in the Neurological Department of Columbia University* 1 (1918): 108. See also Michael Osnato, "A Critical Review of the Pathogenesis of Dementia Praecox with a Discussion of the Relation of Psychoanalytic Principles," *American Journal of Insanity* 75 (1919): 411–431. These two papers provide some of the sharpest critiques of the psychogenetic theories of the Meyerians and psychoanalysts to be published in that era.

49. Karl Menninger to Frederick P. Gay, 9 March 1935, Elmer E. Southard Papers, Harvard Medical Library in the Francis A. Countway Library of Medicine, Boston.

50. Edward Shorter, *A History of Psychiatry: From the Era of the Asylum to the Age of Prozac* (New York: Wiley, 1997), 111; Abbott, "The Emergence of American Psychiatry," 389. According to Abbott, "American nervous and mental disease institutions were extremely centralized by 1915 and

remained so thereafter. They were in fact so centralized that the scientific whims of men as influential as Meyer and White could sway the intellectual structure of the whole field" (356–357).

51. Meyer. "Fundamental Conceptions," 437; Adolf Meyer, "The Dynamic Interpretation of Dementia Praecox (1909)," in *Collected Papers,* 2:451.

52. Meyer, "Dynamic," 437.

53. C. Macfie Campbell, "A Modern Conception of Dementia Praecox: With Five Illustrative Cases," *Proceedings of the American Medico-Psychological Association* 16 (1909): 410–412.

54. *Fifth Annual Report of the Board of Managers of the Manhattan State Hospital to the State Commission in Lunacy for the Year Ending September 30, 1909* (Albany, NY: J. B. Lyon, 1910), 19–20. This trend would reverse in the 1912–13 fiscal year. In the year ending 30 September 1914 dementia praecox cases made up 21 percent of all new admissions. "Approximately 60 percent of the cases of dementia praecox show clearly a shut-in type of personality." By the end of that year the hospital had more than five thousand patients. See *Tenth Annual Report of the Board of Managers of the Manhattan State Hospital to the State Hospital Commission for the Year Ending September 30, 1914* (Albany, NY: J. B. Lyon, 1915), 38.

55. This is evident in an exchange of letters between Hoch and Meyer in late December 1904. Hoch is exploring a new view of dementia praecox based on "dissociation" (a splitting of consciousness) analogous to dreaming, delirium, and hysteria. This is similar to the metaphors of dementia praecox and schizophrenia that Jung and Bleuler would propose in publications in 1907 and 1908. See Gerald N. Grob, *The Inner World of American Psychiatry, 1890–1940: Selected Correspondence* (New Brunswick, NJ: Rutgers University Press, 1985), 22. Hoch was no doubt familiar with the "splitting" metaphor that had entered philosophy, neurology, psychology, and popular culture (for example, "Dr. Jekyll and Mr. Hyde") in the nineteenth century, and may have been familiar with its application to dementia praecox by the Austrian alienists Erwin Stransky (1877–1962) and Otto Gross (1877–1920). It was in 1904 that Stansky proposed his "intrataxic ataxia" concept and Gross his "dementia sejunctiva" as splitting metaphors for the intellectual, emotional, and behavioral disturbances in dementia praecox. Both authors distanced themselves from a neurologically-based splitting mechanism called "sejunction" by Carl Wernicke (1848–1905), but Wernicke did not use this concept specifically for dementia praecox, which he did not accept as a discrete disease entity. On this see German E. Berrios, Rogelio Lueque, and José M. Villagrán, "Schizophrenia: A Conceptual History," *International Journal of Psychology and Psychological Therapy* 3 (2003): 119, 130–131.

56. August Hoch, "The Psychogenic Factors in Some Paranoiac Conditions, with Suggestions for Prophylaxis and Treatment," *Medical Record* 71 (1907): 708–711.

57. August Hoch, "The Psychogenic Factors in the Development of Psychoses," *Psychological Bulletin* 4 (1907): 161–169.

58. August Hoch, "The Psychogenesis in Dementia Praecox," *Medical Record* 73 (1908): 452–454.

59. August Hoch, "The Manageable Causes of Insanity," *State Hospitals Bulletin* 2 (1909): 359.

60. August Hoch, "Constitutional Factors in the Dementia Praecox Group," *Review of Neurology and Psychiatry* 8 (1910): 466.

61. Ibid., 466–467. For his other writings on the psychogenesis of dementia praecox and other mental diseases, see the following by August Hoch: "A Study of the Mental Make-up in the Functional Psychoses," *Journal of Nervous and Mental Disease* 36 (1909): 230–236; "On Some of the Mental Mechanisms in Dementia Praecox," *Journal of Abnormal Psychology* 5 (1911): 255–273; "Personality and Psychosis," *State Hospitals Bulletin* 6 (1913–1914): 220–240; "Precipitating Mental Causes in Dementia Praecox," *American Journal of Insanity* (1914): 637–647; "Suggestions for the Further Systematization of Psychiatric Research in Our Hospitals," *State Hospitals Bulletin* 3 (1911): 477–493. For the personality research questionnaire that was developed at Bloomingdale Hospital, see August Hoch and George S. Amsden, "A Guide to the Descriptive Study of the Personality, with Special Reference to the Taking of Anamneses of Cases with Psychosis," *Review of Neurology and Psychiatry* 577–587. Similar views were illustrated with case histories by Hoch's second in command at the Institute: George H. Kirby, "Dementia Praecox Deteriorations without Trends," *State Hospitals Bulletin* 7 (November 1912): 1–12. For Hoch's integration of Kraepelinian and Freudian influences in his personality research, see Shirley A. Martin, "Between Kraepelin and Freud: The Integrative Psychiatry of August Hoch," *History of Psychiatry* 18 (2007): 267–273.

62. Walter L. Treadway, "Some Observations on Dementia Praecox," *Journal of Nervous and Mental Disease* 42 (1915): 300. Treadway made these remarks at a meeting of the New York Neurological Society.

63. August Hoch, "Early Manifestations of Mental Disorders," in *Proceedings of the Mental Hygiene Conference and Exhibit at the City College of New York, November 8–15, 1912* (New York: Committee on Mental Hygiene of the State Charities Aid Association, 1912), 201–213; J. R. Ernst, "The Importance of the Early Recognition of the Mental Limitations of the Praecox Type," *Medical Record* 87 (1915): 894. By the 1920s some state agencies concerned with mental hygiene produced public health warnings for parents. See, for example, the thirteen-page pamphlet by Harry M. Mc-

Clellan, *Will Your Boy or Girl Develop Dementia Praecox?* (Columbus: Ohio Department of Public Welfare, 1922).

64. C. B. Farrar, "Some Factors in Schizophrenic Dementia," *Psychiatric Bulletin* 9 (1916): 363–340. In his critique of this proposal, the neurologist Michael Osnato observed, "These groups are widely inclusive and constitute classes in which every child living may be placed" ("A Critical Review," 106). Two of Farrar's types are discussed by Max A. Bahr, "Prepsychotic Manifestations of Dementia Praecox," *Indianapolis Medical Journal* 22 (1919): 107–113.

65. E. Stanley Abbot, "Meyer's Theory of the Psychogenic Origin of Dementia Praecox: A Criticism," *American Journal of Insanity* 68 (1911–1912): 15–22.

66. Earl D. Bond and E. Stanley Abbot, "A Comparison of Personal Characteristics in Dementia Praecox and Manic-Depressive Insanity," *American Journal of Insanity* 68 (January 1912): 364.

67. Earl D. Bond, "Personality and Outcome in Two Hundred Consecutive Cases," *American Journal of Insanity* 69 (1913): 735. On Bond's life, see the memoir by his son, Thomas C. Bond, "Looking Back: The Early Years of Earl D. Bond," *McLean Hospital Journal* 6 (1981): 35–45. See also Kenneth E. Appel, "Memoir of Earl Danforth Bond," *Transactions and Studies of the College of Physicians of Philadelphia* 38 (1970): 112–117; Jack D. Pressman, "Making Psychiatry Respectable: Earl Bond, Edward Strecker, Kenneth Appel, and the Institute of Pennsylvania Hospital," *Transactions and Studies of the College of Physicians of Philadelphia* 13 (1991): 425–443.

68. H. D. Singer, "Dementia Praecox," *Journal of Nervous and Mental Disease* 39 (1912): 821. As the state alienist of Illinois, Singer was not alone among Chicago physicians in their suspicion of, or outright rejection of, psychoanalysis. Other skeptics in the Chicago medical community in 1911–1920 were the surgeon Bayard Taylor Holmes (see Chapter 7); Sidney Kuh (1866–1934), a Heidelberg-trained neurologist at the Cook County Hospital; Julius Grinker (1868–?), a professor of clinical neurology at Northwestern University; and Percival Bailey (1892–1973), then a medical student but later a prominent neurologist and neurosurgeon in Boston. See Percival Bailey, *Up from Little Egypt* (Chicago: Buckskin Press, 1969), 204–207.

69. One of the earliest uses of the term "psychiatrist" in this self-referential way can be found in G. Alder Blumer, "The Coming of Psychasthenia," *Journal of Nervous and Mental Disease* 33 (May 1906): 338. This was pointed out in 1971 by Hale, *Freud and the Americans,* 163. See also J. T. Searcy, "Have We a Specialty?," *American Journal of Insanity* 70 (1913): 263–272.

70. E. E. Southard, "Alienists and Psychiatrists: Notes on Divisions and Nomenclature of Mental Hygiene," *Mental Hygiene* 1 (1917): 567–571.

71. Shorter, *A History of Psychiatry,* 162.

72. See, for example, C. Macfie Campbell, "The Form and Content of the Psychosis: The Role of Psychoanalysis in Psychiatry," *State Hospitals Bulletin* 3 (1910): 4. Macfie Campbell would provide an extensively detailed explanation of his method of symbolic interpretation, as well as another polemical poke at the "biochemical hypothesis" of the autointoxicationists, in C. Macfie Campbell, "The Treatment of Dementia Praecox and Allied Conditions," in *The Modern Treatment of Nervous and Mental Diseases,* Vol. 1, ed. William A. White and Smith Ely Jelliffe (Philadelphia: Lea and Febiger, 1913), 1:590–613.

73. Using the word association test method, Jung and his collaborators produced a sizable body of experimental work in the first decade of the twentieth century. See Herbert Read, Michael Fordham, Gerhard Adler, and William McGuire, *The Collected Works of C. G. Jung.* Vol. 2, *Experimental Researches,* trans. Leopold Stein (Princeton: Princeton University Press, 1973).

74. C. G. Jung, "On Psychophysical Relations of the Association Experiment," *Journal of Abnormal Psychology* 2 (1907): 250–260; Frederick Peterson and C. G. Jung, "Psycho-Physical Investigations with the Galvanometer and Pneumograph in Normal and Insane Individuals," *Brain* 30 (1907): 153–218. Two American alienists at the Binghamton State Hospital in New York subsequently took up Jung's methods. See Edward Gillespie and Ross McClure Chapman, "A Study of Dementia Praecox and Allied Conditions by Means of Psychoanalysis and Association Tests," *State Hospitals Bulletin* 3 (1910): 30–38.

75. Carl Gustav Jung, *Über die Psychologie der Dementia praecox* (Halle: Marhold, 1907); Carl Gustav Jung, *The Psychology of Dementia Praecox,* trans. A. A. Brill and Frederick Peterson (New York: Journal of Nervous and Mental Disease Publishing, 1909).

76. John C. Burnham, *Jelliffe: American Psychoanalyst and Physician and His Correspondence with Sigmund Freud and C. G. Jung,* ed. William McGuire (Chicago: University of Chicago Press, 1983), 49. See also John C. Burnham, "Patterns in Transmitting German Psychiatry to the United States: Smith Ely Jelliffe and the Impact of World War I," in *International Relations in Psychiatry: Britain, Germany, and the United States to World War II,* ed. Volker Roelcke, Paul J. Weindling, and Louise Westwood (Rochester, NY: University of Rochester Press, 2010), 91–110.

77. Adolf Meyer, "Thirty-Five Years of Psychiatry in the United States and Our Present Outlook," *American Journal of Psychiatry* 8 (1928): 12.

78. On the eclecticism of American psychiatry in the Progressive Era, see John C. Burnham, "From Avant-Garde to Specialism: Psychoanalysis in America," *Journal of the History of the Behavioral Sciences* 15 (1979): 128–134.

79. On White's life and work, see William Alanson White, *The Autobiography of a Purpose* (New York: Doubleday, Doran, 1938); Archangelo R. T. D'Amore, ed., *William Alanson White: The Washington Years, 1903–1937* (Washington, DC: U.S. Department of Health, Education and Welfare, 1976).

80. For a complete bibliography of Jelliffe's considerable publication on all facets of neurology and psychiatry, see Burnham, *Jelliffe*, 291–309. The textbook that became the standard in American psychiatry for many years was *Outlines of Psychiatry* (New York: Journal of Nervous and Mental Disease Publishing, 1907). White first incorporated psychoanalytic views in the 1909 second edition.

81. Quoted in Burnham, *Jelliffe*, 48. For a summary of Jelliffe's training excursions to Europe, see 48–53.

82. Smith Ely Jelliffe, "The Signs of Pre–Dementia Praecox: Their Significance and Pedagogic Prophylaxis," *American Journal of the Medical Sciences* 137 (August 1907): 159.

83. Ibid., 165.

84. Ibid., 168, 170.

85. On the "two wings"—positive and negative—of the American eugenics movement in the early twentieth century, see Elof Axel Carlson, *The Unfit: A History of a Bad Idea* (Cold Spring Harbor, NY: Cold Spring Harbor Laboratory Press, 2001), 231–245.

86. Smith Ely Jelliffe, "Predementia Praecox: The Hereditary and Constitutional Features of the Dementia Praecox Make-up," *Journal of Nervous and Mental Disease* 38 (1911): 19.

87. Adolf Meyer, Smith Ely Jelliffe, and August Hoch, *Dementia Praecox: A Monograph* (Boston: Richard G. Badger, Gorham Press, 1911), 23.

88. For Meyer's rationale for not conducting follow-up studies, see Adolf Meyer, "Constructive Formulation of Schizophrenia [1921]," in *The Collected Papers*, 2:472.

89. See E. E. Southard, "Diagnosis per Exclusionem in Ordinem," *Journal of Laboratory and Clinical Medicine* 4 (1918): 31–54.

90. J. K. Hall, "Dementia Praecox: Some Neglected Phases," *Charlotte Medical Journal* 62 (1910): 93–97.

91. The place of dementia praecox in the propaganda of the huge literature of the mental hygiene movement is tangential to the narrative I am creating here. The focus of the literature of that movement was on mental "diseases" (plural), and the prophylaxis of dementia praecox was treated no differently from suggestions for the prevention of other psychiatric conditions. Many were vague, general warnings and echoed statements such as this one by a Canadian psychiatrist: "The point I wish to make is, that it may be of great importance to make clear distinctions between disease

and defect at the earliest possible moment. Certainly any marked change of character in early youth must be looked on with grave suspicion, and the children who are moody, introspective and erratic must be scrutinized with care." C. K. Clarke, "The Early Diagnosis of Dementia Praecox," *Canadian Journal of Medicine and Surgery* 37 (1915): 13–14. On the mental hygiene movement, perhaps the best and most comprehensive treatment is by Johannes Coenraad Pols, "Managing the Mind: The Culture of American Mental Hygiene, 1910–1950," PhD diss., University of Pennsylvania, 1997. See also Gerald N. Grob, *Mental Illness and American Society, 1875–1940* (Princeton: Princeton University Press, 1983), 144–78; Sicherman, *The Quest for Mental Health in America;* Norman Dain, *Clifford W. Beers: Advocate for the Insane* (Pittsburgh: University of Pittsburgh Press, 1980).

92. See, for example, Ann-Louise Silver, "Psychoanalysis and Psychosis: Players and History in the United States," *Psychoanalysis and History* 4 (2002): 45–66.

93. Smith Ely Jelliffe and William Alanson White, *Diseases of the Nervous System: A Text-Book of Neurology and Psychiatry* (Philadelphia: Lea and Febiger, 1915), iii.

94. For a contemporary account of the psychogenesis of dementia praecox out of premorbid "pre–dementia praecox" personality types during combat in the First World War, see D. K. Henderson, "War Neuroses—Dementia Praecox in Wartime," *Review of Neurology and Psychiatry* 16 (1918): 353–380. See also the two classic articles that indicated that war trauma–induced dementia praecox was reversible: Karl A. Mannheim, "Psychosis Associated with Influenza, I. General Data: Statistical Analysis," *Journal of the American Medical Association* 72 (1919): 235–241; Karl A. Mannheim, "Influenza and Schizophrenia: An Analysis of Post-Influenzal 'Dementia Praecox' as of 1918, and Five Years Later: Further Studies of the Psychiatric Aspects of Influenza," *American Journal of Psychiatry* 5 (1926): 469–529. On the elevation of neuropsychiatry during World War II, see Hans Pols, "Waking up to Shell Shock: Psychiatry in the U.S. Military during World War II," *Endeavour* 30 (2006): 144–149.

95. Smith Ely Jelliffe, "The Vegetative Nervous System and Dementia Praecox," *New York Medical Journal* 105 (26 May 1917): 968–971.

96. William Alanson White, *Outlines of Psychiatry,* 7th ed. (Washington, DC: Nervous and Mental Disease Publishing, 1919), 183.

97. Edward J. Kempf, "Autobiographical Fragment (1959)," in *Edward J. Kempf: Selected Papers,* ed. Dorothy Clarke Kempf and John C. Burnham (Bloomington: Indiana University Press, 1974), 7–8. On Kempf, see also Milton Engel, "Psychoanalysis and Psychosis: The Contributions of Edward Kempf," *Journal of the American Academy of Psychoanalysis* 18 (1990): 167–184.

98. Edward J. Kempf, "The Social and Sexual Behavior of Infrahuman Primates with Comparable Facts in Human Behavior," in *Edward J. Kempf,* 68–95. His inspiration for this study was G. V. Hamilton, "A Study of Sexual Tendencies in Monkeys and Baboons," *Journal of Animal Behavior* 4 (1914): 295–318.

99. Edward J. Kempf, *The Autonomic Functions of the Personality* (New York: Nervous and Mental Disease Publishing, 1918).

100. Edward J. Kempf, *Psychopathology* (St. Louis: C. V. Mosby, 1920). Compare C. G. Jung, *The Psychology of the Unconscious: A Study of the Transformations and Symbolisms of the Libido. A Contribution to the History of the Evolution of Thought,* trans. Beatrice M. Hinkle (New York: Moffat, Yard, 1916).

7. Bayard Taylor Holmes and Radically Rational Treatments

1. Gerald N. Grob, *Mental Illness and American Society, 1987–1940* (Princeton: Princeton University Press, 1983), vii.

2. This is the expression used by the parents of Ralph Loring Holmes on the elegantly printed 3x5-inch linen card announcing his death: "Ralph Loring Holmes / son of / Dr. Bayard T. Holmes and Agnes A. George Holmes / born May 25th 1887 in Chicago / Became sick February 6th 1905 in Jena / Died in Chicago May 23rd 1916." Adolf Meyer Collection, Alan Mason Chesney Medical Archives of the Johns Hopkins Medical Institutions, Baltimore (hereafter abbreviated as AMC).

3. Bayard Holmes to Adolf Meyer, 19 February 1912. AMC.

4. State of Illinois, State Board of Health, Bureau of Vital Statistics, Standard Certificate of Death, Registered No. 15352. This certificate indicates that Ralph Loring Holmes died at 1 a.m. on 23 May 1916 at Lakeside Hospital in Chicago. He had been attended there from 16 May to 23 May by A. R. Johnstone, M.D., who signed the death certificate. The cause of death was listed as "dementia precox." But under the section for "contributory (secondary)" causes of death, Johnstone wrote, "Cecostomy—acute dilatation of stomach (Duration) 4ds."

5. Biographical details on Holmes can be found in the following: D. Malone, ed., *The Dictionary of American Biography* (New York: Charles Scribner's Sons, 1932), 9:161; W. K. Beatty, "Bayard Taylor Holmes—A Forgotten Man," *Proceedings of the Medical Institute of Chicago* 34 (1981): 120–123; Richard Noll, "Chicago's Dr. Bayard Taylor Holmes: A Forgotten Pioneer in Biological Psychiatry," *Chicago Medicine* 109 (2006): 28–32. Holmes had a keen interest in the history of medicine and contributed biographical as well as autobiographical pieces to the monthly journal *Medical Life,* edited by Victor Robinson, M.D. The July 1924 issue (volume 31, issue 46) was designated the "Bayard Holmes number" and contains two autobiographical papers by him.

This chapter is based on my own publications on Holmes and the treatment of dementia praecox with surgery and organotherapy. See Richard Noll, "Infectious Insanities, Surgical Solutions: Bayard Taylor Holmes, Dementia Praecox and Laboratory Science in Early 20th-Century America. Part 1," *History of Psychiatry* 17 (2006): 183–204, and "Part 2," *History of Psychiatry* 17 (2006): 299–312; "Kraepelin's 'Lost Biological Psychiatry?' Autointoxication, Organotherapy and Surgery for Dementia Praecox," *History of Psychiatry* 18 (2007): 301–320.

6. Bayard Taylor Holmes, "A Guide to the Documents in Evidence of the Toxaemia of Dementia Praecox," *Dementia Praecox Studies* 3 (1920): 23–107.

7. Andrew Scull, *Madhouse: A Tragic Tale of Megalomania and Modern Medicine* (New Haven, CT: Yale University Press, 2005). See also Andrew Scull, "Focal Infection," in *A Century of Psychiatry,* ed. Hugh Freeman (London: Mosby, 1999), 79–81. On a British physician who also practiced surgical solutions for the problem of insanity, see Andrew Scull, "Focal Sepsis and Psychosis: The Career of Thomas Chivers Graves, BSc, MD, FRCS, MRCVS (1883–1964)," in *150 Years of British Psychiatry.* Vol. 2, *The Aftermath,* ed. Hugh Freeman and German E. Berrios (London: Athlone Press, 1996).

8. Bayard Holmes, "Dementia Praecox—The Insanity of the Young," *Dementia Praecox Studies* 4 (1921): 137.

9. Scull, *Madhouse,* 58.

10. Joel Braslow, *Mental Ills and Bodily Cures: Psychiatric Treatment in the First Half of the Twentieth Century* (Berkeley: University of California Press, 1997), 4.

11. Bayard Holmes to Adolf Meyer, 19 February 1912. AMC.

12. Adolf Meyer to Bayard Holmes, 17 February 1912. AMC.

13. Bayard Holmes, "Some Reflections on the Social Significance of Dementia Praecox apropos Dr. Furbush's Statistics," *Dementia Praecox Studies* 5 (1922): 120.

14. Bayard Holmes, "The Family Substance and Coincident Sicknesses of Blood Relatives," in *The Insanity of Youth and Other Essays* (Cincinnati: Lancet-Clinic Publishing, 1915), 96.

15. Edward J. Kempf, *Psychopathology* (St. Louis: C. V. Mosby, 1920), 734–735.

16. Bayard Holmes to Adolf Meyer, 19 February 1912. AMC.

17. Bayard Holmes, "Public Education in Regard to Dementia Praecox," *American Journal of Clinical Medicine* 23 (1916): 983.

18. See James Herrick, "Christian Fenger as I Knew Him, 1885 to 1902: A Study in Personality," *Proceedings of the Institute of Medicine of Chicago* 13 (1941): 318–329.

19. Ludwig Hektoen, "Early Pathology in Chicago and Christian Fenger," *Proceedings of the Medical Institute of Chicago* 11 (1937): 5.

20. Beatty, "Bayard Taylor Holmes," 123.

21. Christian Fenger and Bayard Holmes, "Antisepsis in Abdominal Operations: Synopsis of a Series of Bacteriological Studies," *Journal of the American Medical Association* 9 (1887): 444–470.

22. Bayard Holmes to John Spurgeon, 31 March 1916, Crerar Ms. 099. Special Collections Research Center, University of Chicago Library (hereafter abbreviated as SCRC).

23. Bayard Holmes, "The Apology to the Reader," *Dementia Praecox Studies* 1 (1918): 5.

24. Bayard Holmes to Adolf Meyer, 19 February 1912. AMC. Meyer told Holmes in subsequent correspondence that he didn't remember where he had first heard of Ralph's illness, and offered to review Ralph's treatment records from the Psychopathic Ward of the University of Michigan Hospital in Ann Arbor. Both Holmes and Meyer then contacted its director, Albert M. Barrett, for his clinical notes on the case. See Adolf Meyer to Bayard Holmes, 21 February 1912; Holmes to Meyer, 24 February 1912; Meyer to Holmes, 27 February 1912, all Crerar Ms. 093, SCRC.

25. Bayard Holmes, "Dementia Praecox, the Insanity of the Young," *Dementia Praecox Studies* 4 (1921): 120.

26. Bayard Holmes to Adolf Meyer, 19 February 1912. AMC.

27. Bayard Holmes, "Is It Desirable and Practicable in Medical Schools to Teach Methods of Investigation in Medical Literature?," *Medical News* 63 (1893): 171–173.

28. See the unidentified and undated clippings from a Chicago newspaper, "He Is a Man of Moods—Dr. Bayard Holmes, the Populist Candidate Is a Remarkable Person," in the scrapbook Holmes compiled containing flyers for political events, newspaper clippings, and other memorabilia from his unsuccessful 1895 Chicago mayoral campaign in Crerar Ms. 096, SCRC.

29. Bayard Holmes, "The Clinical 'Late Chloroform Poisoning' and Adolescent Insanity," *Medical Progress* 24 (1908): 357.

30. See W. D. Tigertt, "An Annotated Life of Edgerton Yorrick Davis, M.D., an Intimate of Sir William Osler," *Journal of the History of Medicine and Allied Sciences* 38 (1983): 259–297.

31. Bayard Holmes, *The Friends of the Insane, the Soul of Medical Education, and Other Essays* (Cincinnati: The Lancet-Clinic Publishing, 1911); Holmes, *The Insanity of Youth and Other Essays.*

32. Bayard Holmes, ed., *Alienists and Neurologists: Proceedings of the Sixth Annual Meeting* (Chicago: Chicago Medical Society, 1917).

33. Bayard Holmes, "Prospectus of Dementia Praecox Studies," *Dementia Praecox Studies* 1 (1918): ii.

34. Ibid.

35. Holmes, "Dementia Praecox, the Insanity of the Young," 121.

36. Holmes had argued for the application of modern serological techniques in psychiatry in two early essays: "Serology in Psychiatry" and "The Condition of the Blood in the Insane" in *The Insanity of Youth*, 37–42, 43–50. For the serological framing of newly specified diseases in general medicine, some of which did not survive, see Keith Wailoo, *Drawing Blood: Technology and Disease Identity in Twentieth-Century America* (Baltimore: Johns Hopkins University Press, 1997).

37. Halvar Lundvall, "Blood-Changes in Dementia Praecox and Artificial Leukocytosis in Its Treatment," *American Journal of Clinical Medicine* 22 (1915): 115–120.

38. For a review of the literature on this experimental treatment for dementia praecox, see Bayard Holmes, "The Use of Sodium Nucleate in Dementia Praecox, Including a Review of the Subject from a Clinical Standpoint and an Extensive Bibliography," *Chicago Medical Recorder* 37 (1915): 500–516. In Munich around this time Kraepelin also experimented with injections of sodium nucleinate (or "nucleate") as a treatment for dementia praecox. Reporting the results of other researchers who had tried this method, he wrote, "Nothing was obtained; the same is true of some similar attempts, which I made myself." Emil Kraepelin, *Dementia Praecox and Paraphrenia*, ed. George M. Robertson, trans. R. Mary Barclay (Edinburgh: E. & S. Livingstone, 1919), 282.

39. Gunnar Kahlmeter, "Blutuntersuchungen bei einem Fall von Dementia praecox mit periodischen Verlauf," *Zeitschrift für die gesamte Neurologie und Psychiatrie* 24 (1914): 483–500.

40. Bayard Holmes, "Some Recent Researches in Dementia Praecox," *Official Bulletin of the Chicago Medical Society* 16 (1916): 14–15.

41. Willi Schmidt, "Adrenalin unempfindlichkeit der Dementia praecox," *Münchner medizinische Wochenschrift* 61 (1914): 366–368.

42. Bayard Holmes, "Adrenalin: A New Diagnostic Test for Dementia Praecox," *Alienist and Neurologist* 25 (1915): 449–460.

43. Bayard Holmes and P. G. Kitterman, *Medicine in Ancient Egypt: The Hieratic Material* (Cincinnati: Lancet-Clinic Press, 1914).

44. Bayard Holmes, "Dementia Praecox Studies: Report of One Year of Work in Research in Dementia Praecox," in "First Annual Report of Dementia Precox Studies Conducted by Bayard Holmes, M.D., Chicago, December 21, 1915," unpublished typescript, 55 pages, John Crerar Library, University of Chicago, 2. Other contributions to this report are Julius Retinger, "Report of Laboratory Work from August 1st to December 30, 1915," 8–21; W. H. Solle, "Literary Propaganda," 22–29.

45. Bayard Holmes, "The Abderhalden Reaction Applied to Diagnosis in Psychiatry," *Boston Medical and Surgical Journal* 170 (12 February 1914): 250. The rise and fall of the Abderhalden defensive ferments reaction test is detailed in Chapter 5.

46. Julius Retinger to Adolf Meyer, 13 November 1917, AMC. In his 15 November 1917 reply to Retinger, Meyer writes, "[My colleagues and I] have done some work with the Abderhalden method and I am very much interested in it."

47. Holmes, "First Annual Report . . . December 21, 1915," 2, 5.

48. Although the five-story, three-hundred-bed unit was to follow the trend of psychopathic hospitals such as those in Ann Arbor and Boston and provide innovative acute care and research, the Psychopathic Hospital of Cook County Hospital never realized its full potential. See "Report of the Committee on the Psychopathic Hospital from the City Club of Chicago, 1920," unpublished typescript, Crerar Ms. 092, folder 8, SCRC.

49. Retinger, "Report of Laboratory Work from August 1st to December 30, 1915," 11.

50. Bayard Holmes, "A Plea for Research into the Possibility of the Cure of Dementia Praecox by the Use of Serum Containing the Defensive Ferment," *Medical Recorder* 86 (1914): 870–872.

51. Bayard Holmes, "The Insanity of Youth: The Abderhalden Reaction and Halvar Lundvall's Remedy," in *The Insanity of Youth and Other Essays,* 9–22.

52. Bayard Holmes, "The Relations between Dementia Praecox and Certain Toxic Amines," *American Journal of Clinical Medicine* 22 (1915): 514–517.

53. Holmes, "Dementia Praecox, the Insanity of the Young," 130. See also Bayard Holmes and Julius Retinger, "Clinical Dementia Praecox without Known Disturbed Periods, Scant Adrenalin Mydriasis, and Diminished Pressor Adrenalin Reaction: Typical Defensive Ferment Reactions, Cecal Stasis, Large Load of Betaiminazolylethylamine in the Stool," *Illinois Medical Journal* 29 (1916): 12–19.

54. Bayard Holmes, "Symptomatic Toxaemia from Local Infections," *The Lancet-Clinic* 99 (1908): 5–8.

55. Bayard Holmes and Julius Retinger, "The Relation of Cecal Stasis to Dementia Praecox," *The Lancet-Clinic* 116 (1916): 147.

56. Frank Billings, *Focal Infection: The Lane Medical Lectures* (New York: D. Appleton, 1916).

57. See E. F. Hirsch, *Frank Billings: The Architect of Medical Education, an Apostle of Excellence in Clinical Practice, a Leader in Chicago Medicine* (Chicago: University of Chicago Press, 1966).

58. "Contract of the Cooperative Research Laboratory at Chicago State Hospital," document dated 3 April 1916, Crerar Ms. 093, SCRC.

59. Bayard Holmes to David Galloway, 14 April 1917, Crerar Ms. 099, SCRC.

60. Bayard Holmes, "Outline of the Proposed Laboratory of Research into Cause, Cure and Prevention of Conditions for Which Custody and Confinement Are Furnished by Department of Public Welfare," *Dementia Praecox Studies* 5 (1922): 133.

61. See Bayard Holmes, "The Laboratory for Psychiatry," in *The Friends of the Insane,* 135–146.

62. Holmes, "Dementia Praecox, the Insanity of the Young," 137.

63. Bayard Holmes, "A Personal View of the Victim of Dementia Praecox," *Dementia Praecox Studies* 1 (1918): 48.

64. See Ann Dally, *Fantasy Surgery 1880–1930: With Special Reference to Sir William Arbuthnot Lane* (Amsterdam: Rodopi, 1996). Other than surgery to remove intestinal autointoxications, the removal of normal ovaries was conducted on insane women in asylums in the United States and Britain in the 1880s and 1890s. See Lawrence D. Longo, "The Rise and Fall of Battey's Operation: A Fashion in Surgery," *Bulletin of the History of Medicine* 53 (1979): 244–267; Joseph Price, "Operative Interference for the Relief of the Insane," *Columbus Medical Journal* 18 (1896): 435–438; William Goodell, "Clinical Notes on the Extirpation of Ovaries for Insanity," *American Journal of Insanity* 38 (1882): 294–302; Robert A. Kitto, "Ovariotomy as a Prophylaxis and Cure for Insanity," *Journal of the American Medical Association* 16 (1891): 516–517; and Andrew Scull and Diane Favreau, "A Chance to Cut is a Chance to Cure: Sexual Surgery for Psychosis in Three Nineteenth-Century Societies," *Research in Law, Deviance and Social Control* 8 (1986): 3–39.

65. Roy Porter, *The Greatest Benefit to Mankind: A Medical History of Humanity* (New York: Norton, 1997), 601.

66. Bayard Taylor Holmes, *The Surgery of the Abdomen. Part I. Appendicitis and Other Diseases about the Appendix* (New York: D. Appleton, 1904), xv.

67. Bayard Holmes, "Dementia Praecox, the Insanity of the Young," *Dementia Praecox Studies* 5 (1922): 80.

68. Ibid., 80–81.

69. Bayard Holmes, "The Arrest and Cure of Dementia Praecox," *Medical Recorder* 100 (1921): 233.

70. Scull, *Madhouse,* 45–46, 57.

71. Bayard Holmes, "Histories of Recovered Patients," *Dementia Praecox Studies* 2 (1919): 180–184; "Dementia Praecox, the Insanity of the Young," 5 (1922), 82.

72. Bayard Holmes, "Dementia Praecox Studies: The Treatment of the Toxemia of Dementia Praecox," *American Medicine* 11 (1916), 702.

73. Bayard Holmes, "Second Annual Report of Dementia Praecox Studies Conducted by Dr. Bayard Holmes at the Psychopathic Hospital, Chicago, under the Direction of Dr. Adam Szwajkart, and with the Assistance of Julius Retinger, Ph.D., Leipzig, 1913. Milton Hanke, Ph.D., Chicago 1916. Emil Bunta, M.D. Will E. Solle. December 31st, 1916. 12 copies—This copy No. 6," unpublished typescript, Harvard Medical Library in the Francis A. Countway Library of Medicine, Boston.

74. Holmes, "Dementia Praecox, the Insanity of the Young" (1922), 87–88.

75. Bayard Holmes, "Notes from the Histories of Recovered Patients," *Dementia Praecox Studies* 1 (1918): 49–55. As a medical student in Chicago, the noted neurologist and neurosurgeon Percival Bailey (1892–1973) met Holmes, whom he described as "an extraordinary character" and "an interesting man." Bailey was intrigued by the experimental treatment program for dementia praecox at the Cook County Psychopathic Hospital: "I was . . . interested in his experiments and the possibilities they envisaged of surgical treatment for psychiatric disorders." Bailey's memoir also contains a vivid description of his attempt to have sexual intercourse with a sow when he was an adolescent and his activities at an orgy at the Bicêtre asylum outside Paris in the early 1920s. As far as medical memoirs go, this one is in a class of its own. See Percival Bailey, *Up from Little Egypt* (Chicago: Buckskin Press, 1969), 208, 227. His interest in surgical treatments for psychiatric conditions was put into practice in 1926–28, when he was an attending neurologist at the outpatient clinic of the Boston Dispensary, where "he saw many thyroid glands removed from anxious neurotics" (8).

76. Bayard Holmes to Julius Retinger, 4 June 1917, Crerar Ms. 099, SCRC.

77. Bayard Holmes to George Fuller, 23 December 1917, Crerar Ms. 099, SCRC. Within a year after his termination Retinger found a biochemist position in Chicago at the Durand Hospital of the John McCormick Institute for Infectious Diseases. See Julius Retinger to Adolf Meyer, 1 November 1918, AMC.

78. Bayard Holmes to Adam Szwajkart, 5 September 1917, Crerar Ms. 099, SCRC.

79. H. M. Jones to Adolf Meyer, 7 September 1917, AMC.

80. H. M. Jones, "A Determination of the Numbers of Histadin Decarcoxylating Organisms in the Feces of Dementia Praecox as Compared with the Numbers in Normal Feces," *Journal of Infectious Diseases* 22 (1918): 125–132.

81. Bayard Holmes, "The Yankton Experiment," *Dementia Praecox Studies* 2 (1919): 173–177.

82. This number is based on the initial May 1916 experiment that killed Ralph Loring Holmes, the five appendicostomies or cecostomies Holmes reported he and others performed between July and December 1916, the eight dementia praecox patients operated on during the tenure of the Psychopathic Research Laboratory from April 1917 to February 1918, the seven persons operated on as part of the "Yankton Experiment" in November 1917, and a single case of a twenty-four-year-old male operated on in Orlando, Florida, by surgeon Clyde Brady on 1 August 1919 under instructions from Holmes.

83. Scull, *Madhouse,* 308.

84. For the full text of a report by Phyllis Greenacre suppressed by Adolf Meyer that documented the true horrors of Cotton's experimental surgeries, see Gil Honigfeld, *Dead End: The Lives of Henry Cotton* (Princeton, NJ: Gil Honigfeld, 2009). Copies can be obtained from the author at honigfeld.gil@gmail.com.

85. According to his annual reports, Cotton used the Abderhalden test at his institution from 1914 to 1917, but discontinued its use in 1918 after being convinced of the loci of infections in the body. See Henry A. Cotton, "Medical Director's Report," in *Annual Report of the Board of Managers of the New Jersey State Hospital at Trenton, N.J., for the Year Ending October 31st 1914* (Union Hill, NJ: Dispatch Printing,), 20. See also Henry A Cotton, "The Abderhalden Reaction in Mental Diseases," *Journal of Nervous and Mental Diseases* 12 (1917): 144–148.

86. Holmes, "Dementia Praecox, the Insanity of the Young" (1921), 137.

87. Bayard Holmes, "The End of This Effort to Promote Research into the Causes of Dementia Praecox," *Chicago Medical Recorder* 46 (1924): 235.

88. Bayard Holmes to Victor Robinson, 1 January 1923, Bayard Taylor Holmes Papers, History of Medicine Division, National Library of Medicine, Bethesda, Maryland.

89. "Dr. Bayard Holmes Passes to Rest," *Fairhope (Alabama) Courier,* 11 April 1924, 1, Bayard Taylor Holmes Papers.

90. Linda B. Robertson to Victor Robinson, 2 August 1924, Bayard Taylor Holmes Papers.

91. Adolf Meyer to Bayard Holmes, 30 May 1916, draft of the letter on Meyer's personal stationary, with stenographic shorthand, AMC.

92. Charles Eucharist de Medici Sajous, *The Internal Secretions and the Principles of Medicine,* 9th ed. (Philadelphia: F. A. Davis, 1921), 1:716. On organotherapy in general, see Merriley Borrell, "Organotherapy, British Physiology, and the Discovery of Internal Secretions," *Journal of the History of Biology* 9 (1976): 235–268; Merriley Borrell, "Brown-Séquard's Organotherapy and Its Appearance in America at the End of the Nineteenth Century," *Bulletin of the History of Medicine* 50 (1976): 309–320.

93. Henry J. Berkeley, "Studies of the Lesions Induced by Action of Certain Poisons. VII. Poisoning with the Preparations of the Thyroid Glands," *Bulletin of the Johns Hopkins Hospital* 8 (July 1897): 76–89.

94. "Editorial: Dr. Berkley's Experiments," *Journal of Zoöphily* 10 (February 1901): 20.

95. Susan E. Lederer, *Subjected to Science: Human Experimentation in America before the Second World War* (Baltimore: Johns Hopkins University Press, 1995), 63.

96. Newdigate Owensby would later become one of the first psychiatrists to practice in the state of Georgia. He still maintains a certain notoriety to this day for a 1940 study in which he used aggressive "metrazol storm" drug treatments and electroshock therapy to cure homosexuality. See Newdigate M. Owensby, "Homosexuality and Lesbianism Treated with Metrazol," *Journal of Nervous and Mental Disease* 92 (1940): 65–66.

97. The discussion of these Bay View experiments is based on the report in Henry J. Berkeley, Richard H. Follis, N. M. Owensby, and W. K. Schwartz, "An Investigation into the Merits of Thyroidectomy and Thyro-Lechithin in the Treatment of Catatonia," *American Journal of Insanity* 65 (January 1909): 413–469. See also Randolph Winslow, "Partial Thyroidectomy in Dementia Praecox," *Journal of the American Medical Association* 15 (1910): 1195–96. A later review of this line of treatment can be found in J. R. Eastman and N. Eastman, "Thyroid Surgery and Dementia Praecox Syndrome," *Annals of Surgery* 76 (1922): 438–443.

98. Sajous, *The Internal Secretions,* 1921. See also C. E. M. Sajous, "The Ductless Glands in Cardiovascular Disease and Dementia Praecox," *Medical Record* 91 (13 January 1917): 82–84; Harvey Cushing, "Psychic Disturbances Associated with Disorders of the Ductless Glands," *American Journal of Insanity* 69 (1913): 965–990.

99. Emil Kraepelin, *Dementia Praecox and Paraphrenia,* trans. R. Mary Barclay (Edinburgh: Livingstone, 1919) 278.

100. M. Stern, R. P. Folsom, and I. S. Ritter, "Vasectomy and Its Influence upon 100 Cases of Dementia Praecox Studied at the Manhattan State Hospital," *State Hospital Quarterly* 10 (1924–1925): 404–412.

8. The Rise of Schizophrenia in America, 1912–1927

1. August Hoch, "Review of Bleuler's Schizophrenia," *Review of Neurology and Psychiatry* 10 (1912): 259–287. For the German psychiatric community's recognition of the differences between Kraepelin and Bleuler, see Hans W. Gruhle, "Bleulers Schizophrenie und Kraepelins Dementia praecox," *Zeitschrift für die gesammelte Neurologie und Psychiatrie* 17 (1913): 114–133.

2. These reminiscences, from late 1918 or early 1919, were from a letter sent to Elmer E. Southard and are reproduced in Richard Noll, "'Non-Dementia Non-Praecox: Note on the Advantages to Mental Hygiene of Extirpating a Term,' by E. E. Southard [1919] (Classic Text No. 72)," *History of Psychiatry* 18 (2007): 501–502.

3. A. A. Brill, "A Case of Schizophrenia (Dementia Praecox)," *American Journal of Insanity* 66 (July 1909): 69; I. W. Eggleston, "A Brief History of Dementia Praecox," *State Hospitals Bulletin* 3 (1910–1911): 23–29. Whether Brill actually used the term "schizophrenia" as a diagnosis at the Vanderbilt Clinic or at Bellevue Hospital beginning in 1909 is an open question. Dementia praecox was a relatively uncommon (but increasingly frequent) diagnosis for the outpatients at the Vanderbilt Clinic between January 1900 and December 1909, constituting only 168 out of 18,285 diagnosable medical cases. Only about 10 percent of the Vanderbilt outpatients (1,900 individuals) were "mental cases." See Smith Ely Jelliffe and A. A. Brill, "Statistical Summary of Cases in the Department of Neurology, Vanderbilt Clinic, for Ten Years—1900 to 1909," *Journal of Nervous and Mental Disease* 38 (July 1911): 391–412.

4. Eugen Bleuler, "Die Prognose der Dementia Praecox—Schizophreniegruppe," *Allgemeine Zeitschrift für Psychiatrie* 65 (1908): 436–464. An edited English translation of this seminal paper appeared as Eugen Bleuler, "The Prognosis of Dementia Praecox: The Group of Schizophrenias," in *The Clinical Roots of the Schizophrenia Concept: Translations of Seminal European Contributions to Schizophrenia,* ed. John Cutting and M. Shepherd (Cambridge: Cambridge University Press, 1987), 59–74. The monograph is Eugen Bleuler, *Dementia Praecox oder Gruppe der Schizophrenien* (Leipzig: FranzDeuticke, 1911). The English translation did not appear until decades later: Eugen Bleuler, *Dementia Praecox or the Group of Schizophrenias,* trans. Joseph Zinkin (New York: International Universities Press, 1950).

5. The best treatments of the life and work of Eugen Bleuler can be found in the publications of Daniel Hell, since 1991 a successor to Bleuler as medical director of the Burghölzli, and his colleagues. See Daniel Hell, Christian Scharfetter, and Arnulf Möller, eds., *Eugen Bleuler: Leben und Werk* (Bern: Huber, 2001); Arnulf Moller, Christian Scharfetter, and Daniel Hell, "Development and Termination of the Working Relationship of C. G. Jung and Eugen Bleuler, 1900–1909," *History of Psychiatry* 13 (2002): 445–453; Daniel Hell, "Eugen Bleulers Seelenverständnis und die Moderne," in *Das Unbewusste in Zürich: Literatur und Tiefenpsychologie um 1900—Sigmund Freud, Thomas Mann und C. G. Jung,* ed. Thomas Sprecher (Zurich: Verlag Neue Zürcher Zeitung, 2000), 39–52; Christian Scharfetter, *Eugen Bleuler 1857–1939: Polyphrenie und Schizophrenie*

(Zurich: vdf Hochschulverlag, 2006). For other biographical information on Bleuler and his views on schizophrenia, Freud, and psychopathology in general, see the following: Manfred Bleuler, "Eugen Bleuler," *Archives of Neurology and Psychiatry* 26 (1934): 610–628; Manfred Bleuler, "Schizophrenia: Review of the Work of Prof. Eugen Bleuler," *Archives of Neurology and Psychiatry* 26 (1931): 610–627; Henri Ellenberger, *The Discovery of the Unconscious: The History and Evolution of Dynamic Psychiatry* (New York: Basic Books, 1970), 666–667; Henri Ellenberger, "The Scope of Swiss Psychology," in *Beyond the Unconscious: Essays of Henri Ellenberger in the History of Psychiatry,* ed. Mark S. Micale (Princeton: Princeton University Press, 1993), 177–179; Peter Loewenberg, "The Creation of a Scientific Community: The Burghölzli, 1902–1914," in *Fantasy and Reality in History* (New York: Oxford University Press, 1995), 53–70; Paolo Fusar-Poli and Pierluigi Politi, "Paul Eugen Bleuler and the Birth of Schizophrenia (1908)," *American Journal of Psychiatry* 165 (2008): 1407; G. Stoltz-Ingenlath, "Epistemological Aspects of Eugen Bleuler's Conception of Schizophrenia in 1911," *Medicine, Health Care and Philosophy* 3 (2000): 153–159; Ernst Falzelder, "The Story of an Ambivalent Relationship: Sigmund Freud and Eugen Bleuler," *Journal of Analytical Psychology* 52 (2007): 343–368; Ernst M. Falzelder and John C. Burnham, "A Perfectly Staged 'Concerted Action' against Psychoanalysis: The 1913 Congress of German Psychiatry," *International Journal of Psychoanalysis* 88 (2007): 1223–44; Thomas G. Dalzell, "Eugen Bleuler 150: Bleuler's Reception of Freud," *History of Psychiatry* 18 (2007): 471–482; Thomas G. Dalzell, "The Reception of Eugen Bleuler in British Psychiatry, 1892–1954," *History of Psychiatry* 21 (2010): 325–339; R. Kuhn, "Eugen Bleuler's Concepts of Psychopathology," *History of Psychiatry* 15 (2004): 361–366. For American and British misreadings of Bleuler and his schizophrenia concept, see Kiernan McNally, "Schizophrenia as Split Personality/Jekyll and Hyde: The Origins of the Informal Usage in the English Language," *Journal of the History of the Behavioral Sciences* 43 (2007): 69–79; Kiernan McNally, "Eugen Bleuler's Four A's," *History of Psychology* 12 (2009): 43–59. Bleuler's metaphysical turn in the 1920s was heralded by Eugen Bleuler, *Naturgeschichte der Seele und ihres Bewusstwerdens: Eine Elementarpsychologie* (Berlin: J. Springer, 1921). A vivid description of Bleuler and Jung's relationship can be found in the early chapters of the definitive biography of the latter by Deidre Bair, *Jung: A Biography* (Boston: Little, Brown, 2003). On Jung's integration of metaphors from the classical scholarship of his day on Hellenistic (Aryan) mystery cults, see Richard Noll, *The Jung Cult: Origins of a Charismatic Religion* (Princeton: Princeton University Press, 1994); Carrie Dohe, "The Wandering Archetype:

C. G. Jung and Germanic-Aryan Spirituality circa 1871–1945," PhD diss., University of Chicago, forthcoming. For background to Bleuler's and Jung's fascination with spiritualism and the occult, see Heather Wolffram, *The Stepchildren of Science: Psychical Research and Parapsychology in Germany, c. 1870–1939* (Clio Medica/Wellcome Institute Series in the History of Medicine) (Amsterdam: Rodopi, 2009).

6. Bleuler, "The Prognosis," 62

7. Ibid., 65.

8. Ibid., 67–68.

9. I am indebted to German E. Berrios for this observation about Bleuler's core mechanisms. See G. E. Berrios, "Introduction. 1911: Eugen Bleuler, The Fundamental Symptoms in Dementia Praecox or the Group of Schizophrenias," in *The Origins of Modern Psychiatry*, ed. C. Thompson (New York: Wiley, 1987), 181. On the relation of Bleuler's "splitting" to nineteenth century "faculty psychology," and the popularity of the "splitting" metaphor in that century to explain unusual or unpredictable human behavior, see Berrios, "Introduction," 167–169; German E. Berrios, Rogelio Luque, and José M. Villagran, "Schizophrenia: A Conceptual History," *International Journal of Psychology and Psychological Theory* 3 (2003): 118–119. The assumptions of British associationist psychology and philosophy are also posited as precursors to Bleuler's concept.

10. Bleuler, "The Prognosis," 59

11. Bleuler, Dementia Praecox or the Group," 53.

12. Otto Diem, "Die einfach demente Form der dementia praecox," *Archiv für Psychiatrie und Nervenkrankheiten* 37 91903), 111–187. An English translation can be found in Cutting and Shepherd, *The Clinical Roots*, 25–36.

13. Bleuler, "Dementia Praecox or the Group," 236.

14. Ibid., 239.

15. Ibid.

16. See Hoch, "Review," 260–261.

17. F. W. Mott, "The Huxley Lecture on Hereditary Aspects of Nervous and Mental Diseases," *British Medical Journal* 2 (October 1910): 1018. On the eugenics movement and the Eugenics Record Office, see Daniel J. Kevles, *In the Name of Eugenics: Genetics and the Uses of Human Heredity* (Berkley: University of California Press, 1985); and especially Elof Axel Carlson, *The Unfit: A History of a Bad Idea* (Cold Spring Harbor, NY: Cold Spring Harbor Laboratory Press, 2001). With respect to psychiatry, see Ian Dowbiggin, *Keeping America Sane: Psychiatry and Eugenics in the United States and Canada, 1880–1940* (Ithaca, NY: Cornell University Press, 1997).

18. The earliest pedigree charts of dementia praecox to appear in an American journal may be found in A. J. Rosanoff and Florence J. Orr, "A Study

of Heredity in Insanity in the Light of the Mendelian Theory," *American Journal of Insanity* 68 (1911): 221–261.

19. Michael Willrich, "The Two Percent Solution: Eugenic Jurisprudence and the Socialization of American Law, 1900–1910," *Law and History Review* 16 (1998): 63–111.

20. Ibid., 82.

21. William J. Hickson, "The Relation of Propfhebephrenia and Dementia Praecox to Crime," *Illinois Medical Journal* 28 (1915): 262.

22. Ibid., 264. For Hickson's reports on the activities of the Psychopathology Laboratory, see Municipal Court of Chicago, *Tenth and Eleventh Annual Reports of the Municipal Court of Chicago for the Years December 6, 1915 to December 2, 1917, Inclusive* (Chicago: Fred Klein, 1918), 124–180; Municipal Court of Chicago, *Twelfth, Thirteenth and Fourteenth Annual Reports of the Municipal Court of Chicago for the Years December 2, 1917 to December 6, 1920 Inclusive* (Chicago: Fred Klein, 1921), 29–42.

23. See Harry Olson, "The Municipal Court of Chicago and Its Psychopathic Laboratory," in *Report of the Proceedings of the Thirty-Eighth Annual Meeting of the Missouri Bar Association Held at St. Louis, Missouri, December 3 and 4, 1920* (St. Louis: Missouri Bar Association, 1920), 62. Hickson's remarks on dementia praecox as the causative factor in crime are found in his massive initial report: Municipal Court of Chicago, *Report of the Psychopathic Laboratory of the Municipal Court of Chicago, May 1, 1914, to April 30, 1917* (Chicago: Fred Klein, 1917), 21, 28–48.

24. Harry Hamilton Laughlin, *Eugenical Sterilization in the United States* (Chicago: Psychopathic Laboratory of the Municipal Court of Chicago, December 1922). Olson wrote the introduction to this volume.

25. *Tenth Annual Report of the Board of Managers of the Manhattan State Hospital to the State Hospital Commission for the Year Ending September 30, 1914* (Albany: J. B. Lyon, 1915), 38.

26. *Eleventh Annual Report of the Board of Managers of the Manhattan State Hospital to the State Hospital Commission for the Year Ending September 30, 1915* (Albany: J. B. Lyon, 1915), 20.

27. David Kennedy Henderson, *The Evolution of Psychiatry in Scotland* (Edinburgh: E. & S. Livingstone, 1964), 181.

28. See Henderson, *Evolution,* 183. Also Adolf Meyer, "Plans for Work in the Phipps Psychiatric Clinic (1913)," in *The Collected Papers of Adolf Meyer.* Vol. 2, *Psychiatry,* ed. Eunice E. Winters (Baltimore: The Johns Hopkins University Press, 1951), 185–192.

29. August Hoch, "Personality and Psychosis," *American Journal of Insanity* 69 (1913): 887–897.

30. Eugen Bleuler, "Autism," *American Journal of Insanity* 69 (1913): 871–886.

31. Henderson, *Evolution,* 182.
32. Adolf Meyer, "Organization of the Work of the Henry Phipps Psychiatric Clinic, Johns Hopkins Hospital, with Special Reference to the First Year's Work (1914)," in *Collected Papers,* 2:207. For an innovation (yet another form) that Meyer introduced around 1915 as a method for charting the psychobiological facts of a patient's life, see Ruth Leys, "Types of One: Adolf Meyer's Life Chart and the Representation of Individuality," *Representations* 34 (1991): 1–28.
33. David K. Henderson [1915], unpublished, untitled typescript with hand corrections, 15 pages, Adolf Meyer Collection, Box I/1659/18, Alan Mason Chesney Medical Archives, Johns Hopkins University, Baltimore, 4–5.
34. J. H. Stephens, K. Y. Ota, W. W. Moore, J. W. Schafer, and L. Covi, "Inpatient Diagnoses during Adolf Meyer's Tenure as Director of the Henry Phipps Psychiatric Clinic, 1913–1940," *Journal of Nervous and Mental Disease* 174 (1986): 750. A portion of these data were analyzed by Thomas A. C. Rennie, "Follow-up Study of Five Hundred Patients with Schizophrenia Admitted to the Hospital from 1913 to 1923," *Archives of Neurology and Psychiatry* 42 (1939): 877–891. An example of the primacy of Meyerian case history detailing over comparative analysis and methods of quantification can be found in Gladys C. Terry and Thomas A. C. Rennie, *Analysis of Parergasia* (New York: Nervous and Mental Disease Monographs, 1938). An appendix to this volume containing "seventeen individually coded and charted case histories illustrative of six clinical reaction patterns" is very revealing about Meyer's actual "treatment" for parergasia at the Phipps Psychiatric Clinic: almost all patients so diagnosed were drugged with sedatives (primarily the barbiturates barbital and luminal, but also paraldehyde, sedormid, and "white oil"). Despite his public propaganda about the need for mental hygiene "habit training" for the largely psychogenic "reactions" of dementia praecox and schizophrenia, in practice Meyer relied heavily on pharmacologic treatment as his primary therapy. He also administered pituitary or thyroid extract to some patients in addition to hydrotherapy, cold wet packs, nutritional supplements, massage, exercise, enemas, and "attempts to rouse and encourage utilization of interests" (181).
35. E. E. Southard, "General Psychopathology," *Psychological Bulletin* 12 (15 July 1915): 249.
36. F. X. Dercum, "The Story of Dementia Praecox," *New York Medical Journal* 104 (12 August 1916): 293.
37. Smith Ely Jelliffe, "The Treatment of the Schizophrenic (Dementia Praecox) Patient," *International Clinics: A Quarterly of Clinical Lectures* 27 (1917): 163–174.

38. Gerald N. Grob, *Mental Illness and American Society, 1875–1940* (Princeton: Princeton University Press, 1983), 187.

39. On the history of the development of psychiatric epidemiology in the United States, see Gerald Grob, "The Origins of American Psychiatric Epidemiology," *American Journal of Public Health* 75 (1985): 226–236. This article contains information on several figures who played a key role in making the dementia praecox construct a real disease by making it an object of their published statistical analyses, primarily in the work of Horatio M. Pollock and Benjamin Malzberg of the New York State Hospital Commission and Edith M. Furbush of the National Committee for Mental Hygiene. See Horatio M. Pollock, "Geographical Distribution of Dementia Praecox in New York State," *State Hospital Quarterly* 4 (1918): 312–323; Horatio M. Pollock and William Nolan, "Sex, Age and Nativity of Dementia Praecox First Admissions to the New York State Hospitals 1912 to 1918," *State Hospital Quarterly* 4 (1918): 498–516; Horatio M. Pollock, "Dementia Praecox as a Social Problem," *Mental Hygiene* 4 (1919): 575–579; Horatio M. Pollock and Edith M. Furbush, "Annual Census of the Insane, Feebleminded, Epileptics and Inebriates in Institutions in the United States, January 1 1918," *Mental Hygiene* 3 (1919): 78–107; Horatio M. Pollock and Edith M. Furbush, "Comparative Statistics of State Hospitals for Mental Diseases, 1918," *Mental Hygiene* 4 (1920): 137–191; Horatio M. Pollock and Edith M. Furbush, "Mental Diseases in Twelve States," *Mental Hygiene* 5 (1921): 353–389; Horatio M. Pollock and Edith M. Furbush, "Patients with Mental Disease, Mental Defect, Epilepsy, Alcoholism and Drug Addiction in the Institutions in the United States, January 1, 1920," *Mental Hygiene* 5 (1921): 139–169; Horatio M. Pollock, "The Future of Mental Disease From a Statistical Standpoint," *American Journal of Psychiatry* 80 (1924), 423–434; Horatio M. Pollock, "Frequency of Dementia Praecox in Relation to Sex, Age, Environment, Nativity, and Race," *Mental Hygiene* 10 (1926): 596–611; Horatio M. Pollock, Benjamin Malzberg, and Raymond G. Fuller, *Hereditary and Environmental Factors in the Causation of Manic-Depressive Psychoses and Dementia Praecox* (Utica, NY: State Hospitals Press, 1939).

    Perhaps the earliest attempt at an epidemiological study of dementia praecox in the American medical literature was W. W. Coles and S. C. Fuller, "A Statistical Study of One Hundred and Nine Cases of Dementia Praecox in Men," *Journal of the American Institute of Homeopathy* (1909): 322–327. Also of note is William J. Nolan, "Occupation and Dementia Praecox," *State Hospital Quarterly* 3 (1917): 127–154.

40. James V. May, "Statistical Studies of the Insane," *American Journal of Insanity* 70 (1913): 429.

41. On Salmon's life, see the hagiographic biography by Earl D. Bond, *Thomas W. Salmon, Psychiatrist* (New York: Norton, 1950).

42. "Report of the Committee on Statistics of the American Medico-Psychological Association," *American Journal of Insanity* (October 1917): 255.

43. Ibid., 258.

44. Ibid., 257.

45. Ibid., 256.

46. "The trouble with Meyerian open-mindedness, of course, was that it never gave any answers, even *pro tem* answers, to general questions. For Meyer, everything was a matter of individual cases. This made him a great clinician, and excellent and influential trainer of young physicians, but a poor theoretician. . . . By the 1920s American psychiatry had Meyer's problem writ large. . . . There was much writing, but little thought; much theory, but little systematic investigation." Andrew Delano Abbott, "The Emergence of American Psychiatry, 1880–1930," PhD diss., University of Chicago, 1982, 247. Despite Abbott's reluctance as a sociologist to resort to "great man" theories of historical causation, he nonetheless concluded that much of the process of "derationalization" that characterized the profession of American psychiatry from 1900 to 1930 could indeed be attributed to the exceptional influence of Meyer (and to a lesser extent E. E. Southard). In opposition to Meyer (and to those who denied the cohesiveness of psychiatric opinion), Southard argued that the new uniform classification scheme reflected the "extraordinary unanimity" of opinion about nosology already reflected in his "favorite textbooks" (those by DeFursac, Dercum, Diefendorf, Knapp, Church and Peterson, and White). See E. E. Southard, "Recent American Classifications of Mental Diseases," *American Journal of Insanity* 75 (January 1919): 334–335.

47. Adolf Meyer, "The Aims and Meaning of Psychiatric Diagnosis (1917)," in *The Collected Papers of Adolf Meyer*. Vol. 3, *Medical Teaching,* ed. Eunice E. Winters (Baltimore: The Johns Hopkins University Press, 1951), 51.

48. See Lawrence C. Kolb and Leon Roizin, *The First Psychiatric Institute: How Research and Education Changed Practice* (Washington, DC: American Psychiatric Press, 1993), 57.

49. Committee on Statistics, American Medico-Psychological Association and the National Committee for Mental Hygiene, Bureau of Statistics, *Statistical Manual for the Use of Institutions for the Insane* (New York: AMPA and NCMH, 1918), 24–25. The funding source for the statistical project of the NCMH (as well as Thomas Salmon's salary) was the Rockefeller Foundation. However, after Alan Gregg assumed control over targeted

grants in 1931, Foundation funding for the NCMH was reduced and then cut off in 1939. The manual was revised repeatedly under a new title: *The Statistical Manual for the Use of Institutions for Mental Diseases,* 2nd ed., revised (Utica, NY: State Hospitals Press, 1920); 3rd ed., revised (1923); 4th ed., revised (1927); 5th ed., revised (1930); 6th ed., revised (1934); 7th ed., revised (1937); 8th ed., revised (1938); 9th ed., revised (1939); 10th ed., revised (1945).

50. According to German E. Berrios and his colleagues, the current definition of schizophrenia in the *Diagnostic and Statistical Manual of Mental Disorders, 4th ed., Text Revision (DSM-IV-TR)* (Washington, DC: American Psychiatric Press, 2000), as well as in all editions going back to the third edition of 1980 *(DSM-III),* is a convergence that "is closely linked to post-Fisherian standards of statistical significance, genetics and neuroimaging," whereas Kraepelin's dementia praecox concept was based on "descriptivism, microscopy and neuropathology" and Bleuler's schizophrenia concept was based on a convergence of Kraepelin's dementia praecox concept, British associationism, and Herbartian "faculty psychology." See Berrios et al., "Schizophrenia,"), 114.

51. See the letter of 4 November 1921 from Albert M. Barrett to Adolf Meyer in Gerald N. Grob, *The Inner World of American Psychiatry, 1890–1940: Selected Correspondence* (New Brunswick, NJ: Rutgers University Press, 1985), 31–33. See also Horatio M. Pollock, "Uniform Statistics of Mental Diseases," *American Journal of Public Health* 8 (1918): 229–231.

52. E. E. Southard, "Cross-Sections of Mental Hygiene, 1844, 1869, 1894," *American Journal of Psychiatry* 76 (1919): 107.

53. E. E. Southard, "Applications of the Pragmatic Method in Psychiatry," *Journal of Laboratory and Clinical Medicine* 5 (1919): 139–145.

54. These letters are reproduced in Grob, *The Inner World,* 28–29.

55. The full text of Southard's unpublished lecture, and the responses to his queries about dementia praecox versus schizophrenia from George Kirby, A. M. Barrett, August Hoch, and Adolf Meyer are reproduced in full in Noll, "Non-Dementia Non-Praecox," 483–502.

56. Emil Kraepelin, *Dementia Praecox and Paraphrenia,* trans. R. Mary Barclay (Edinburgh: E. & S. Livingstone, 1919). For Southard's review of the complete four-volume work, see E. E. Southard, "General Psychopathology," *Psychological Bulletin* 13 (1916): 229–257. For an earlier review, see George H. Kirby, "Dementia Praecox, Paraphrenia and Paranoia: Review of Kraepelin's Latest Conception," *American Journal of Insanity* 71 (October 1914): 349–359.

57. Cited in Noll, "Non-Dementia," 499–500.

58. Cited in ibid., 501.

59. Adolf Meyer, "Constructive Formulation of Schizophrenia," in *The Collected Papers,* 2:471–476.

60. Cited in Noll, "Non-Dementia," 502.

61. Cited in ibid., 500–501.

62. Elizabeth Lunbeck, *The Psychiatric Persuasion: Knowledge, Gender and Power in Modern America* (Princeton: Princeton University Press, 1994), 147.

63. C. Macfie Campbell, "A Discussion of Some Errors in the Diagnosis of Schizophrenia," in *Schizophrenia: Statistical Studies from the Boston Psychopathic Hospital (1925–1934),* ed. C. Macfie Campbell and Edwin B. Wilson (Boston: Boston Psychopathic Hospital, 1934), 43. These remarks were delivered in an address to the New York Academy of Medicine on 9 December 1929. Earlier Southard had proposed that an "empathic index" could be used to differentially diagnose patients. Empathy depended upon "how far we *read or feel ourselves into* the person, group nation or race." Persons representing different diagnostic categories would evoke different empathetic responses. The "schizophrenic (dementia praecox)" group is "strange," and "the victim of dementia praecox" will "give one an impression of queerness that probably no other phenomena can give." E. E. Southard, "The Empathic Index in the Diagnosis of Mental Diseases," *Journal of Abnormal Psychology* 8 (1918): 200, 211. The diagnostically significant gut feeling in a psychiatrist evoked by a person with dementia praecox was later given the name "praecox feeling" ("Praecox Gefühl") by a Dutch psychiatrist. See H. C. Rümke, "Das Kernsyndrom der Schizophrenie und das 'Praecox Gefühl,'" *Zentralblatt gesamte Neurologie und Psychiatrie* 102 (1941): 168–169.

64. E. S. Abbot, "Forms of Insanity in Five Years Admissions to, and Discharged from, the Hospitals for the Insane in Massachusetts," *Proceedings of the American Medico-Psychological Association* 16 (1909): 159–170.

65. Lunbeck, *Psychiatric Persuasion,* 120, 147. Lawson G. Lowry, who was a pathologist at the Danvers State Hospital and an instructor in neuropathology at Harvard in 1918 before joining the Boston Psychopathic Hospital, wrote extensively on this issue: "Differential Diagnosis in Psychiatry: A Comparison of Symptoms in Various Disease States," *Boston Medical and Surgical Journal* 178 (23 May 1918): 703–708; "An Analysis of the Accuracy of Psychopathic Hospital Diagnoses," *American Journal of Insanity* 75 (1918–1919): 351–370; "A Study of the Diagnoses in Cases Seen at the Psychopathic Department and Hospital Department at the Boston State Hospital," *American Journal of Insanity* 77 (1920–1921): 437–439; "Variations in the Diagnosis of Dementia Praecox and Manic-Depressive Psychosis," *Journal of Nervous and Mental Disease* 58 (1923):

33–39. An earlier anecdotal discussion of the issue is found in H. H. Drysdale, "The Manic-Depressive and Dementia Praecox Psychoses: Their Differential Symptomatology," *Proceedings of the American Medico-Psychological Association* 223 (1916): 225–236.

66. Dominic Beer, "'The Manifestations of Insanity' by Emil Kraepelin [1920]," (Classic Text No. 12; introduction and translation), *History of Psychiatry* 3 (1992): 527, 523, 528.

67. Ibid., 528–529. The original is Emil Kraepelin, "Die Erscheinungsformen des Irreseins," *Zeitschrift für die gesamte Neurologie und Psychiatrie* 62 (1920): 1–29.

68. Paul Hoff, "Kraepelin: Clinical Section—Part I," in *A History of Clinical Psychiatry: The Origin and History of Psychiatric Disorders,* ed. German Berrios and Roy Porter (London: Athlone Press, 1995), 268. On the apparent shift in 1913 in the importance given to psychopathology over neuropathology as a central diagnostic structure for dementia praecox, see Paul Hoff, *Emil Kraepelin und die Psychiatrie als klinische Wissenschaft* (Berlin: Springer-Verlag, 1994), 124–125. This prioritizing unbalanced Kraepelin's position on the mind-body problem, that of psychophysical parallelism. Given Kraepelin's bias against anecdotal historical evidence, it is not surprising that he would have low regard for the emphasis on the individual case study as clinical evidence promoted by the followers of Meyer and Freud. For his alleged involvement in preventing the influence of psychoanalysis in German psychiatry, see Falzelder and Burnham, "A Perfectly Staged 'Concerted Action,'" 1223–44.

69. In his 1982 doctoral dissertation, Andrew Delano Abbott ("The Emergence," 324–331, 410) provides the most extensive evidence of the initial (1900–1909), then waning interest in Kraepelin's writings. Abbott's evidence should serve as another reminder that Kraepelin has been more widely read, analyzed, and discussed since about 1980 than he ever was in early twentieth-century America.

70. Emil Kraepelin, *Dementia Praecox and Paraphrenia,* ed. George M. Robertson, trans. R. Mary Barclay (Edinburgh: E. & S. Livingstone, 1919), 76. For a view of how Adolf Meyer and his staff were employing a similar (but not identical) use of the term "schizophrenic" at the Henry Phipps Psychiatric Clinic in 1918, see Phyllis Greenacre, "The Content of the Schizophrenic Characteristics, Occurring in Affective Disorders," *Proceedings of the American Medico-Psychological Association* 25 (1918): 161–166.

71. See the reproduction of the checklist in Lawson G. Lowrey, "On the Indexing of Case Records.—An Analysis of the Methods Used at the Danvers State Hospital," *Bulletin of the Massachusetts Commission on Mental*

Disorders 2 (April 1918): 314. As noted earlier, after formally leaving his position there in 1909, Southard continued to rely on the symptom-index data collection at Danvers and attempted to modify its categories. See his remarks in the *Sixteenth Annual Report of the State Board of Insanity of the Commonwealth of Massachusetts for the Year Ending November 30, 1914* (Boston: Wright and Potter, 1915), 233–234.

72. The web address is www.indexcat.nlm.nih.gov.

73. Leopold Bellak, *Dementia Praecox: The Past Decade's Work and Present Status. A Review and Evaluation* (New York: Grune and Stratton, 1948). Like Nolan D. C. Lewis's volume in 1936, Bellak's extensive literature review was funded by the Scottish Rite of Freemasonry (Thirty-third Degree) for the Northern Masonic jurisdiction of the United States of America. Bellak's conclusion after reviewing 3,200 papers in multiple languages was that "dementia praecox is not a disease entity" but *"a syndrome or a reaction type."* However, "patients usually subsumed under that diagnosis have in common a more or less similar type of reaction to various etiological factors ranging from hypothetically completely organic to hypothetically completely psychogenic ones." In essence, this is the familiar dimensional view of mental illness that, through the Meyerians and Freudians, dominated American eclecticism at that time. Bellak proposed *"differentiating definitely between schizophrenia and dementia praecox,"* with the former representing the psychogenic end of the spectrum and the latter representing the organic end of the spectrum (5, 444–445).

74. Eugen Bleuler, *Textbook of Psychiatry,* trans. A. A. Brill (New York: Macmillan, 1924).

75. George H. Kirby to Adolf Meyer, 27 March 1925, Adolf Meyer Collection, Box I/2188/2, Alan Mason Chesney Medical Archives, Johns Hopkins Medical Institutions. Emil Kraepelin visited the United States twice, once in 1908 and again for several months in 1925 to evaluate Stanley McCormick, a wealthy member of the McCormick family of Chicago. He was diagnosed both times by Kraepelin with the catatonic type of dementia praecox. McCormick had been living at his Riven Rock estate in Montecito, near Santa Barbara, California. A series of prominent alienists had lived with him to provide constant care. After August Hoch retired from the New York State Psychiatric Institute on 1 October 1917; he was the next to move to the Riven Rock estate. Hoch died in 1919 while attending a conference in nearby San Francisco. See Richard Noll, "Styles of Psychiatric Practice, 1906–1925: Clinical Evaluations of the Same Patient by James Jackson Putnam, Adolf Meyer, August Hoch, Emil Kraepelin and Smith Ely Jelliffe," *History of Psychiatry* 10 (1999): 145–190. For a more nuanced treatment of Kraepelin's German national-

ism and its impact on his international colleagues (and seeming lack thereof on the Rockefeller Foundation, which gave his institute money anyway), see Eric J. Engstrom, "Organizing Psychiatric Research in Munich (1903–1925): A Psychiatric Zoon Politicon between State Bureaucracy and American Philanthropy," in *International Relations in Psychiatry: Britain, Germany and the United States through World War II*, ed. Volker Roelcke, Paul J. Weindling, and Louise Westwood (Rochester, NY: University of Rochester Press 2010), 48–66.

76. Adolf Meyer, "The Evolution of the Dementia Praecox Concept," in Association for Research in Nervous and Mental Disease, *Schizophrenia (Dementia Praecox)* (New York: Paul Hoeber, 1928), 13.

77. "More Dementia Praecox: So Says Dr. Pollock, Who Declares Most Cases Are Harmless," *New York Times,* 29 December 1925, 25.

78. See the transcript of the discussion following Karl M. Bowman, "Endocrine and Biochemical Studies in Schizophrenia," in Association for Research in Nervous and Mental Disease, *Schizophrenia (Dementia Praecox),* 277. To be fair to Jelliffe, his remark was an attempt to merge the symbolic meaning, and causal force, of Freudian mechanisms with the "fight or flight" response of the vegetative (autonomic) nervous system— still his pet theory of dementia praecox.

79. Abbott, "The Emergence," 409.

80. Smith Ely Jelliffe, "The Mental Pictures in Schizophrenia and in Epidemic Encephalitis," in Association for Research in Nervous and Mental Disease, *Schizophrenia (Dementia Praecox),* 205–209. Jelliffe, who was fluent in German, had been following the long debate in Germany concerning Kraepelin's claims about the status of natural disease entities in psychiatry. Two of the sharpest critics were Alfred Hoche (1865– 1943) and Oswald Bumke (1877–1950). For an interesting reassessment of this debate, see Volker Roelcke, "Biologizing Social Facts: An Early 20th Century Debate on Kraepelin's Concepts of Culture, Neurasthenia, and Degeneration," *Culture, Medicine and Psychiatry* 21 (1997): 383–403.

81. See George Kirby, Thomas K. Davis, and Henry Alsop Riley, *Schizophrenia (Dementia Praecox): An Investigation of the Most Recent Advances* (Baltimore: Williams and Wilkins, 1931).

82. Nolan D. C. Lewis, *Research in Dementia Praecox (Past Attainments, Present Trends and Future Possibilities)* (New York: National Committee for Mental Hygiene, 1936), 28–29, 212.

83. C. Macfie Campbell, "On the Definition or Delimitation of the Schizophrenic Type of Reaction," in Association for Research in Nervous and Mental Disease, *Schizophrenia (Dementia Praecox),* 29, 17.

84. Macfie Campbell, "A Discussion of Some Errors," 43; C. Macfie Camp-
    bell to C. M. Hincks, 14 December 1934, in Grob, *The Inner World*, 48.
    The limits, indeed the failure, of classification, statistical quantifica-
    tion, and biomedical laboratory research methods in psychiatry contin-
    ued to be stressed by this most ardent pupil of Adolf Meyer in Charles
    Macfie Campbell, *Towards Mental Health: The Schizophrenic Problem*
    (Cambridge, MA: Harvard University Press, 1933). On Macfie Camb-
    pell's life see Harry C. Solomon and Stanley Cobb, "Charles Macfie
    Campbell, M.D. 1876–1943," *Journal of Nervous and Mental Disease* 98
    (1943): 561–563.

85. As discussed in Chapter 4, these were the remarks of Edward C. Runge,
    superintendent of the City Asylum in St. Louis. See Gershom H. Hill,
    "Dementia Praecox," *Proceedings of the American Medico-Psychological Asso-
    ciation* 7 (1900): 288.

86. Edward Shorter, *A History of Psychiatry: From the Era of the Asylum to the
    Age of Prozac* (New York: Wiley, 1997), 106.

87. Eugen Bleuler, "The Physiogenic and the Psychogenic in Schizophre-
    nia," *American Journal of Psychiatry* 10 (1930): 203, 208.

88. M. Bleuler, "Schizophrenia," 610, 616–617, 625. Manfred Bleuler origi-
    nally wanted to be a surgeon but eventually became a psychiatrist like his
    father. After his father's death in 1939, he assumed his father's former
    position as chief in 1942. He trained in the United States on and off be-
    tween 1929 and 1933 at the Boston Hospital, the Boston Psychiatric
    Hospital, and the Bloomingdale Hospital in New York.

89. Although the Institute was officially formed in 1917 it was not until April
    1918 that clinical and scientific activity began. On the men and activities
    led by Kraepelin in Munich, see Hanns Hippius and Norbert Müller, "The
    Work of Emil Kraepelin and His Research Group in München," *European
    Archives of Psychiatry and Clinical Neuroscience* 258 (2008): 3–11. For a broader
    historical perspective, including a history of the Institute, see Hanns Hip-
    pius, Jürgen Möller, Norbert Müller, and Gabriele Neundörfer-Kohl, *The
    University Department of Psychiatry in Munich: From Kraepelin and His Predeces-
    sors to Molecular Psychiatry* (Berlin: Springer, 2008). See also Engstrom,
    "Organizing Psychiatric Research in Munich."

90. Per Dalen, "The Dissolution of Dementia Praecox [1924] by Oswald
    Bumke," (Classic Text No. 13) trans. and introduction, *History of Psychiatry*
    4 (1993), 137–138. The original is Bumke, "Die Auflösung der Dementia
    Praecox," *Klinische Wochenschrift* 3 (1924): 437–440, which appeared three
    weeks before Bumke started his new position in Munich on 1 April 1924.

91. Hippius, et al., *The University Department of Psychiatry*, 242. I wish to
    thank Norbert Müller for graciously sharing his unpublished data which

documents the use of schizophrenia and the decline of dementia praecox before Kraepelin's departure from the Munich clilnic.

92. The details of Kraepelin's contact with the Rockefeller Foundation, including English translations of his letters and those of his colleagues and daughter, can be found in a massive report written and edited in 1928 by Alan Gregg for Richard M. Pearce, the director of the Medical Sciences Division in the Rockefeller Foundation, and the Foundation's Board of Trustees. Pearce died in 1930, and in January 1931 Gregg was promoted to his position. The document comprises 274 pages of analysis, correspondence, budgets, blueprints, field reports, and chronologies pertaining to the endowment of Kraepelin's German Research Institute for Psychiatry. It includes Gregg's original field report from 1926, in which he submitted diary entries concerning his conversations with Kraepelin, Bumke, and others in Munich. It can be found in the collections of the Rockefeller Archive Center in Sleepy Hollow (formerly North Tarrytown), New York. I was able to consult and obtain copies of this document during a memorable blizzard in January 1996 and have been forever grateful for the generosity of the staff, who kept the Center open just for me. This document is Alan Gregg, "Historical Record: Forschungsanstalt für Psychiatrie, Munich (Institute for Psychiatric Research). (1925–1928)," Rockefeller Archive Center, Foundation Archive Collection 1.1 Projects, Record Group 717 Germany, Series 717A, Sub-Series Forschungsanstalt, Box 9, Folder 54. The quotations from Gregg's diary and correspondence to Gregg and Pearce are from this document. See also William H. Schneider, "The Men Who Followed Flexner: Richard Pearce, Alan Gregg, and the Rockefeller Foundation Medical Divisions, 1919–1950," in *Rockefeller Philanthropy and Modern Biomedicine: International Initiatives from World War I to the Cold War,* ed. William H. Schneider (Indianapolis: Indiana University Press, 2002), 39–40, 59n116.

93. Gregg, "Historical Record," 1.

94. Ibid., 79.

95. Felix Plaut to Alan Gregg, 9 October 1926, in ibid., 183.

96. Ibid.

97. Dr. F. Schmidt-Kraepelin to Alan Gregg, 16 October 1926, in ibid., 184.

98. American Psychiatric Association, *Diagnostic and Statistical Manual: Mental Disorders* (Washington, DC: American Psychiatric Association, 1952). On the origins of this new system of classification and nomenclature, see Gerald N. Grob, "Origins of DSM-I: A Study in Appearance and Reality," *American Journal of Psychiatry* 148 (1991): 421–430.

99. See Charles P. Peters, "Concepts of Schizophrenia after Kraepelin and Bleuler," in *The Concept of Schizophrenia: Historical Perspectives,* ed. John G. Howells (Washington, DC: American Psychiatric Press, 1991), 98. For a chronological survey of dementia praecox and schizophrenia concepts, including their transformations in the various editions of the *DSM,* see Edward Shorter, *A Historical Dictionary of Psychiatry* (New York: Oxford University Press, 2005), 267–279.

100. "Medicine: Man's Madness," *Time* (18 May 1936).

101. Adolf Meyer, "The Evolution of the Dementia Praecox Concept (1925)," in *The Collected Papers,* 2:477.

Epilogue

The epigraph is from Charles E. Rosenberg, *Our Present Complaint: American Medicine, Then and Now* (Baltimore: The Johns Hopkins University Press, 2007), 32. As should be clear to those who know his work, Rosenberg's perspective has had a deep influence not only on the shaping of my own thinking about dementia praecox and schizophrenia, but also on my interest in failed theories and medical treatments of the past that have become invisible to us.

1. The best treatment of the character of American eclecticism in the psychiatry of the 1920s, 1930s, and 1940s can be found in Jack D. Pressman, *Last Resort: Psychosurgery and the Limits of Medicine* (Cambridge: Cambridge University Press, 1998). Pressman beings his narrative with the year 1921, which heralded "psychiatry's renaissance," a period that he ends at the year 1935. I would argue that 1918 would be a better starting point.

2. For an example of the absence of Meyer and American eclecticism in the histories of dementia praecox and schizophrenia that focus on Kraepelin, Bleuler, and Freud, see Hannah Decker, "The Historical Evolution of Dementia Praecox," in *Phenomenology and Treatment of Schizophrenia,* ed. William E. Fann, Ismet Karacan, Alex D. Pokorny, and Robert L. Williams (New York: Spectrum, 1978), 301–310.

3. Harold Bloom, *Anxiety of Influence: A Theory of Poetry* (Oxford: Oxford University Press, 1975).

4. The psychiatrist Gerald Klerman (1928–1992) outlined a famous nine-point "neo-Kraepelinian credo" in 1978, which affirmed that psychiatry was a branch of medicine, that there is a boundary between the normal and the sick, that there are discrete mental illnesses, and that psychiatry should focus on classification, diagnosis, and biological research. See Gerald L. Klerman, "The Evolution of the Scientific Nosology," in *Schizophrenia: Science and Practice,* ed. J. D. Shershow (Cambridge,

MA: Harvard University Press, 1978), 99–121. For background, see Roger K. Blashfield, *The Classification of Psychopathology: Neo-Kraepelinian and Quantitative Approaches* (New York: Plenum Press, 1984); Hannah S. Decker, "How Kraepelinian Was Kraepelin? How Kraepelinian Are the Neo- Kraepelinians?—From Emil Kraepelin to *DSM-III*," *History of Psychiatry* 18 (2007): 337–360.

5. The path of disease specification for schizophrenia is chronicled in the successive editions of S. R. Hirsch and Daniel Weinberger, *Schizophrenia*, 2nd ed. (Oxford: Blackwell Science, 2003). Weinberger (in 1986) and the British psychiatrist R. M. Murray (in 1985) were the originators of the current neurodevelopmental model of schizophrenia. See R. M. Murray, "Neurodevelopmental Schizophrenia: The Rediscovery of Dementia Praecox," *British Journal of Psychiatry* 165 (1994): 6–12. The classic book that everyone who works with people with schizophrenia *actually* reads is the various editions of E. Fuller Torrey, *Surviving Schizophrenia: A Manual for Families, Patients and Providers*, 5th ed. (New York: Harper: 2006). When the first edition appeared in 1983 it quickly became the central source of information about schizophrenia for state hospital workers— psychiatrists, psychologists, nurses, social workers, attendants, and administrators. Through the widely available successive editions of *Surviving Schizophrenia*, Torrey has almost single-handedly convinced the American public that "schizophrenia is a brain disease." I remember how shocked I was to read such a bold and clear statement of opinion in 1985. Times have changed.

6. Charles E. Rosenberg, "The Crisis in Psychiatric Legitimacy: Reflections on Psychiatry, Medicine and Public Policy," in *American Psychiatry, Past, Present and Future: Papers Presented on the Occasion of the 200th Anniversary of the Establishment of the First State-Supported Mental Hospital in America*, ed. George Kriegman, Robert D. Gardner, and D. Wilfred Abse (Charlottesville: University Press of Virginia, 1975), 147; Samuel Guze, *Why Psychiatry Is a Branch of Medicine* (New York: Oxford University Press, 1992). Samuel Guze (1923–2000) was one of the primary architects of the biological psychiatry of the late twentieth century. On his significance, see the biographical entry for him in Edward Shorter, *A Historical Dictionary of Psychiatry* (Oxford: Oxford University Press, 2005), 121. For a triumphal acknowledgment of the paradigm shift that he helped bring about, see Samuel Guze, "Biological Psychiatry: Is There Any Other Kind?," *Psychological Medicine* 19 (1989): 315–323. According to a recent article in the *New York Times*, a 2005 government study found that only eleven percent of the 48,000 psychiatrists in the United States provide psychotherapy to their patients, and this number is expected

to decline even further. In 2009 the median annual compensation for psychiatrists was approximately $191,000. A continual reduction in reimbursement fees by insurance company providers has led to an increase in the volume of services provided. Many see forty or more patients a day for medication monitoring. Psychiatrists no longer want to hear the personal narratives of their patients. See Gardiner Harris, "Talk Doesn't Pay, So Psychiatry Turns Instead to Drug Therapy," *New York Times* (5 March 2011).

7. The pendulum may indeed be swinging back toward a position that Meyer would recognize: "reactive" conditions that are a better fit with dimensional rather that categorical concepts. See Hermann M. van Praag, "Kraepelin, Biological Psychiatry, and Beyond," *European Archives of Psychiatry and Clinical Neuroscience* 258 (2008): 29; Allan V. Horwitz and Jerome C. Wakefield, *The Loss of Sadness: How Psychiatry Transformed Normal Sorrow into Depressive Disorder* (Oxford: Oxford University Press, 2007), 113. Recently the argument has been put forth that eclecticism still lies at the heart of psychiatric practice, although it must be kept in check. See S. Nassir Ghaemi, *The Rise and Fall of the Biopsychosocial Model: Reconciling Art and Science in Psychiatry* (Baltimore: The Johns Hopkins University Press, 2009). Some of the methodological problems awaiting biological psychiatry if it opens its diagnostic manuals to dimensional "reactive" conditions are exemplified in the problematic history of stress research (a natural descendent of Meyerian "reaction type" concerns). See Andrew Abbott, *Chaos of Disciplines* (Chicago: University of Chicago Press, 2001), 34–59. For a more optimistic view of the value of dimensional approaches in psychiatry, see Jules Angst, "Psychiatric Diagnosis: The Weak Component of Modern Research," *World Psychiatry* 6 (2007): 94–95. For a pointed critique of dimensional diagnosis of psychotic symptoms see Stephen M. Lawrie, Jeremy Hall, Andrew M. McIntosh, David G. C. Owens and Eve C. Johnstone, "The 'Continuum of Psychosis': Scientifically Unproven and Clinically Impractical," *British Journal of Psychiatry* 197 (2010): 423–425.

8. See Edward Shorter, *Doctors and Their Patients: A Social History* (New York: Simon and Shuster, 1985).

9. Rosenberg, *Our Present Complaint*, 43, 19.

10. They add, "As paradoxical as it may sound in a Neo-Kraepelinian age, Kraepelin would have agreed with those who sought to 'denosologize' his legacy." Eric J. Engstrom and Matthias M. Weber, " 'The Directions of Psychiatric Research' by Emil Kraepelin" (introduction and translation; Classic text No. 63), *History of Psychiatry* 16 (2005): 346.

11. Ibid., 360–361.

12. Because this book will appear at least two years before the publication of *DSM-5,* the ongoing debates within the American Psychiatric Association may lead to a decision *not* to add a dimensional diagnostic method. For a front-row seat to the process, follow the frequent new postings on www .dsm5.org. The Internet is filled with criticisms of almost every aspect of this process, and many such blogs can be found at the website for *Psychiatric Times.* See especially the scathing critique by Allen Frances, the chief editor of *DSM-IV:* "Opening Pandora's Box: The 19 Worst Suggestions for DSM5," *Psychiatric Times,* 11 February 2010, www.psychiatrictimes.com/ print/article/10168/1522341. For a rousing exchange between Frances and a host of prominent psychiatrists on the *DSM-5* process, see the entire issue of the *Association for the Advancement of Philosophy and Psychiatry Bulletin* 17 (2) (2010). In his opening salvo, Frances appeared to be channeling the spirits of Adolph Meyer, Charles Macfie Campbell, and Karl Menninger when he wrote, ". . . mental disorders don't really live 'out there' waiting to be explained. They are constructs we have made up—and often not very compelling ones at that. . . . alas, I have read dozens of definitions of mental disorder (and helped to write one) and I can't say that any have the slightest value whatsoever. . . . Indeed, the concept of mental disorder is so amorphous, protean, and heterogeneous that it inherently defies definition. This is a hole at the center of psychiatric classification." See Allen Frances, "DSM in Philosophyland: Curiouser and Curiouser," *AAPP Bulletin* 17 (2) (2010):21. Through reading comments like this one, by such a distinguished American psychiatrist, one is tempted to conclude that American psychiatry is in the midst of an epistemic meltdown.

13. E. Fuller Torrey, *Surviving Schizophrenia: A Manual for Families, Patients and Providers,* 5th ed. (New York: Harper Paperbacks, 2006), 100–103. Torrey introduced this term in April 1999 at a conference that explored the possibility that schizophrenia and bipolar disorder might share the same underlying disease process.

14. On this issue, see Tayla Greene, "The Kraepelinian Dichotomy: The Twin Pillars Crumbling?," *History of Psychiatry* 18 (2007): 361–379. For a recent linkage of dimensional symptoms—not categories of mental disorder—to genes, see T. Reitkerk, M. P. M. Boks, I. E. Sommer, et al., "The Genetics of Symptom Dimensions of Schizophrenia: Review and Meta-Analysis," *Schizophrenia Research* 102 (2008): 197–205. See also The International Schizophrenia Consortium, "Common Polygenic Variation Contributes to the Risk of Schizophrenia and Bipolar Disorder," *Nature* 460 (2009):748–752.

15. Frances, "Opening Pandora's Box." According to Frances, "The false positive rate would be alarming—70% to 75% in the most careful studies

and likely to be much higher once the diagnosis is official, in general use, and becomes a target for drug companies. . . . There is no proof that the atypical antipsychotics prevent psychotic episodes, but they do most certainly cause large and rapid weight gains (see the recent FDA warning) and are associated with reduced life expectancy—to say nothing about their high cost, other side effects, and stigma." In the past several years criticism has been mounting against the way psychiatric drugs are approved and marketed, with particular attention paid to possible adverse side effects. Because the professional identity of psychiatrists is fused with their role as societal gatekeepers who allow or deny access to these drugs, it will be interesting to see what effect these critiques have on the profession. For an example of the kinds of anomalous evidence that is being catalogued as part of the challenge to biological psychiatry's dominant treatment modality, see Peter Breggin, *Brain-Disabling Treatments in Psychiatry*, 2nd ed. (New York: Springer, 2008). Evidence in favor of an attenuated or potentially pre-psychotic personality construct known as "schizotypy" is presented by psychologist Mark Lenzenweger, *Schizotypy and Schizophrenia: The View From Experimental Psychopathology* (New York: Guilford, 2010). Further evidence for "psychosis risk" predictors can be found in T. O. Cannon et al., "Prediction of Psychosis in Youth at High Clinical Risk: A Multisite Longitudinal Study in North America," *Archives of General Psychiatry* 65 (2008): 28–37.

16. See the many contributions of the psychiatrist and historian David Healy on this issue. A particularly accessible discussion can be found in David Healy, *Mania: A Short History of Bipolar Disorder* (Baltimore: The Johns Hopkins University Press, 2008), 185–252. As a consequence of the efforts of corporations to create new markets for their products, Healy and other critics have employed the term "disease mongering" as the cause of a future "Pharmageddon." See also the epilogue in Gerald N. Grob and Allan V. Horwitz, *Diagnosis, Therapy and Evidence: Conundrums in Modern American Medicine* (New Brunswick, NJ: Rutgers University Press, 2010), 192–197.

17. Currently "bizarre delusions" are the heaviest weighted criterion for diagnosing schizophrenia according to *DSM-IV-TR* (2000). A symptom term that may seem to be obvious to everyone is in fact not. See Michel Cermolacce, Louis Sass, and Josef Parnas, "What Is Bizarre in Bizarre Delusions? A Critical Review," *Schizophrenia Bulletin* 36 (2010): 667–679. On the hyperreflexivity of consciousness at the core of schizophrenia and modern society, see Louis A. Sass, "The Consciousness Machine: Self and Subjectivity in Schizophrenia and Modern Culture," in *The Conceptual Self in Context: Culture, Experience, Self-Understanding*, ed. Ulrich Neisser

and David A. Jopling (Cambridge: Cambridge University Press, 1997), 203–232.

18. For schizophrenia, see Hirsch and Weinberger, *Schizophrenia*. Also see the website for the Schizophrenia Research Forum, which has weekly updates from the world of schizophrenia research. Of particular value is their "Current Papers" section, which provides links to the abstracts of the 100 to 200 new clinical and biological studies published *every week*. Thanks to the Internet, we can watch disease specification operate in real time. A paradigmatic shift away from recent emphases on schizophrenia as a brain or neurotransmitter disorder towards views, similar to Kraepelin's, that dementia praecox or schizophrenia may be the end result of long-term systemic ("whole body") metabolic or peripheral disease processes, is especially evident in the work of Sabine Bahn and her laboratory colleagues at the Institute of Biotechnology at the University of Cambridge. See M. Herberth et al., "Impaired Glycolytic Response in Peripheral Blood Mononuclear Cells of First-Onset Antipsychotic-Naïve Schizophrenia Patients," *Molecular Psychiatry* (2010):1–12. Also relevant to this paradigm shift has been the work of Norbert Müller and his colleagues at Kraeeplin's former university clinic in Munich. See Norbert Müller and Markus Schwarz, "Immune System and Schizophrenia," *Current Immunology Review* 6 (2010): 213–220. For bipolar disorder, see Frederick K. Goodwin and Kay Redfield Jamison, *Manic-Depressive Illness: Bipolar Disorders and Recurrent Depression,* 2nd ed. (Oxford: Oxford University Press, 2007). For melancholia, see Edward Shorter and Max Fink, *Endocrine Psychiatry: Solving the Riddle of Melancholia* (Oxford: Oxford University Press, 2010); Michael Allan Taylor and Max Fink, *Melancholia: The Diagnosis, Pathophysiology and Treatment of Depressive Illness* (Cambridge: Cambridge University Press, 2010).

ACKNOWLEDGMENTS

This could have been a very different book.

My treatment of dementia praecox could have been a dense, theory-laden exercise in the sociology of medicine and science, perhaps an exposition on its function as one of Ludwig Fleck's "thought styles" or as a Foucauldian social construct (with an emphasis on its tragic effects as such), or an illustration of Georges Canguilhem's insights about the relationship of institutional power to historically contingent notions of health and disease and the formation of biological concepts, or a Thomas Kuhn–like conceptualist credo delegitimizing the view that scientific investigations converge on the "truth," especially in the history of psychiatry. In this book there are strains of all these, but mostly none of these. Instead I just wanted to tell a story. I'm old-fashioned. I wanted to communicate my excitement about the history of psychiatry in a descriptive narrative style that would attract new readers to this fascinating domain. To serve this end I have deliberately kept my interpretative framework to a minimum. And so, restraining myself from my Teutonic impulse to display the (presumed) depth and breadth of my knowledge by bloating the number and size of footnotes with (too many) tangential references, I have tried to keep things simple. Maybe I *am* simple. That will be for the reader to judge.

This may not have been a book.

If it were not for the years of financial and moral support showered on me by Dr. Karen Walton, the provost and vice president for academic affairs at DeSales University, I could not have completed the research for this project. Thank you, Karen.

For the granting of a sabbatical in the fall of 2009 so I could complete the writing of this book, I would like to thank my dear friend and department chair at the time, Dr. Katharine Ramsland; Fr. Bernard O'Connor, president of DeSales University; Dr. Robert Blumenstein, dean of undergraduate studies; and the Board of Trustees of my institution. Phyllis Vogel of the Trexler Library at DeSales University hunted down numerous obscure articles and books for me through interlibrary loan, and I cannot thank her enough for the important role she played in my research.

My editor, Elizabeth Knoll, is a gem. Patient, cogent, and a true colleague on this project.

Gerry Grob, Fuller Torrey, Eric Engstrom, David Healy, William Carpenter, Sabine Bahn, Susan Lamb, Jamie Walkup, and Gil Honigfeld all read drafts of sections of this work. Eric and Gil read through the entire manuscript and made valuable suggestions for improvement, especially when they disagreed with me. I am grateful for their assistance in making this a much better book than it would have been. All of its remaining deficits are, of course, due entirely to me. Also useful were the detailed comments and criticisms from the two anonymous reviewers of the final manuscript, and from the committee members of the Board of Syndics of Harvard University Press who approved its publication by the Press.

Hans Pols of the University of Sydney graciously invited me to present the preliminary findings of my research at a conference held at the Australian National University in Canberra in July 2007. Thank you, Hans and Stephanie, for your many kindnesses. I also presented my research on dementia praecox and schizophrenia at the Institute of Health, Health Care Policy, and Aging Research at Rutgers University in New Brunswick, NJ, in October 2006, and was treated graciously by Gerry Grob, Allan Horwitz, Louis Sass, and Jamie Walkup.

I wish to thank German E. Berrios, editor of *History of Psychiatry*, for granting me permission to use portions of material I previously published in the following articles: "Infectious Insanities, Surgical Solutions: Bayard Taylor Holmes, Dementia Praecox and Laboratory Science in Early 20th-Century America, Part I," *History of Psychiatry* 17 (2006): 183–204, and "Part II," 299–312; "The Blood of the Insane," *History of Psychiatry* 17 (2006): 395–418; "Kraepelin's 'Lost Biological Psychiatry'? Autointoxication, Organotherapy and Surgery for Dementia Praecox," *History of Psychiatry* 18 (2007): 301–320; " 'Non-Dementia Non-Praecox: Note on the Advantages to Mental Hygiene of Extirpating a Term,' by E. E. Southard [1919]," *History of Psychiatry* 18 (2007): 483–502.

Much needed moral and intellectual support during this long project was provided by Leonard George, Hugh and Charlotte Gallagher, Norka Karina Morales, Heather Granitz, Jim Pawlik, Margee Stout and John Zamarripa, Sam Martineau, Larry Chapp, Rodney Howsare, Boyce Jubilan, Amy Saborsky, Andrew Essig, Todd Bricker, Jennifer Moore, Al Sproule, Colleen Petrick, Kristin Bremer, Susan Naylor-Emlen, and my sisters, Linda, Lori, Barbara, and Beverley. Jason Pompilio, fellow aficionado of psychosis, always provided libations at just the right time. Catherine John and the Cleveland clan—Joan, Joyce, Majid, Amir, and Jamal—kept me sane when I needed it most.

Jessica McCabe was given the torturous assignment of sifting through Adolf Meyer's writings on dementia praecox, and she survived the ordeal—I think.

Janis Kaghazwala was enormously supportive during the revision process. I couldn't have done it without you, Jan.

Revenants of the patients and staff of Ancora Psychiatric Hospital in Hammonton, New Jersey, with whom I shared my daily existence between 1984 and 1988, emerged from the chambers of my memory palace during the years of researching and writing this book. Sometimes, to my surprise, they visited my dreams. The intellectual and emotional seeds of this project can be traced to my experiences as a psychologist on the wards of that state hospital. I will always be grateful for the wisdom imparted to me by the patients, their families, and my colleagues.

I would like to dedicate this book to the memory of my parents and to Wolfgang Noll, my beautiful boy of twelve summers, a true hypercosmic son. *Nama, sol invictus.* No wonder his favorite Greek god is Helios. And one more thing:

This is the book I wanted to write.

This is the book I've *always* wanted to read.

INDEX

Abbott, Andrew Delano, 21, 174, 266, 291n14, 296n27, 303nn27,28, 339n21, 342n50, 364n46, 367n69

Abbot, Edward Stanley, 127, 259; critique of Meyer and Hoch, 179–181

Abderhalden, Emil, 133–137

Abderhalden defensive ferments reaction test, 133–137

Abderhalden-Fauser reaction, 136

Adolescent insanity, 101, 336n2

Alienists, 11; as distinct from neurologists, 15–18; use of term by both asylum physicians and neurologists, 17; asylum practice of, 18–35; training of, 19–23; learned helplessness of, 35, 41, 70; distinct from psychiatrist, 181

Allen, George, 32

Alzheimer, Alois, 83, 138, 139, 164, 330n68; personality and physique, 340–341n36

American eclectic framing of dementia praecox, 186, 187–189, 276–277; difference from views of Jung and Bleuler, 188, 241; in first American classification system, 252–253; and psychoanalysis, 264–268

American Medical Association, 14, 24

American Medico-Psychological Association (AMPA), 18, 21, 22, 24, 25, 44, 45, 78, 84, 85, 86, 95, 102, 150, 156, 181, 246, 249, 254, 261

American Neurological Association, 101, 150

American Psychiatric Association, 24, 154, 181, 252, 274

American Psychological Association, 77

Amsden, George S., 177–178

Association for Research in Nervous and Mental Disease, 263

Association for the Study of Internal Secretions, 121

Association of Medical Superintendants of American Institutions for the Insane, 24

Attendants and nurses in asylums, 33–35

Autism, 238, 246

Autointoxication as a possible cause of dementia praecox: accepted by Kraepelin, 71, 73, 77, 94, 121–124; rejected by Meyer, 73, 75; Dunton, 116; Weygant, 123; Jung, 123–124, 183; Bleuler, 124; Campbell, 130–131; Dercum, 131; White, 131; Southard, 321n12

Harvard University Press is a member of Green Press Initiative (greenpressinitiative.org), a nonprofit organization working to help publishers and printers increase their use of recycled paper and decrease their use of fiber derived from endangered forests. This book was printed on recycled paper containing 30% post-consumer waste and processed chlorine free.